Success in Practical/Vocational Nursing

From Student to Leader

Fourth Edition

Signe S. Hill, RN, BSN, MA
Formerly Instructor, Practical Nurse Program
Northeast Wisconsin Technical College
Green Bay, Wisconsin

Helen Stephens Howlett, RN, BSN, MS
Formerly Instructor, Practical Nurse Program
Northeast Wisconsin Technical College
Green Bay, Wisconsin

W.B. Saunders Company
A Harcourt Health Sciences Company
Philadelphia London New York St. Louis Sydney Toronto

W.B. SAUNDERS COMPANY
A Harcourt Health Sciences Company

The Curtis Center
Independence Square West
Philadelphia, Pennsylvania 19106

Library of Congress Cataloging-in-Publication Data

Hill, Signe S.
   Success in practical/vocational nursing: from student to leader/Signe S. Hill, Helen
Stephens Howlett.—4th ed.

     p. cm.

   Includes index.

   Previous eds. published under the title: Success in practical nursing: personal and
vocational issues.

   ISBN 0–7216–9059–9

    1. Practical nursing—Vocational guidance. I. Howlett, Helen A. II. Hill, Signe S.
Success in practical nursing. III. Title.

RT62.H45 2001

610.73′06′93--dc21   00-058339

Vice President, Nursing Editorial Director: Sally Schrefer
Senior Editor: Terri Wood
Developmental Editor: Catherine Ott
Production Manager: Pete Faber
Project Manager: Tina Rebane
Illustration Specialist: Rita Martello
Illustrator: Robert Yancey

SUCCESS IN PRACTICAL/VOCATIONAL NURSING: From Student to Leader   ISBN 0–7216–9059–9

Printed in the United States of America.

Last digit is the print number: 9   8   7   6   5   4   3   2

To Frank,
For the lessons you have taught me
about love, friendship,
and being a partner.

    Signe S. Hill

In loving memory of my mom,
Helen E. Stephens, 1912–1999.
To George,
For all you do, this book's for you.

    Helen Stephens Howlett

Contributor

Michael S. Hill, MS, CRC, ABDA
Case Manager
Preferred Works, Inc.
St. Paul, Minnesota

Reviewers

Verna Benner Carson, PhD, RN, CS-P
Tender Loving Care—
Staff Builders Home Health Care

Brenda Hempen, RN, BSN
Hawkeye Community College
Waterloo, Iowa

Lynda Maurer, RN, BSN, MS
Lebanon County Career and Technology Center
Lebanon, Pennsylvania

Janet Tompkins McMahon, RN, MSN
Pennsylvania College of Technology
Williamsport, Pennsylvania

Carol E. Pool, RN, BA
Valley Grande College
Weslaco, Texas

Donna J. Quam, RN, BSN, PHN
Fergus Falls Community College
Fergus Falls, Minnesota

Jonette Inge Talbott, RN, BSN
Southside Virginia Community College
John H. Daniel Campus
Keysville, Virginia

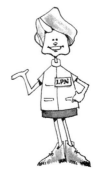

Preface

Dear Student Practical/Vocational Nurse and Instructor,

We appreciate the opportunity to work with you. This entire text is completely revised. At the request of practical/vocational nursing instructors, we have greatly expanded the content on both leadership and management. Chapter 13, Developing Leadership Skills, includes a discussion of five core areas and three specific areas in which knowledge and skill are needed to be an effective leader. Chapter 14, Management, Supervision, and Charge Nurse Skills for Practical/Vocational Nurses, helps prepare practical/vocational nurses for management/supervisory roles in nursing homes and for extended care units as LP/VN charge nurses. A detailed discussion on delegation is included, and the official paper on delegation by the NCSBN can be found in Appendix H. A detailed section on how to assign tasks is included.

A completely new Chapter 8, Straightforward Communication Skills, focuses on practical, real-life issues in nursing. Affective communication, male/female differences, life span communication, and communicating with instructors and staff are discussed.

Chapter 18, Nursing Ethics and the Law, discusses legal aspects related to specific ethical principles. In response to legal questions posed by reviewers, a quick reference section on dealing with potential legal situations and how to document the nursing action has been added.

Other updates include Internet job search, electronic resumes, multistate licensure, a separate chapter on health care settings, a discussion of Eastern religions, NIC and NOC, the Internet as a learning resource, career opportunities including certifications recognized in many states, and more.

Each chapter is written to stand alone and can be used in the order desired to meet program needs. The two-column format is easy to read, interactive, and filled with need-to-know information. Numerous examples and suggestions provide a 1–2–3 approach for applying the concepts presented. Throughout the text, learning exercises challenge the student to think critically. End-of-chapter review questions have been added, with the answers provided on the inside back cover of this book. An Instructor's Manual with over 350 multiple-choice test questions is available free to adopters of the text.

Please share your comments and suggestions with us by writing to the Nursing Books Division in care of the W.B. Saunders Company. We look forward to hearing from you.

Signe S. Hill
Helen Stephens Howlett

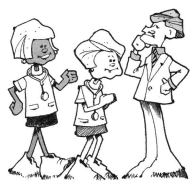

*Illustrations by
Robert Yancey,
Luxemburg, Wisconsin.*

Acknowledgments

So many assisted with making the fourth edition of *Success in Practical/Vocational Nursing: From Student to Leader* a reality. The authors are deeply indebted to the following: Terri Wood, Senior Editor, who foresaw the need to expand the information on nursing leadership/management and supervision skills. She both challenged and facilitated our way through a maze of reviewer suggestions, content additions, and deletions and was actively involved throughout the process.

Catherine Ott, Developmental Editor, responded to our requests with promptness, accuracy, and humor. Her role as liaison with other departments and individuals was invaluable, as was her active involvement throughout the manuscript preparation.

Special thanks to our Marketing Manager, Linda Morris, for her commitment to this edition.

We would like to thank Michael Hill for updating Chapter 20, Finding a Job. Mr. Hill has approximately 20 years of vocational rehabilitation experience, including job placement/marketing, transferable skills analysis, state and federal workers' compensation expertise, administration of short- and long-term disability plans, and employee consultation regarding the Federal Medical Leave Act and Americans with Disabilities Act Programs.

Mary Parrott, Library Services Manager at Northeastern Wisconsin Technical College in Green Bay, Wisconsin, continues to be supportive of our textbook. We appreciate her updates on CD-ROM and computerized learning resources.

Thanks to Mona Kempfert for her availability and computer expertise.

Family and friends were simply there, periodically inquiring about progress, deadlines, and when there would be time for more extensive contact. We deeply appreciate their support.

Finally, as always, we acknowledge each other in our continuing effort to bring you the most up-to-date, need-to-know personal/vocational issues text. We work together and separately and always critique each other's writing, mindful of the text's purpose for class and as a post-graduate reference.

Signe S. Hill
Helen Stephens Howlett

Contents

APPENDICES

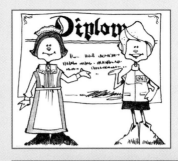

PART **ONE**

Knowing Yourself

Chapter 1

How Practical/Vocational Nursing Evolved

Outline

Early Western Cultures
Age of Christianity
The Renaissance
Age of Industrialization
Seventeenth and Eighteenth Centuries

Nineteenth Century
First School of Nursing
Florence Nightingale
Civil War
Formal Training: Practical Nursing

Twentieth Century: Organization/Law/
   Licensing
Nursing Organizations
You Have Come a Long Way

Key Terms

almshouses
ALPNA
Barton, Clara
Dix, Dorothea Lynde
Gamp, Sairey
Mississippi, 1914

NAPNES
NFLPN
Nightingale, Florence
NLN
Phoebe

Prig, Betsy
self-proclaimed nurse
Semmelweis, Ignaz Philipp
Sisters of Charity
Wald, Lillian

Objectives

Upon completing this chapter you will
be able to:
1. Describe the role of self-defined
   practical nurses throughout history.
2. Discuss four major events that influenced changes in practical
   nursing.

3. Identify the year in which the first
   school of practical nursing was
   founded.
4. Name the year in which licensing
   for practical nursing first began.

5. Present the rationale for your personal stand on entry into nursing
   practice.
6. Discuss the purpose of NAPNES,
   NFLPN, NLN, and ALPNA.

The length of the course for the modern trained practical (or vocational) nurse* is approximately one year in most states, with some variation in the actual number of weeks. Historically speaking, nurses had less educational preparation for their work than do current trained practical nurses.

In reviewing the varied and colorful evolution of this vocation, practical nurses are referred to in a broad sense as those who from the beginning of time chose to or were appointed to care for individuals who were ill, injured, dying, or having babies. Names used to designate this person have included attendant, wet nurse, **self-proclaimed nurse,** midwife, trained nurse, and practical nurse. Most often, the individual doing this work was someone who seemed to have a "gift" or "touch" for helping others during a medical crisis. Some "nurses" learned from others in an apprenticeship setting, and others extended their "mothering" skills to the care of the sick. The practical nurse was the original home health nurse and visiting nurse. Much of the care was offered in the home. They were on call for the needy.

It is worth noting that as early practical nurse training programs became available, they carefully limited their teaching to those things that would be known by a good homemaker or a competent maid. Training included information that would in no way compete with that of the physicians of the time, who themselves had limited knowledge and training. It is also interesting to realize that nursing history does not parallel medical history. When medicine advanced, nursing did not. When medical advances slowed down, nursing progressed.

Nursing has experienced many changes throughout its history, and the changes are not yet over. A major change that has occurred in practical nursing is a gradual increase in the required formal knowledge base and a requirement for licensing to practice practical nursing. Unlike the historically untrained or poorly trained practical nurse, who had unlimited and unsupervised freedom to practice, the present practical nurse is now often a hybrid who is being taught basic skills during the educational program. After graduation, the licensed practical/vocational nurse (LP/VN) is permitted to perform complex nursing skills as delegated by the registered nurse (RN) and allowed by the nurse practice act. Delegation is allowed as long as the RN is willing to teach the skill, observe the return demonstration, and document the teaching or learning process for the LP/VN's file in the place of employment. In addition, most nurse practice acts call for *direct* supervision by RNs for all complex nursing tasks delegated by them. See Chapter 14 for information on delegation.

Reading about nursing history can be enjoyable and can help you see your place among the many centuries of women and men who have given care, relief, and support to the sick. In this chapter we provide a broad overview of the role of nursing during different periods of history. By knowing about the changes that occurred in nursing in the past, you will be ready to better understand and adapt to possible changes in the future. Currently, you are the future of nursing. Years later, you will be part of nursing's rich and varied history.

Early Western Cultures

Recorded nursing history is about one and a half centuries old, but it is interesting to speculate about what might have occurred before that time. It is known that primitive cultures looked on illness as a direct reflection of a personal relationship with the gods. Ill fortune, as it applied to health, was regarded as a sign of disfavor because of behavior that was not pleasing to the gods. Among these cultures there was generally a wise person (medicine man) who possessed magical powers that allowed him to get in touch with and deal with the angered gods. For example, some pagan cultures had a shaman (holy man) who would go into a trance. While in the trance he would "slip into a crack in the earth" to travel down the river to the "valley of the dead." There he would bargain with

---

*The term licensed vocational nurse is the legally recognized term in California and Texas; all other states in the United States use the term licensed practical nurse.

the gods to find out what was needed from the one who was ill or if indeed the ill person would die. Stories of these customs were passed on through song.

Ancient Egypt

Although no direct evidence exists of nursing in Egypt, written records of procedures used in ancient Egypt were probably those of the attendants (nurses) who assisted the priests in caring for the ill. Temples became sanitariums where diseased people were treated. It is thought that Egyptian physicians and attendants 4000 years ago had an extensive list of treatments for specific illnesses. They differed rather remarkably from medicines used today. Interesting evidence was found in the tomb of an eleventh-dynasty queen, whose tomb included a medicine chest complete with vases, spoons, medicines, and herbs. "Lizard's blood, swine's ears and teeth, putrid meat and fat, tortoise brains, old books boiled in oil, milk of a lying-in woman, water of a chaste woman, lice and excreta of men, donkeys, dogs, lions, and cats are examples of some of the ingredients that were used" (Kalish and Kalish, 1995, p. 3).

Egyptian physicians were considered skillful at treating fractures. The custom of embalming enabled the Egyptians to become well acquainted with organs of the body. From clinical observation they learned to recognize some 250 different diseases. To treat them they developed a number of drugs and procedures such as surgery (Deloughery, 1998, p. 4). There is evidence of detailed instructions for daily nursing care, which included recording the pulse, using splints and bandages, and using hollow reeds for urinary catheters.

Ancient Hebrews

The ancient Hebrews had houses for the sick and homes for the aged and began many practices of personal hygiene and public sanitation. Once again, the close association between religion and medicine

was seen, as priests functioned in the role of major health officer.

The Old Testament has many passages that refer to wet nurses and to those who nursed the sick or acted as companions. The passages include Numbers 11:12, Exodus 2:7 and 2:9, II Kings 4:4, and Genesis 24:59 and 35:8.

Ancient Greece

In the fifth century BC, the greatest civilization of the time, ancient Greece, gave the world *Hippocrates, Socrates, Plato,* and *Aristotle* and a system of logical thought that paved the way for the rational treatment of illness, rather than people accepting illness as god-inflicted.

Hippocrates, the "father of modern medicine," translated teachings that were once the secrets of priests into a textbook of medicine and introduced a system of observing symptoms and applying carefully reasoned principles to care. These observations replaced the superstitions and illogical concepts of primitive medicine. "The writings of Hippocrates refer to procedures that today would be undertaken in modern hospitals by nurses but do not refer to the nursing vocation as such. He labeled the health care provider a *physician.* His use of this word should not be confused with modern usage. In fact, much of the ancient Greek physician's craft falls under what modern nurses would claim as their practice" (Deloughery, 1998, p. 5). However, many of Hippocrates' teachings were discarded because of the previously established beliefs. The Hippocratic oath is the ethical code of modern medical practice.

 Critical Thinking Exercise

Obtain a copy of the Hippocratic Oath. Note that Hippocrates referred to all health care workers as physicians. Does the oath apply to the work you will do as a LP/VN?

Aristotle provided additional knowledge about the heart and blood vessels, but because it was forbidden to touch the dead, his knowledge was not widely used.

Women did not become trained nurses in Greece because they occupied a low position in society. They were not considered worthy to be trained in medicine or nursing. Household nursing and child care were done by domestics or servants. The Hippocratic nursing procedures for the sick were carried out by the physician or the physician's students.

Age of Christianity (First to Fifth Centuries AD)

Greece's power and prestige declined. The Roman empire was the dominant power at the time of Christ's birth. Rome established military hospitals, and much of the practical nursing of the day was done by relatives and friends. Much of the knowledge of medicine and nursing gained in the Greek era of power was lost. Few could read and understand the works of Hippocrates and other great thinkers of his time.

As Christianity grew through the centuries, nursing developed as a form of Christian charity. Christian nurses included both men and women, each caring for members of their own sex. St. Paul, of Biblical fame, introduced a woman named Phoebe, an ordained deaconess, to Rome about 30 years after the Crucifixion. **Phoebe,** a practical nurse, is known as the *first visiting nurse.* In addition to the order founded by the deaconess, other orders were established that ministered to the sick and the poor.

Dark Ages and Middle Ages (476–1000 and 1000–1475 AD)

When the power of the Roman empire declined, invading tribes brought violence and chaos to Europe. The period from 476 to 1000 AD has been called the Dark Ages to reflect the loss of widespread education and learning in Europe. The Christian church retreated behind the walls of convents and monasteries. Learning was kept alive within these walls. In the Middle Ages (1000–1475), both men and women were involved in nursing because monks and nuns continued the custom of necessary practical nursing of the sick. An interesting group of monks was the *Knights Hospitalers,* a military order trained to fight as well as to tend the sick and wounded.

One of the nursing brotherhoods founded during this time was the *Alexian Brothers,* which exists today in a dual religious and nursing role. The history of nursing during this period includes stories of highborn women who renounced their heritage to care for the sick. Someone needed to do the nursing because the Middle Ages were a time of horrible epidemics, such as that of the infamous bubonic plague, which killed millions of people. At the end of the Middle Ages, Europe seemed to be old and worn out. Religious fervor was replaced by cynicism and despair. Religious orders no longer assumed as much responsibility for care of the sick.

The Renaissance (1400–1600)

The Renaissance (1400–1600) was a time of rebirth of learning. The information of the ancient Greeks and Romans was sought and put to use.

The scientific method of the Greeks was employed again. The disciplines of anatomy, physiology, and scientific healing were developed. Nursing declined and was all but forgotten until the nineteenth century. It is thought that the religious Reformation, in which the church split into Catholic and Protestant factions, contributed to the decline in organized nursing. In Protestant countries, such as England and Germany, monasticism nearly ended, and with it, nursing. Greater personal freedom may have been achieved during the Renaissance, but with it the tradition of unselfish service to humanity almost disappeared. It was a cruel age, marked by neglect of the poor, homeless, and ill. It is worth noting that one man, St. Vincent de Paul, almost single-handedly organized the **Sisters of Charity** in France to care for the poor and nurse the sick.

Age of Industrialization (Eighteenth and Nineteenth Centuries)

As industrialization became more widespread in the eighteenth century, so did problems with disease. The movement of people to cities, the unhealthy working conditions, child labor, and overcrowding all had an impact on health care during the Industrial Revolution. Hospitals did not offer good care to patients, but they grew in number, as did their mortality rates. Many patients shared the same bed amid unsanitary conditions. The practice of asepsis had not yet became a part of medical and nursing knowledge. Once inside the hospital, patients frequently contracted more diseases than those they had when they came to the hospital. Home care continued without benefit of training, although the chances for survival were probably better in the home than in the hospital. In Vienna during this time, women in labor begged to be allowed to deliver in the street rather than in the hospital. To be admitted meant sure death because the mortality rate at times was 100%.

Not until 1847 were *antiseptic methods* first developed and used. **Ignaz Philipp Semmelweis,** a Hungarian obstetrician, began to study what was called *childbed fever.* When a physician friend died following a cut on the finger during an autopsy, Semmelweis recognized that his friend had died from essentially the same disease that killed women who had babies. He identified the cause of the childbed (puerperal) fevers as septic materials carried to the mothers on the hands of medical students directly from the autopsy room. As a result, he insisted that medical students and physicians wash their hands in a solution of *chloride of lime* before entering the obstetric ward. Antisepsis soon included the instruments and utensils used in the ward. As a result, the rate of death from childbed fever dropped dramatically in that ward.

Seventeenth and Eighteenth Centuries

Meanwhile, back in the North American colonies during the seventeenth and early eighteenth centuries, hospital care did not exist; family members cared for those who became ill. What did exist were **almshouses** for the poor and pesthouses for those with contagious diseases. The motivation for building the pesthouses was to protect the public, not to treat the sick.

Medicine in America was less developed than that in Europe. Colonial physicians were poorly trained except for the few who obtained their education in England. Nursing continued to be done by untrained persons as well as those in a few religious orders whose mission was to care for the sick. The *first real hospital in America* was built in Philadelphia in the mid-1700s at the urging of *Benjamin Franklin.* All the early American hospitals emulated French and English hospitals and made hospitalization available to the poor for a small fee.

Hospitals obtained medical services by permitting teaching on the wards. Medical advances were slow. The treatment of choice for many diseases was brandy, whiskey, emetics, purgatives, and bleeding. Illustrations in this chapter depict historical nursing settings.

Nineteenth Century

Early nineteenth-century American hospitals were places of confinement where one picked up additional diseases. The hospital wards were dirty, unventilated, and filled with patients with discharging wounds. Perfume was used to cover up offensive odors. Nurses of that time used snuff as a way of trying to make their work conditions bearable. Pain, hemorrhage, infections, and gangrene were the order of the day. Nursing was considered an inferior, undesirable occupation. Religious attendants (nurses) were replaced by lay people often drawn from the criminal population. They exploited and abused patients. Supervision was nonexistent, and

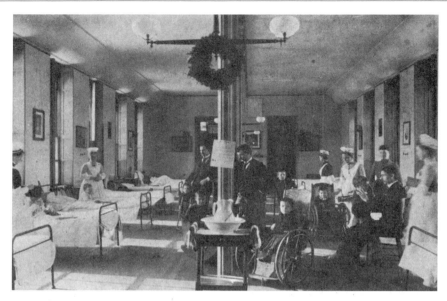

FIGURE 1–1. A pediatric unit under the aegis of the Connecticut Training School (ca. 1878). Note that there are two faculty members supervising three students. (Courtesy of Yale Medical Library.) (From Dolan JA, Fitzpatrick ML, Herrmann EK. *Nursing in Society: A Historical Perspective.* 15th ed. Philadelphia: W.B. Saunders, 1983.)

there was little or no nursing service at night, unless a delivery or a death was expected. For that, a "watcher" was hired.

Nurses were often widows with large families. Drinking on duty and accepting bribes from patients and families were commonplace. "Vice was rampant among these women, who sometimes aided the dying by removing pillows and bed clothes and by performing other morbid activities to hasten the end" (Kalish and Kalish, 1995, p. 26).

In Europe, nursing in secular institutions had become nonexistent, especially in Protestant countries, where the services of the Sisters of Charity were not available. Typical of the hospital nurse at the time were the ignorant, gin-soaked nurse midwives such as **Sairey Gamp** and **Betsy Prig** in Charles Dickens' 1849 novel, *Martin Chuzzlewit.*

Nursing care in America was every bit as bad. An excerpt describing the cholera epidemic in the Philadelphia General Hospital in 1833 painted a picture of overcrowding and demands for increased

wages. Nurses drank the stimulants intended for the sick and were seen drunk and fighting over the dead. Finally, an appeal was made to the Bishop for the services of the Sisters of Charity. They came, restored order, and nursed the sick.

First School of Nursing (1836)

In *1836,* the *first real school of nursing* was founded. In that year a German pastor established a hospital in his parish in Kaiserswerth, Germany. The purpose of the program was to teach the principles of nursing care to the Lutheran Order of Deaconesses. Many of the graduates of the Kaiserswerth Deaconess Institute settled in other parts of the world and established similar programs. The most famous pupil was the Englishwoman **Florence Nightingale,** founder of modern nursing, who attended the school for three months.

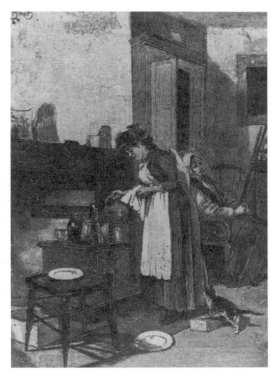

FIGURE 1–2. Caring for a sick person in a tenement house. (From Dolan JA, Fitzpatrick ML, Herrmann EK. *Nursing in Society: A Historical Perspective.* 15th ed. Philadelphia: W.B. Saunders, 1983.)

Florence Nightingale (1820–1910)

Florence Nightingale had an unusual background for a nurse of that period. She had wealthy and influential parents, was well educated before pursuing nursing, and had been presented at Court, indicating her social standing. In her day, women were considered intellectually inferior to men. Education for middle and upper class women often consisted only of lessons in etiquette, dancing, music, deportment, embroidery, painting, and modern languages. Instead of being tutored by governesses or in a private school, her father tutored Miss Nightingale in modern and ancient languages, history, composi-

tion, and philosophy. He was a strict taskmaster; she was an eager student (LeVasseur, 1998, p. 281). She had to beg her parents to be permitted to take nurses' training, because nursing was seen as a job suitable only for the Sairey Gamp type of woman.

Shortly after the start of the 1853 Crimean War (in which Britain, France, Turkey, and Sardinia fought Russia for control of access to the Mediterranean from the Black Sea), information about the neglect and poor care of casualties began to reach England. A correspondent for the London *Times* wrote vivid accounts of the deplorable conditions and lack of medical and nursing care for the British troops. He noted that Russian troops were tended by the Sisters of Mercy, the French were tended by the Sisters of Charity, and the wounded of England were almost completely neglected. So persistent were his charges that a commission was sent to investigate. As a result, the Secretary of War decided that England, too, should have a group of women nurses to tend the war casualties.

He contacted Florence Nightingale and explained the situation to her. Because she had both nursing and administrative experience, the Secretary of War perceived her as the one nurse in England capable of organizing and supervising care in a foreign land.

Being appointed to the task of organization and supervision of nurses during the Crimean War gave Miss Nightingale an unexpected opportunity for achievement. She left England for Crimea with 38 self-proclaimed nurses of limited experience, of whom 24 were nuns. Upon arrival, they found overcrowded, filthy hospitals with no beds, no furniture, no eating utensils, no medical supplies, no blankets, no soap, no linens, and no lamps. The barracks hospital, meant for 1700 patients, packed in 3000 to 4000 patients.

The wounded lay on the floor in their battle uniforms, in filth. Florence Nightingale took charge, using the supplies she had brought, and she raised funds to purchase supplies that the doctors could not obtain for the army. She hired people to clean up the "hospitals" and established laundries to wash linens and uniforms. She expected a great deal of

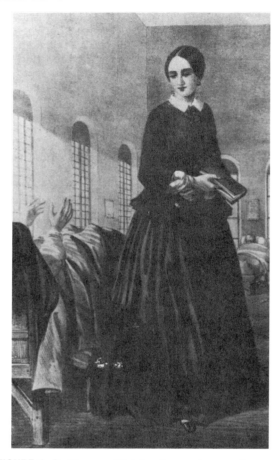

FIGURE 1–3. Florence Nightingale carrying out the "nursing process." (*Nursing Mirror* photograph.) (From Dolan JA, Fitzpatrick ML, Herrmann EK. *Nursing in Society: A Historical Perspective.* 15th ed. Philadelphia: W.B. Saunders, 1983.)

nurses were those who were of good character, experienced a sense of calling, and were well trained to meet the physical needs of patients. Often after hours, it was said, Miss Nightingale could be seen making additional rounds with her lamp to check on the patients, earning her the title "The Lady with the Lamp."

Miss Nightingale had help during many of those nights. Mary Seacole, a black nurse from Jamaica, West Indies, played an important role. She used her own money to build a lodging house and turned the second floor of it into a hospital. She was especially knowledgeable about tropical medicine and used herbs and natural plant medicines to treat patients with cholera, yellow fever, malaria, and diarrhea. At the end of her day she would go to the barracks hospital and offer her help to Miss Nightingale. They worked side by side caring for the soldiers. Both Miss Seacole's government and the British Commonwealth honored her for the lives she saved (Cherry and Jacob, 1999, Chapter 1).

By the end of six months, it was obvious that the efforts of Miss Nightingale and her nurses were paying off. The death rate among the wounded dropped from 420 deaths per 1000 casualties to 22 per 1000. She stayed through the war and was the last to leave. Many of her nurses had become ill during the war and were sent home to recover. Miss Nightingale herself became ill with Crimean fever, probably typhus, and almost died. When she returned home she was decorated by Queen Victoria.

Santa Filomena*

Whene'er a noble deed is wrought,
Whene'er is spoken a noble thought,
   Our hearts, in glad surprise,
   To higher levels rise.
The tidal wave of deeper souls
Into our inmost being rolls,
   And lifts us unawares
   Out of all meaner cares.
Honour to those whose words or deeds

herself and those who worked with her. It was not an easy task, and a major prejudice that had to be overcome was that of the medical officers, who considered the nurses intruders.

The hours were long and difficult for Miss Nightingale and her nurses. She was concerned too that sometimes the nurses became more involved in converting patients to their particular faith than in giving general care. She believed that the best

*Henry Wadsworth Longfellow's tribute to Florence Nightingale, "Saint of the Crimea." Published in the first number of the *Atlantic Monthly,* November, 1857.

Thus help us in our daily needs,
   And by their overflow
   Raise us from what is low!
Thus thought I, as by night I read
Of the great army of the dead,
   The trenches cold and damp,
   The starved and frozen camp—
The wounded from the battle plain,
In dreary hospitals of pain—
   The cheerless corridors,
   The cold and stony floors.
Lo! In that house of misery,
A lady with a lamp I see
   Pass through the glimmering gloom,
   And flit from room to room.
And slow, as in a dream of bliss,
The speechless sufferer turns to kiss
   Her shadow, as it falls
   Upon the darkening walls.
As if a door in heaven should be
Opened, and then closed suddenly,
   The vision came and went—
   The light shone and was spent.
On England's annals, through the long
Hereafter of her speech and song,
   That light its rays shall cast
   From portals of the past.
A lady with a lamp shall stand
In the great history of the land,
   A noble type of good,
   Heroic womanhood.
Nor even shall be wanting here
The palm, the lily, and the spear,
   The symbols that of yore
Saint Filomena bore.

One of Florence Nightingale's major goals was to establish a school of nursing in England. An overwhelming number of physicians opposed such a school on the basis that "because nurses occupied much the same positions as housemaids, they needed little instruction beyond poultice making, the enforcement of cleanliness, and attention to their patients' personal needs" (Kalish and Kalish, 1995, p. 36).

Miss Nightingale did establish a school of nursing in 1860 in England and wrote several books on nursing. Her most famous book was *Notes on Nursing*. She believed nurses should work only in hospi-

tals, not on private duty. She emphasized high moral character in addition to technical skills. Her personal and nursing decisions showed the influence of Plato's and Hippocrates' works. Examples include her decision to remain single, her sense of mission, concern with patient environment, focus on the whole patient, the need for keen observation, and assisting nature to heal the patient (LeVasseur, 1998, p. 282). The core of her spirituality was a belief in perfection.

To her, nursing was a sacred calling, a commitment to work for mankind, not a business. Other Victorian women like her shared the sense of the sacredness of time and the belief that wasting it was a sin. Nursing became a way for Florence Nightingale to work toward the perfection of mankind and her personal salvation. She was against licensure because she thought that was too much like nurses' being in a union. Her major contributions were the elimination of prejudice against a better class of women entering nursing and creating a push toward development of nursing as a respectable vocation. She was intelligent, well educated, and skeptical. This combination made her the foremost critical thinker, in nursing, of its meaning and its role.

Miss Nightingale continued to be involved in health policy well into her eighties. She was the first woman to receive the Order of Merit from the King of England. Although it was proposed that she be buried in Westminster Abbey, her wish to be buried in the family burial place in Willows, Hampshire, was honored. The Nightingale Pledge was written by Lystra Gretter, principal of Farrand Training School in Detroit, in 1893. It continues to be recited in many schools during graduation.

 Critical Thinking Exercise

Review the pledge. Does it apply to the practical nurse in the twenty-first century?

In the spring of 1989, the Florence Nightingale Museum opened in London, England, on the grounds of St. Thomas Hospital, the site of the Nightingale School of Nursing. The Museum is a tribute to this nursing leader despite the fact that she wrote before her death: "I do not wish to be remembered when I am gone" (quote from Miss Nightingale's journal as found in the museum). In spite of her great and courageous contributions to nursing, Florence Nightingale saw only her own faults and her failures.

Critical Thinking Exercise

What would Florence Nightingale say to nursing applicants today who say they are entering nursing to "help" people, to get a job, or to make money? Have we matured as a vocation or as a profession? What do you think?

Civil War (1861–1865)

During the same time period in America, when the country embarked on the Civil War in 1861, there was no such thing as a trained nurse. In the South, especially, there was a great deal of prejudice about women working in hospitals. There was general male opposition, but especially opposition from the medical profession. As a southern woman put it, "It seems strange that what the aristocratic women of Great Britain have done with honor is a disgrace for their sisters on this side of the Atlantic to do" (Kalish and Kalish, 1995, p. 38).

Casualties were high on both sides. Many soldiers died right on the field. Others died because of a poorly trained medical corps. Southern women offered their services as volunteers, but most of the nursing was done by infantrymen assigned to do a task they did not want to do. It was many months before southern women were recognized by the Confederate government for their contribution.

In the North, women offered their services as nurses to the government. One hundred women were selected to take a short training course from doctors in New York City. **Dorothea Lynde Dix,** a teacher by profession and a long-time advocate for better conditions for mental patients, was appointed Superintendent of Nurses. Her task was to organize a corps of female nurses. She requested women under 30 years of age, plain-looking, wearing simple brown or black dresses, without bows, curls, jewelry, or hoop skirts. Women who did not meet the criteria nursed anyway but without official recognition or pay from the government. Eventually, through Miss Dix's efforts, the first hospitals for the mentally ill were also established.

In evaluating the nursing of the Civil War, doctors decided that the nursing system was defective. They did not approve of the women. However, it was a success in the eyes of the wounded soldiers.

Clara Barton, a teacher by profession, was one of the first civilians in the Civil War to round up army supplies. She rented a warehouse, filled market baskets, and encouraged friends to send comforts for the soldiers. Her efforts resulted in her being appointed Superintendent of the Department of Nurses for the Army in 1864. Clara Barton's efforts frequently found her on the front lines, and she nearly lost her life on two occasions. After the war, President Andrew Johnson commissioned her to do what she wanted to do—find missing prisoners of war. Later, while visiting in Europe for health reasons, she met J. Henri Dunant, founder of the *International Red Cross.* He asked for her help in introducing the Red Cross to America. Finally in 1881, through Clara Barton's efforts, the first chapter of the *American Red Cross* was established in Danville, New York.

As often happens, something good emerges out of something not so good. Many of Florence Nightingale's books and ideas had made their way to America but had been ignored. The Civil War experience was the force needed to develop nurse-training schools. The first training schools were separate from hospitals, with the intent being to educate nurses. Soon, hospital-based schools of nursing sprang up. In many hospitals, schools became a cost-effective way of providing a nursing labor force, that is, free. After graduation, nurses generally worked in patients' homes.

Being a student nurse in the 1870s was a difficult experience. Living conditions, working hours, and responsibilities required a great deal of physical and emotional endurance. Not only did these students work long hours, they were also required to sign contracts in return for a course of lectures, on-the-job training, and minimal allowances.

Formal Training: Practical Nursing

The first class for formal training of practical nurses was offered in *1892* at the YWCA in Brooklyn, New York. The focus was on training nurses to offer home health care for patients with chronic illness, the aged, and children. The course was three months in length. It was considered successful, and because of this, other similar programs were developed. Programs that have been identified include an 1892 course in Boston offered by the Massachusetts Emergency and Hygiene Association, the Ballard School in New York in 1897, and the Thompson School for Practical Nursing in Brattleboro, Vermont in 1907. The course of study included cooking, care of the house, dietetics, simple science, and simple nursing procedures.

Until World War I, most nursing done by practical nurses was home nursing, primarily because most people were cared for in the home. Even operations were performed in the home. There is some truth in the way old Western movies portrayed surgery being done on the kitchen table. The nurse's 24-hour schedule included such procedures as cupping and applying leeches; preparing stupes for relief of abdominal distention, mustard plasters for relief of congestion, and poultices for drawing out pus from infections; and administering enemas. These were often nutritive enemas containing eggnog with brandy or chicken broth. Remember, there were no intravenous solutions then. Some practical nurses also assumed the then-accepted role of mid-

wife and taught new mothers the basics of cleanliness, diet, and care of the child. In New York City in 1919 approximately 1700 midwives attended 30% of all births in the city.

By the end of the nineteenth century there was a renewed interest in charitable work and concern for the sick. Practical nursing began to expand from home nursing to public health nursing, care of patients in the slums, school nursing, industrial nursing, and well-baby care. Once again, practical nurses pioneered in this new public health movement.

One of the best-known centers in 1893 was the *Henry Street Settlement* in New York. It was founded by **Lillian Wald,** a social worker who graduated from nursing school and intended to become a doctor. She taught home nursing to immigrants and was so impressed by their need for medical care that she left medical school to begin a nursing service, the Henry Street Settlement. Practical nurses who were members of the Henry Street Settlement taught families in New York slums the basics of cleanliness and control of communicable diseases. There was a decrease in school absenteeism because the spread of childhood illness was reduced. School nurses visited schools and new mothers and their babies. They taught mothers the basics of preventing the summertime killer of infants—cholera infantum. It was estimated that their efforts resulted in survival of 1200 more babies than usual during the summer heat wave. Another original contribution of the nurses was the development of "Little Mother Leagues" in the slums, in which all girls over eight years old were taught how to take care of their younger siblings, including the infants.

Twentieth Century: Organization/Law/Licensing

By 1903, states began to take steps that ultimately led to monitoring of practical nursing. During this period, nursing organizations were developed. Certainly the most influential step was taken by the

TABLE 1–1: Practical Nursing Milestones

Period in History	Event
Ancient Egypt	Midwives delivered babies Untrained attendants assisted priests in caring for the ill
Ancient Hebrews	Wet nurses and attendants nursed the sick and acted as companions
Ancient Greece (Fifth Century BC)	Household nursing and child care were done by domestics and servants
Age of Christianity (First to Fifth Centuries)	Both men and women were nurses; each cared for members of own sex *Phoebe*—The first visiting nurse
Dark Ages (476–1000)	Monks and nuns continued to do practical nursing *Knights Hospitalers*—A military order trained to fight as well as to tend the sick and wounded
Middle Ages (1000–1475)	Time of epidemics. Highborn women renounced their heritage to care for the sick *Alexian Brothers* founded—a nursing brotherhood that still exists in a dual religious and nursing role At the end of the Middle Ages, religious orders no longer assumed as much responsibility for care of the sick
Renaissance (1400–1600)	Scientific methods of the Greeks were employed again, but nursing declined until the nineteenth century
Age of Industrialization (Eighteenth and Nineteenth Centuries)	Deplorable, unsanitary conditions Untrained care givers *Semmelweis*—Developed antiseptic methods (1847)
Seventeenth and Eighteenth Centuries (American Colonies)	Almshouses and pesthouses Nursing done by untrained persons
Nineteenth-Century America	Nursing considered an inferior, undesirable occupation. Care given by untrained lay people often drawn from the criminal population Charles Dickens' novel *Martin Chuzzlewit* (1849) introduced Sairey Gamp and Betsy Prig as the nurse prototype of that period
1836	First real school of nursing, in Kaiserswerth, Germany. *Florence Nightingale* attended for three months Eighteen years later, after start of Crimean War, she nursed wounded with 38 self-identified (untrained) nurses
1860	Florence Nightingale established a school of nursing in England. She wrote several books. The most famous was *Notes on Nursing*
Civil War (1861–1865)	In the South: Most nursing done by infantrymen assigned to the task. Southern women volunteered services In the North: *Dorothea Lynde Dix*, a teacher, was appointed Superintendent of Nurses and organized a corps of female nurses (untrained)
1864	*Clara Barton*, a teacher, collected supplies for soldiers. This led to her appointment as Superintendent of the Department of Nurses for the Army

continued

Period in History	Event
1881	Clara Barton established the first chapter of the American Red Cross in Danville, New York
1892	First class for formal training of practical nursing: YWCA, Brooklyn, New York
1893	Nightingale Pledge written by Canada-born Lystra Gretter, principal of Farrand Training School in Detroit *Henry Street Settlement* founded by Lillian Wald, a social worker, who graduated from a nursing program *Practical nurses* pioneered in this new public health movement. They went into homes and taught the basics of cleanliness and control of communicable diseases to families in New York slums
1897	Ballard School for Practical Nursing opened in New York
1907	Thompson School for Practical Nursing opened in Brattleboro, Vermont
1914	*Mississippi* is the first state to pass a law to license practical nurses
1917	*Standardization* of nursing requirements for practical nursing by National League of Nursing Education (now the National League for Nursing [NLN])
World War I	Shortage of practical nurses. Army School of Nursing established. *Smith Hughes Act* of 1917 provided money for developing additional schools of practical nursing
1920s	Acute shortage of practical nurses Many did not return to nursing after the war
1920–1940	Most practical nursing limited to public health agencies and visiting nurse associations
1938	New York only state to have mandatory licensure
World War II	At home, practical nurses worked in clinics, health departments, industries, hospitals. In the war, they ventured into hardship tours in Europe, North Africa, and the Pacific. The number of practical nurses peaked in 1940 at 159,009
1941	*NAPNES* (National Association of Practical Nurse Education and Service), the nation's professional organization dedicated exclusively to practical nursing, was founded
1944	Comprehensive study of practical nursing by U.S. Department of Vocational Education. This was the first time that tasks of practical nursing were agreed upon
End of World War II	Nursing shortage saw movement of practical nurses into hospitals and gradually increasing responsibilities
1949	NFLPN (National Federation for Licensed Practical Nurses) organized

continued

TABLE 1–1 continued	
Period in History	**Event**
1949	Joint Committee on Practical Nurses and Auxiliary Workers in Nursing Services recommended use of the title *licensed practical nurse* and differentiated between tasks of registered nurses and LPNs
1951	*Journal of Practical Nursing* published by NAPNES (now *Practical Nursing Today*)
1952	Approximately 60% of the nurse work force was made up of practical nurses
1955	All states had licensure laws for practical/vocational nurses
1957	NLN established a Council of Practical Nursing Programs
1961	NLN began offering accrediting services for practical nursing programs
1965	ANA (American Nurses Association) first moves toward two distinct levels in nursing—professional and technical
1979	NLN published first list of competencies for practical/vocational nursing programs
1980s	Resurgence of ANA's move toward two distinct levels of nursing. This resulted in some states adopting two levels of nursing and then rescinding their decision because of the nursing shortage
1984	Creation of ALPNA (American Licensed Practical Nurses Association)
1989	The American Medical Association (AMA) initiated and subsequently dropped the Registered Care Technician (RCT) proposal
1990s	Unlicensed personnel are used for client care. The number of hospital jobs has decreased. The primary employment site has moved into the community
1994	First computerized adaptive test (NCLEX-PN) available to practical/vocational nursing graduates
1995	Full-time nursing positions in hospitals decreased. Client/nurse ratios increased. Primary employment in community continues
1996	Long-term care certification examinations for LP/VNs by National Council of State Boards of Nursing with the National Association for Practical Nurse Education available
2000	Increased demand for LP/VNs in nursing homes and extended care; demand down in hospitals

National League of Nursing Education (now the National League for Nursing, or NLN), which in 1917 developed a nationwide system of standardization of nursing requirements for practical nursing.

In **1914, Mississippi** was the first state to pass a law licensing practical nurses. This was an important event because the public had no way of knowing who was providing nursing care. Remember that for centuries, self-proclaimed nurses were responsible for the majority of the nursing that was done. Licensing, however, was not mandatory, and by 1938 New York was the *only state to have mandatory licensure.*

Critical Thinking Exercise

Does your state have mandatory licensure? What year did it begin?

At the onset of World War I, there were few practical nurses and few schools of practical nursing. Hurriedly "trained" nurses were rushed to the battlefront. An army school of nursing was established to combat the severe nursing shortage and to improve the overall quality of care. Many nurses looking for glamor and excitement found superhuman demands made of them during the war.

The home front was facing a battle of its own in 1917–1918, with a major epidemic of pneumonia in 1917 and a worldwide epidemic of Spanish influenza in 1918. The mortality rate was high, especially in 1918. The *Smith Hughes Act of 1917* provided money for developing additional schools of practical nursing. The first high school vocational practical nursing program opened at the Minneapolis, Minnesota, Girls Vocational High School in 1919. However, the new schools could not supply nurses quickly enough to meet the severe shortage in the United States.

After the war, many nurses did not continue nursing, so there was an acute shortage of nurses in the 1920s. Many more hospitals opened schools of nursing, but their real purpose was to provide staffing. Hospitals without schools were staffed heavily with untrained help.

In the period between the two World Wars, 1920–1940, six states had laws licensing practical nurses, but there were few practical nursing schools throughout the country. Much of their work continued to be done through public health agencies and through visiting nurse associations.

During the Depression of the 1930s, many nurses lost their jobs or worked in hospitals for room and board rather than a salary. When it became fairly obvious that America was becoming involved in World War II, nursing leaders began to prepare for the need for all kinds of nurses. They did not want to face the nursing shortage experienced during World War I. This was a monumental task, because nursing had decreased in popularity as a vocation.

Practical nurses played a significant role both at home and in the war. At home, practical nurses worked in clinics, health departments, industry, and hospitals. At the battlefields, nurses could be found in Europe, North Africa, and the Pacific. One of the most widespread diseases they fought was malaria in the East Indies, the Philippines, and southern Asiatic countries. The number of practical nurses in America peaked in 1940 at 159,009 and by 1944 was already experiencing a decline.

Nursing Organizations

The National Association for Practical Nurse Education and Service, Inc. (**NAPNES**), was founded in 1941. The multidisciplinary composition of its membership includes licensed practical nurses (LPNs), registered nurses (RNs), physicians, hospital and nursing home administrators, students, and public members. It was the first organization formed to promote practical nursing schools and continuing education for LP/VNs. The membership fee includes a subscription to *The Journal of Practical Nursing,* the official magazine of NAPNES. Membership is open to anyone concerned with the advancement of practical/vocational nursing.

This association was the first to be recognized by the U.S. Department of Education as an official accrediting agency for schools of practical nursing. For the past several years, NAPNES has no longer accredited practical nursing programs. (See NAPNES Nursing Practice Standards, Appendix B.)

The end of World War II saw a continuing shortage of nurses. This shortage helped practical

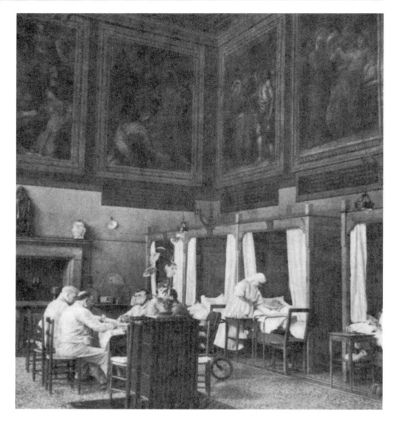

FIGURE 1–4. A Sister at the Hotel Dieu in Beaune giving care to a patient in a room compartment. Ambulatory patients enjoy meals at the table in the center. Note the works of art. (From Dolan JA, Fitzpatrick ML, Herrmann EK. *Nursing in Society: A Historical Perspective.* 15th ed. Philadelphia: W.B. Saunders, 1983.)

nurses play an important part in hospital nursing. Most hospitals gradually increased the responsibilities designated for the practical nurse.

In 1944, the U.S. Department of Vocational Education made a comprehensive study of practical nursing. This was the first time that the tasks of practical nursing were agreed upon. Extensive specific duties were outlined, with an emphasis on maintaining aseptic technique. The terms "to judge," "to appraise," "to recognize," and "to determine" were often used to describe the scope of the practical nurse's job.

Other important changes followed. In 1949, the Joint Committee on Practical Nurses and Auxiliary Workers in Nursing Services recommended use of the title licensed practical nurse. Furthermore, the Committee differentiated between the tasks of the RN and the LPN and saw the LPN as being under the supervision of the RN. The Committee also suggested that practical nurses organize to make decisions on their salary, working conditions, and employment standards.

Because of the work of the Joint Committee, many practical nursing programs were strengthened with regard to content and focused for the first time on the preparation of practical nursing instructors. Up to this point, any graduate nurse was eligible to teach practical nursing.

By 1952, almost 60% of the nursing work force was made up of practical nurses. In many instances, RNs expressed bitterness because hospitals, clinics, and other agencies were hiring practical nurses for less money and assigning tasks to them beyond their educational level. They also expressed concern that the public was unable to differentiate between the levels of nurses because both wore the same type of white uniforms, caps, and pins. Many practical nurses quickly stopped wearing the practical nursing insignia, which was meant to identify the practical nurse. In many agencies, pay continued to be poor, and practical nurses alternately performed tasks belonging to the RN one day and those belonging to nursing aides, for lesser compensation, on other days. Many practical nurses felt trapped in such situations because of their need for employment.

The **NFLPN** (National Federation of Licensed Practical Nurses, Inc.), organized in 1949, is the policy-making body for LPNs and LVNs. NFLPN is made up of LP/VNs, student practical/vocational nurses, and associate members. It was formed by LP/VNs who wanted an organization to work for and speak on behalf of them. Membership includes a publication called *Practical Nursing Today*. The organization

1. keeps its members involved with matters of interest to practical/vocational nursing,
2. makes health, accident, malpractice, and personal liability insurance plans available to its members,
3. works for LP/VN representation on boards of nursing,
4. provides a voice in nursing legislation on a national level,
5. encourages agencies to provide continuing education for practical nurses,
6. provides a statement of functions and qualifications of LPNs,
7. works with other health organizations to promote quality patient care, and
8. provides CEU opportunities.

See NFLPN Nursing Practice Standards for the LP/VN in Appendix C.

The **NLN** (National League for Nursing), created by combining three nursing organizations in 1950, is involved with all types of nursing: consultation; accreditation of nursing education programs; professional testing services; surveys on admissions, enrollments, competencies, graduation, studies on nursing education, and service; information sources on trends in nursing; and conventions, meetings, workshops, and continuing education. NLN membership is open to all nurses and others concerned

with health care. The membership fee includes a subscription to its journal *Nursing and Health Care Perspectives*. See Entry-Level Competencies of Graduates of Educational Programs in Practical Nursing in Appendix D.

In 1961, the NLN established a separate department of practical nursing programs. A major breakthrough was the development of a system for accrediting schools of practical nursing. This was supported by the American Nurses Association (ANA) and the NFLPN. To be accredited by the NLN, a school had to meet standards set by the NLN. With the exception of programs receiving federal funds, it was not, nor is it now, mandatory for schools to be accredited by the NLN, because the major responsibility for approval of nursing programs rests with each state board of nursing. The NLN continues to accredit nursing programs while it challenges the U.S. Department of Education's recommendation to withdraw the NLN's recognition as an accrediting agency. The 1960s brought a move by the ANA to streamline nursing into two distinct levels: the two-year technical and the four-year professional nurse.

The **ALPNA** (American Licensed Practical Nurses Association) was founded in 1984. Its major function is involvement in lobbying and legislative issues that affect the LP/VN. Anyone wanting to promote LP/VN interests is welcome to join.

In 1975 there were 1337 practical nursing programs, graduating a total of 46,080 practical/vocational nurses. Approximately two thirds of the practical nurses were employed in hospitals, 17.3% in nursing homes, 7.5% in private duty, and 6.5% in doctors' offices, clinics, and dental offices. Admission standards in most schools increased, as did the difficulty of the curriculum.

In the 1980s, a resurgence of the ANA movement toward establishing two levels of nursing temporarily gained momentum. Some states worked toward adoption of the ANA recommendation. Because a serious nursing shortage developed in the late 1980s, the ANA movement stalled.

With the goal of easing the nursing shortage, the American Medical Association in the summer of 1989 proposed a new health care worker, the Registered Care Technologist (RCT). The RCT would be trained in one- and two-year programs. Because this new level of health care worker correlated with existing personnel, the practical/vocational nurse and the associate-degree nurse, the RCT proposal was not successful. This event is a gentle reminder for practical/vocational nurses to be strong, organized, and vigilant as a group. Changes in the health care system are occurring daily, as are changes in opportunities for LP/VNs.

If you want a voice in your vocation of nursing, join your vocational organization(s). Additional information can be obtained by writing to the organization headquarters.

NAPNES
1400 Spring St., Suite 330
Silver Spring, MD 20910
(301) 588–2491
e-mail: napnes@bellatlantic.net
NFLPN
893 US Hwy. 70 West, Suite 202
Garner, NC 27529
(919) 779–0046, (800) 948–2511
website: http://www.nflpn.org
NLN
61 Broadway
New York, NY 10006
(212) 363–5555, (800) 669–1656
website: http://www.nln.org
ALPNA
1090 Vermont Ave. NW, Suite 800
Washington, DC 20005
(202) 682–9000

Important Influences in Nursing History

Many RNs influenced the course of nursing and practical nursing history. Table 1–2 identifies some of those registered nurses.

You Have Come a Long Way

As a final note, it may be interesting to compare present practical/vocational nursing tasks with those

that you would have been expected to perform in 1887. Practical/vocational nursing has indeed come a long way.

The following job description was given to floor nurses by a hospital in 1887 (author unknown):

In addition to caring for your 50 patients, each nurse will follow these regulations:

1. Daily sweep and mop the floors of your ward, dust the patient's furniture and window sills. Maintain an even temperature in your ward by bringing in a scuttle of coal for the day's business.
2. Light is important to observe the patient's condition. Therefore, each day fill kerosene lamps, clean chimneys, and trim wicks. Wash the windows once a week.
3. The nurse's notes are important in aiding the physician's work. Make your pens carefully; you may whittle nibs to your individual taste.
4. Each nurse on day duty will report every day at 7 AM and leave at 8 PM, except on the Sabbath, on which day you will be off from 12 noon to 2 PM.
5. Graduate nurses in good standing with the director of nurses will be given an evening off each week for courting purposes or two evenings a week if you go regularly to church.
6. Each nurse should lay aside from each pay day a goodly sum of her earnings for her benefits during her declining years so that she will not become a burden. For example, if you earn $30 a month you should set aside $15.
7. Any nurse who smokes, uses liquor in any form, gets her hair done at a beauty shop, or frequents dance halls will give the director of nurses good reason to suspect her worth, intentions, and integrity.
8. The nurse who performs her labors and serves her patients and doctors without fault for five years will be given an increase of five cents a day, providing there are no hospital debts outstanding.

TABLE 1-2: Some Persons/Events in Nursing History

Mary Robinson	1859	First visiting nurse
Linda Richards	1873	America's first professionally trained nurse (1-year program); organized other training schools; developed a system of written records and orders
Euphemia Van Rensselaer	1876	Introduced first uniform—apron and cap (Bellevue Training School for Nurses)
Mary E. P. Mahoney	1879	First African-American graduate nurse
Clara Barton	1882	Established the American Red Cross
Elizabeth Weston	1888	First Native American nurse. Graduate of Training School of the University of Pennsylvania. Came from Lincoln School for Indian girls in Philadelphia. After graduation returned to care for her people on a Sioux reservation in North Dakota
Emily L. Loveridge	1890	Graduate of Bellevue Training School for Nurses. Went west to establish first school of nursing in the Northwest at Good Samaritan Hospital, Portland, Oregon
Mabel Staupers	1890–1989	First executive director and last president of the National Association of Colored Graduate Nurses. Credited with integration of black nurses into ANA and other nursing organizations. Wrote *No Time For Prejudice*
Isabel Hampton Robb	1893	Wrote first substantial nursing text: *Nursing: Its Principles and Practice for Hospital and Private Use.* Promoted nurses' rights, 3-year training program, 8-hour day, and licensure
Lillian Wald and Mary Brewster	1893	First visiting nurse service for the poor: Nurses Settlement House in slum section, lower East Side, New York City. Later moved to Henry Street and name changed to Henry Street Settlement House
Lavinia L. Dock	1896	First president of forerunner of ANA (Nurses Associated Alumnae of the United States and Canada). Wrote four-volume *History of Nursing* with Adelaide Nutting. Outlined principles on which ANA was founded
Dita H. Kinney	1901	First Superintendent of Nurses of the Army Nurse Corps
Mrs. Bedford Fenwick (Great Britain)	1901	First president of International Council of Nurses. Proposed state registration of nurses

continued

TABLE 1–2 continued		
Adelaide Nutting	1907	First graduate of Johns Hopkins Training School for Nurses. First nurse in the world to hold professorship in a university (Columbia). In 1917, Chair of Committee to Develop National Curriculum
Lillian Wald, Ella Phillips Crandall, Mary Beard, Mary Lent, Edna Foley, Lystra Greiter, Elizabeth G. Fox	1912	Formed National Organization of Public Health Nurses. Lillian Wald, first president
Margaret Sanger	1916	A public health nurse, she spearheaded the birth control movement as a response to high maternal and child mortality. Opened first birth control clinic in America
Annie W. Goodrich	1918	President of ANA. Became Chief Inspecting Nurse for army hospitals at home and abroad. Supported formation of Army School of Nursing, became dean of school
	1924	U.S. Indian Bureau Nursing Service founded
Mary Breckenridge	1925	Organized Frontier Nursing Service of Kentucky
Sage Memorial Hospital School of Nursing, Ganado, Arizona	1930	First school of nursing for American Indians
Lucile Petry	1943	Director of U.S. Cadet Nurses Corps
Esther Lucille Brown, Ph.D., a researcher	1948	"Brown" Study: Advocated movement of nursing education to collegiate setting
Mildred L. Montag	1952	Appointed as first Associate Degree Nursing Program Project Coordinator. Project based on Montag's doctoral thesis, "Education of Nursing Technicians." Project located at Queen's College, New York

Summary

☐ The varied and colorful evolution of practical nursing has been described with limited reference to roles played by RNs in the course of nursing history. This account is an attempt to show practical/vocational nursing students that their vocation began to develop in ancient times and is not an appendage of professional nursing. Practical/vocational nurses can be rightly proud of their own nursing "roots."

☐ The duties of practical/vocational nurses have changed according to the needs present at various times in history. Currently, practical/vocational nurses are taught basic skills during their educational program. According to some states' nurse practice acts, they are allowed to perform complex skills delegated by an RN. However, in these states, the RN must teach the complex skill involved, be satisfied with the LP/VN's performance, and document this for the LP/VN's file. Direct supervision by an RN is also required for performance of complex nursing tasks.

☐ You can have a voice in the decisions affecting practical nursing. Consider the odds faced by these historical figures in nursing:

> Florence Nightingale, founder of modern nursing
> Clara Barton, founder of the American Red Cross
> Lillian Wald, founder of public health nursing
> Dorothea Dix, advocate for the mentally ill

☐ No more frontiers, you say? Don't you believe that. You can, for example, begin by taking a stand through your vocational organization—the local and state practical nurses associations. Valuable support groups exist in the form of nursing organizations. Student membership is available in the NFLPN, and state conventions frequently sponsor a student day. NAPNES continues to fight for the rights of practical nurses and supports continuation of the vocation. The NLN focuses on nursing needs at all levels of nursing and provides broad services for nurses in all areas. Seek out your state LP/VN association to gain a voice in your vocation.

☐ It has been suggested by some that the history of practical nursing sounds depressing. Not so. Practical nurses have always been in the forefront of doing the real, down-to-earth nursing tasks. They have often done what no one else dared or cared to do. In the beginning, most of these "nurses" had little or no training. Consider that Florence Nightingale herself left the Kaiserswerth Deaconess Institute training program after three months of training. It is with this in mind that this chapter has focused on figures in nursing history who had limited nursing education and yet enormous courage to care for patients, most often without glamor or fanfare. What these nurses did have was the gratitude of their patients and the quiet satisfaction of a job well done. We salute you, the new practical/vocational nurses and the nurses who have paved the way for you.

Review Questions

1. How does the education of nurses in early civilizations compare with your education?
   A. "Healing touch" was emphasized.
   B. Nurses were chosen from the upper class.
   C. Physicians were responsible for direct supervision.
   D. Training was limited to what would be done by a competent maid.
2. How did the religious Reformation affect the growth of nursing?
   A. It provided a resurgence of caring for the poor and the sick.
   B. Greater personal freedom resulted

in a decrease of unselfish service to humanity.
   C. Protestants and Catholics challenged each other to provide the best care.
   D. The development of antiseptic methods decreased the death rate.
3. What is Florence Nightingale's contribution to nursing?
   A. Critical thinking, focus on whole patient, importance of patient environment, need for careful observation.
   B. She wrote the first substantial nursing text and promoted nurses' rights, including changing the 12-hour day to 8 hours.

C. She wrote the Nightingale Pledge in 1893 to set guidelines and inspire new nurses upon graduation.

D. She began the first visiting nurse service for the poor in the Nurses' Settlement House in the lower East Side slum section of New York.

4. Where was the first formal training of practical nurses started in the U.S.?
   A. At the YWCA in Brooklyn, New York.
   B. The Thompson School in Brattleboro, Vermont.
   C. The Henry Street Settlement in New York.
   D. The Department of Nurses for the Army.

5. Which nursing organization includes a subscription to *Practical Nursing Today* in the membership fee?
   A. NLN
   B. ANA
   C. NFLPN
   C. NAPNES

References

Cherry B, Jacob S. *Contemporary Nursing Issues, Trends, and Management.* St. Louis: C. V. Mosby, 1999.

Deloughery G. *Issues and Trends in Nursing,* 3rd ed. St. Louis: C. V. Mosby, 1998.

Kalish P, Kalish B. *The Advance of American Nursing,* 3rd ed. Boston: Little, Brown, 1995.

LeVasseur J. *Plato, Nightingale, and Contemporary Nursing.* IMAGE: J of Nursing Scholarship. Vol. 30, No. 3. Indianapolis: Sigma Theta Tau, 1998.

Widerquist J. The spirituality of Florence Nightingale. Nurs Res 41(1):49–55, 1992.

Bibliography

ANA Report. Trained attendants and practical nurses. Am J Nurs 44:7–8, 1944.

Backer B. The Nightingale Pledge: A commitment that survives the passage of time. Nursing and Health Care 14: 3, March 1993.

Brown E. *Nursing for the Future.* New York: Russell Sage Foundation, 1948.

D'Antonio P. Nineteenth century nursing. Reflections. Vol. 3, No. 3. Indianapolis: Sigma Theta Tau, 3rd/4th Quarter, 1997.

Deming D. Practical nurses—A professional responsibility. Am J Nurs 44:36–43, 1944.

Fahy E. Covering the history of nursing. Nursing and Health Care 14:3, March 1993.

Frantz A. Nursing pride: Clara Barton in the Spanish-American War. Am J Nurs 98(10), Oct. 1998.

Goldsmith J. New York's practical nurse program. Am J Nurs 42:1026–1031, 1942.

Kinder J. President NLN. Letter, November 1986.

Longfellow HW. *The Political Works of Longfellow,* Cambridge ed. Boston: Houghton-Mifflin, 1975.

McGuane E, Bullough B. Proud history, promising future. Practical Nurs 40–42, Dec. 1992.

Metules T. Pins and pinning—the traditions continue. RN No. 12, Dec. 1998.

NLN Research and Policy. Practical nursing's role in a community-based health care system. Prism: NLN Research of National League for Nursing 2:1–8, 1994.

Philips E. Practical nurses in a public agency. Am J Nurs 44:974–975, 1944.

Pillitteri A. One nursing curriculum 100 years ago: A retrospective view as a prospective necessity. J Nurs Ed 33(6):286–287, June 1994.

Server S. The story of the lamp. Am J Pract Nurs 5(1), 1998.

Thompson M. *The Cry and the Covenant.* New York: Signet Books, 1955.

Chapter 2

The Health Care Team

Outline

Who is Responsible for Mrs. Brown's Discharge?
    Mrs. Brown's Emergency Care
    The Surgical Experience
    Postanesthesia Care Unit (PACU)
    Intensive Care—A Time of Close Observation
    Surgical Floor—An Eye to Discharge
    Extended Care Unit—On the Road to Rehabilitation
The Health Care Team
    What Is Nursing?
    Nursing's Place on the Health Care Team

Registered Nurses (Professional Nurses)
    Education
    The Role of Registered Nurses
    Education Beyond the Basic Nursing Programs for Registered Nurses
Practical/Vocational Nurses
    Role of the Practical/Vocational Nurse
    Expanded Role of the Practical/Vocational Nurse
Student Nurses
Nursing Assistants
Unlicensed Assistive Personnel (UAP)

Clerk Receptionists (Ward Clerks, Health Unit Clerks, Health Unit Coordinators)
Unit Managers
Delivery of Client Care Services in Acute Care Settings
    Case Method
    Functional Method
    Team Method
    Primary Method (Primary Care)
    Case Management Method
Supply and Demand
Patient-Focused Care: Another System for Delivering Client Care
    What Is Patient-Focused Care?

Key Terms

advanced practice
associate degree nursing
baccalaureate nursing programs
case management method
case method
certification
clerk receptionist
cross training
decentralized

differentiated practice
diploma programs
functional method
independent
interdependent
nursing assistant
patient-focused care
practical/vocational nurse

primary care method
registered nurse
skill mix
standards of care
student nurse
team method
unit manager
unlicensed assistive personnel

Objectives

Upon completing this chapter you will be able to:
1. Explain in your own words the goal of the health care team.
2. List ten members of the health care team (nurses count for one member).
3. Identify the nursing personnel who are part of the health care team according to the following criteria:

    a. education
    b. role and responsibilities
    c. licensing
4. Define nursing.
5. Describe in your own words the following methods used to deliver nursing service:
    a. case method
    b. functional method

    c. team method
    d. primary care
    e. case management method
    e. patient-focused care
6. Describe the practical/vocational nurse's role in the methods used to deliver the nursing services listed in Objective 5.

Who Is Responsible for Mrs. Brown's Discharge?

Mrs. Amelia Brown, aged 75 years, lives with her daughter on a 200-acre farm in rural Wisconsin. While working in the barn, Mrs. Brown fell and broke her right hip. She required surgery to repair the hip. Under general anesthesia during surgery, Mrs. Brown's blood pressure reached dangerously high levels, but it quickly stabilized under the anesthesiologist's interventions. Despite this setback, Mrs. Brown was discharged after six days in the hospital. She and her family agreed that she was not ready to return home at that point in her recovery, so she was discharged to an extended care facility. Here she was given physical therapy to learn how to function at home with her restrictions in ambulation. Two weeks later, Mrs. Brown was discharged from the extended care facility to her home.

Sounds like another success story for nursing, doesn't it? We will follow Mrs. Brown as she progresses through the health care system and then decide who should get credit for Mrs. Brown's discharge back to the farm.

Mrs. Brown's Emergency Care

After Mrs. Brown falls, her daughter calls the emergency squad to transport her mother to the nearest hospital. This hospital is located 20 miles away in a city with a population of 98,000. The three persons manning the emergency squad are **emergency medical technicians (EMTs).** Each EMT has taken a course in basic life support skills of approximately 120 hours. Each has been certified as an EMT by means of a national test. The EMTs are currently taking a five-month paramedic course, which is preparing them to provide more advanced life support skills. On the way to the hospital, the EMTs monitor Mrs. Brown's blood pressure, pulse, respirations, and level of consciousness. They keep her right leg immobilized. The EMTs maintain contact with the hospital emergency room by means of a two-way radio.

On arriving at the emergency room (ER), the EMTs provide the **registered nurse (RN)** with verbal and written reports of Mrs. Brown's status. The **emergency room doctor** examines Mrs. Brown and orders an x-ray film of her right hip. The **x-ray technician** brings the x-ray equipment to the ER and takes an x-ray film of Mrs. Brown's right hip. The x-ray technician has had a minimum of preparation in a two-year program conducted by a hospital or technical college. This technician is prepared to perform diagnostic measures involving radiant energy. The **radiologist** on duty reads the x-ray film of Mrs. Brown's right hip. On the basis of the physical examination and the results of the x-ray, the ER physician diagnoses a fracture of Mrs. Brown's right proximal femur. The ER physician notifies Mrs. Brown's **family physician** and contacts the **orthopedic surgeon** she requests.

The RN receives Mrs. Brown in the ER and assesses her and provides care until she is admitted to the hospital. The RN is a graduate of a diploma or three-year program in nursing. This nurse has passed a national examination to become an RN. RNs who work in the ER participate regularly in continuing education courses at the hospital and at seminars given regionally and nationally for ER nurses. Mrs. Brown is prepared for surgery.

To be qualified to be in charge of the medical care of Mrs. Brown, the family physician has attended four years of college, four years of medical school, one year of internship, and approximately a three-year residency program. Medical school consists of a program that provides the basic knowledge and skills needed to be a medical doctor. Internship involves a program of clinical experiences designed to complete the requirements for licensure as a practicing physician. The residency program prepares physicians for practice in a specialty. The specialty in this situation is family practice. With some exceptions, the ER physician, the radiologist, and the orthopedic surgeon have had the same education as the family physician. The ER physician has completed a residency program in emergency or trauma medicine. The radiologist has completed a residency program in the reading and interpretation of x-ray films. The orthopedic surgeon has completed a three- to five-year residency in performing surgery for problems of bones and joints. Each of these physicians has passed the board examinations, which license them as physicians and allow them to practice under the state medical practice act. Each physician in this scenario is board certified in his or her specialty area.

Laboratory studies are ordered preoperatively. **Lab personnel** draw blood for the studies. Lab personnel have varied educational backgrounds. Some have on-the-job training to obtain blood samples. A medical lab technician has two years of education. A medical technologist (MT) has four-plus years of education and can be certified by a national examination. Lab personnel are responsible for collecting the specimens needed for lab tests, performing the tests, and reporting the results to physicians and staff.

The family requests that their parish priest be contacted to give Mrs. Brown the sacrament of the sick (see Chapter 10). Because surgery is imminent, the pastoral care department is notified. A Roman Catholic **priest,** a member of the pastoral care team, anoints Mrs. Brown with holy oils, prays with her, and gives her Holy Communion. To be able to meet Mrs. Brown's spiritual needs, the priest has had four years of college and four years of theological school before being ordained.

The Surgical Experience

In the ER, the **anesthetist** prepares Mrs. Brown and her family for the anesthesia part of the surgical experience. This health care worker is an RN with a bachelor of science in nursing (BSN). This nurse has studied an additional two to three years in an approved school of anesthesiology after the four-year BSN program. The anesthetist provides anesthesia to clients undergoing surgery. Mrs. Brown is transferred to the surgical suite, where she undergoes a right hip pinning procedure under general anesthesia. This type of anesthesia will put Mrs. Brown in a state of unconsciousness. During surgery, the anesthetist monitors Mrs. Brown's vital signs continuously while she is unconscious. The orthopedic surgeon is assisted by the **surgical tech-**

nician. The surgical technician sets up the sterile environment. This health care worker makes sure the surgeon's instruments and supplies are available when he requests them for the pinning of Mrs. Brown's right hip. The surgical technician is a graduate of a one-year diploma program at the local technical college. The overall functioning of the surgical team is coordinated by the **professional nurse,** who has a minimum qualification of a BSN.

During surgery, the anesthetist notes that Mrs. Brown's blood pressure is rising to a dangerous level. She contacts the **anesthesiologist** STAT (immediately!). The anesthesiologist, a medical doctor with a residency in anesthesiology, orders antihypertensive drugs (drugs that lower the blood pressure). The situation is quickly brought under control. Surgery is completed, and Mrs. Brown is sent to the postanesthesia care unit (PACU).

Postanesthesia Care Unit

The purpose of the PACU is to monitor the client's vital signs, level of consciousness, movement, and any special equipment required by the client after surgery. When the client's condition is stable, he or she is transferred to the hospital room. Mrs. Brown is assessed by a PACU **registered nurse** who is a graduate of a three-year school of nursing. After one and a half hours, Mrs. Brown is assessed as being ready to leave the PACU. Because of the episode involving high blood pressure during surgery, Mrs. Brown's surgeon orders her to go to the intensive care unit (ICU) overnight for closer observation instead of to the postoperative surgical floor. A **transport aide,** who is trained on the job, and a **staff nurse** from the PACU take Mrs. Brown to the ICU.

Intensive Care — A Time of Close Observation

The ICU is staffed by RNs who went to school for either two years (associate degree nurses), three years (diploma nurses), or four years (baccalaureate nurses). Each nurse has taken the same national examination to become an RN. None of these nurses are qualified to work in the ICU immediately on graduation from their nursing programs. Most institutions prepare a nurse for the responsibilities of this unit through in-service classes after a minimum amount of experience or through a postgraduate or continuing education course. Mrs. Brown's nurse is a **two-year graduate** and is responsible for the care and observation of two clients.

The family is unable to answer some additional questions about Mrs. Brown's medical history. The family physician asks the **clerk receptionist (ward clerk)** to obtain Mrs. Brown's medical records from the medical records department. The clerk receptionist assumes the responsibility for many of the clerical duties that are a necessary part of any client care area. The clerk receptionist learns these skills by taking a course that varies in length, depending on the area of the country. The course averages about one semester of theory and clinical experience. The **medical records department** is staffed by personnel who have gone to school for two to six years to learn the skills required for indexing, recording, and storing client records, which are legal documents. Thanks to Mrs. Brown's old records, which are sent to the ICU, the family physician receives answers to his medical questions.

The surgeon writes postoperative orders for Mrs. Brown, including an order for patient-controlled analgesia (PCA) to control postoperative pain. The hospital **pharmacist** has studied for a minimum of four to six years to become licensed to prepare, compound, and dispense drugs prescribed by a physician or dentist. The pharmacist fills the order for Mrs. Brown's drugs and intravenous solutions.

The **respiratory therapy department** is contacted to evaluate Mrs. Brown's respiratory status and suggest treatment to prevent respiratory problems. Respiratory care technicians (CRTTs) are graduates of 18-month programs in respiratory therapy. Respiratory care therapists (RRTs) are graduates of associate degree or four-year college programs in respiratory therapy. Within 24 hours after admission to the ICU, Mrs. Brown is judged to be

in stable condition. She is transferred by a **transport aide** and an ICU **staff member** to the surgical floor.

Surgical Floor — An Eye to Discharge

The **nurse manager** on the surgical floor at this hospital is an RN who has graduated from a four-year nursing program. As manager of the unit, this nurse is responsible for all the care given to clients. Mrs. Brown's **team leader** is an RN from a two-year nursing program. This nurse is responsible for formulating a plan of care for each of the assigned clients and modifying these plans as needed.

The team leader receives a verbal report and the current care plan for Mrs. Brown from the ICU personnel. The team leader begins assessment of her new admission. The **practical/vocational nurse (LP/VN)** helps put Mrs. Brown to bed and immediately takes her vital signs. The LP/VN is a graduate of a one-year vocational program in nursing. The LP/VN has taken a national examination to become licensed as a practical/vocational nurse. The practical/vocational nurse is assigned to give Mrs. Brown bedside care.

A referral is sent to the physical therapy department. The **physical therapist (PT)** assesses the strength of Mrs. Brown's unaffected extremities. The PT sets up a program of exercises and ambulation with no weight-bearing on the right extremity. The goal of treatment is to prevent the development of complications. Physical therapy keeps up the strength of Mrs. Brown's unaffected extremity until she is able to bear weight fully on the right side. The PT has been educated in a four- or five-year college program. Some PTs have a master's degree in physical therapy. The **physical therapy assistant (PTA)** has been educated in a two-year community college or technical school setting. The PTA carries out the plan of care developed by the PT.

Soon after the patient is transferred to the surgical floor, the **social worker** visits Mrs. Brown and her family to discuss discharge plans. The social worker suggests that Mrs. Brown stay in an extended care facility for two weeks to participate in extensive physical therapy before returning to the farm. Social workers help clients and families solve problems with the financial concerns of hospitalization. They arrange for community agencies to provide appropriate care and services needed by clients after discharge from the hospital. Social workers also help the family communicate their health care needs more clearly. Social workers obtain a bachelor's degree in social work in four years and a master's degree in one additional year of college. Mrs. Brown's social worker talks to the PT and the family. All agree that with exercise and skills teaching, the family eventually will be able to care for Mrs. Brown at home.

As the time for discharge to the extended care facility gets closer, a **patient care technologist (PCT)** is assigned to take Mrs. Brown's vital signs. PCTs perform treatments and skills assigned to them by the RN or the LP/VN. PCTs are trained by the hospital for the specific duties they are to perform. Training involves classes (sometimes autotutorial or self-study classes) and a clinical component. The training a PCT gets is short and varies from facility to facility. The job titles "unlicensed assistive personnel" and "patient care assistant" are used in some facilities. The responsibilities of the LP/VN in relation to PCTs are discussed in Chapter 14.

Because Mrs. Brown is 50 pounds overweight, her physician orders a weight reduction diet. The **dietician** teaches Mrs. Brown and her daughter the elements of weight reduction that will be carried out when Mrs. Brown returns to the farm. The dietician is responsible for planning the meals and supplementary feedings for clients and the cafeteria meals for staff. The dietician also supervises the preparation of food and counsels clients and their families about nutritional problems and therapeutic diets. This health professional is educated in a four- to five-year college program, followed by a year of internship in a health care agency.

Every day during Mrs. Brown's stay, the **housekeeper** cleans her room and bathroom. Maintaining cleanliness is an effort to maintain medical asepsis (absence of germs) and provide a pleasant environment. The housekeeper receives training in the needed skills by the employing institution or through a short course in a technical school.

Finally, Mrs. Brown is discharged from the hospital. She leaves by **Medi-Van** and is transported to the extended care facility.

Extended Care Unit — On the Road to Rehabilitation

Mrs. Brown's roommate in the extended care facility is an 80-year-old woman who has had a stroke. She is also preparing to go home after additional physical therapy. The **PT** conducts an initial assessment of Mrs. Brown and incorporates the hospital physical therapy plan of care with her findings. The **PTA** helps Mrs. Brown daily with exercises and ambulation, using a walker and minimum weight-bearing on her right leg. A **nursing assistant (NA)** is assigned to assist Mrs. Brown with her personal care. Nursing assistants are educated to give bedside care through courses of a minimum of 75 hours' duration. Successful completion of this course of study makes the NA eligible to be placed on the state registry of NAs.

A referral is sent to the occupational therapy department. The **occupational therapist (OT)** completes an assessment of Mrs. Brown. The **occupational therapy assistant (OTA)** carries out the plan of care. The goal for Mrs. Brown is to be as independent as possible when she returns to the farm despite her physical limitations. Occupational therapy helps clients restore body function through specific tasks and skills. Educational requirements include a four-year occupational therapy program. Some four-year graduates pursue a master's degree in their field. A two-year program prepares OTAs for their roles.

Mrs. Brown receives her newly prescribed blood pressure medication from the **practical/vocational nurse,** who also is functioning in her expanded role as charge nurse in this facility. The **day supervisor,** an RN with a bachelor of science degree in nursing, checks Mrs. Brown daily to monitor her progress. Ten days later, Mrs. Brown excitedly waits for her family to take her back to the farm. She is pleased with her progress and is confident about going back to her home. She knows that at this time she is unable to gather the eggs each day, but she is anxious to get back in the kitchen.

Critical Thinking Exercise

Who is responsible for Mrs. Brown's return to the farm? After reading Mrs. Brown's story, you can see that it is impossible to give any one member of the health care team credit for sending Mrs. Brown home. Everyone needs to work together!

The Health Care Team

A primary goal of health care is to restore optimal physical, emotional, and spiritual health to clients. This goal is accomplished by promoting health, preventing illness, and restoring health when illness or accident has occurred. Health care includes a large number of specialized services. It is necessary for groups of people to work together to provide clients with all the services they need to maintain comprehensive health care. These groups of health care workers are called the health care team.

For Mrs. Brown to be rehabilitated after her fall, it took a minimum of 123.5 years of education for all the health care workers in this scenario to learn how to perform their respective jobs. The x-ray technician's x-ray film confirmed the presence of a hip fracture. The narcotic pain reliever supplied by the pharmacist relieved pain after the surgical procedure, allowing Mrs. Brown to move more freely and avoid complications. The treatment by the RRT helped prevent pneumonia. The PTs, OTs, and nursing staff all helped restore Mrs. Brown's health and prevent further illness by avoiding complications. The dietician's expertise allowed Mrs. Brown to receive the basic nutrients she needed to maintain her health, heal her fracture, and lose weight. Teaching about weight reduction diets promoted

health by keeping Mrs. Brown's weight within acceptable limits.

As you can see, each member of the health care team, because of his or her specific preparation in a field of study, can increase the quality of health care for a client. It is impossible for one person to provide the knowledge, expertise, and skills that the health care team as a whole can provide.

Each member of the health care team must have good communication skills. Good communication ensures that care is coordinated for the client's benefit (see Chapter 8). Fragmentation of care can be avoided. Each health care team member has to be able to anticipate problems and avoid them when possible (by using critical thinking skills). When problems do occur, the health care team needs to use problem-solving skills to find solutions in the process of delivering care. In this way, the quality of client care is continuously improved. The team must strive continually to keep their care client-oriented. The team needs to realize that a cooperative effort is needed to reach client goals.

What Is Nursing?

What is nursing, and what do nurses on the health care team do? The American Nurses Association (ANA) is a national nursing organization that is recognized as being representative of professional nurses in the United States. This organization defines nursing as dealing with the diagnosis and treatment of human responses to health and illness (American Nurses Association, 1995, p.6).

Another often-used definition of nursing, by Virginia Henderson, complements this one. Henderson states that "the unique function of the nurse is to assist the individual, sick or well, in the performance of those activities contributing to health or its recovery (or to peaceful death) that he would perform if he had the necessary strength, will, or knowledge" (Henderson, 1966, p. 15).

The direction of practical/vocational nursing has been channeled by the two descriptions just given. Both refer to nursing's interest in illness and wellness. It is important for practical/vocational nurses to understand their role in Mrs. Brown's care. An understanding of the education, licensure, roles, and responsibilities of the varied members of the health care team is necessary.

Nursing's Place on the Health Care Team

Nursing staff on the health care team include unit managers, RNs, LP/VNs, student nurses, NAs, and cross-trained staff. Assisting the nursing staff are unlicensed assistive personnel (UAPs). Clerk receptionists, although not nurses, are an important part of the unit staff. The members of the health care team are generally on duty in acute or residential health care organizations 24 hours a day, seven days a week. Some members of the health care team may not be scheduled at night or on weekends or holidays, and some of these persons are available on an on-call basis. In the community, health care workers' hours vary depending on site of employment. Some sites are open only Monday through Friday during day hours. Others also offer services in the evening. And others are open 7 days a week and sometimes 24 hours a day.

Registered Nurses (Professional Nurses)

Education

Today, over 2.6 million RNs are employed in nursing. *Registered nurses* are the largest group of health care workers in the United States. Nursing is a female-dominated profession; approximately 6% of RNs are male. The graduates of the three types of educational programs for professional nurses—two-, three-, and four-year programs—currently take the same licensing examination. On successful completion of this examination, all these graduates hold the title of registered nurse.

- **Associate degree nursing** (ADN) programs are found in community colleges, junior colleges, and technical schools. The ADN educational program includes general education courses, including courses in the biologic, behavioral, and social sciences, as well as nursing theory courses and clinical practice. On graduation, the two-year (associate degree) graduate receives an associate degree in nursing and is eligible to take the national licensure examination for registered nurses (NCLEX-RN) to become a registered nurse.

- Three-year nursing programs (**diploma programs**) are conducted by a hospital-based school of nursing. These nursing programs comprise the same general education courses as two-year programs, with nursing theory courses in addition. Diploma programs traditionally have emphasized clinical experience. The three-year nursing graduate receives a diploma in nursing. Upon graduation, this nurse is eligible to take the NCLEX-RN examination to become a registered nurse.

- Four-year (baccalaureate) nursing programs are found in colleges and universities. **Baccalaureate nursing programs** emphasize course work in the liberal arts, sciences, and nursing theory, including public health. Upon graduation, the four-year nurse receives a BSN and is eligible to take the NCLEX-RN examination to become a registered nurse.

The Role of Registered Nurses

Graduates of all three nursing programs are prepared for general duty staff nursing in a hospital or nursing home. Nursing education programs also prepare graduates of all three programs to function in a community-based, community-focused health care system. Although you may find two- and three-year RNs in supervisory and administrative positions, only baccalaureate graduates have been prepared in their nursing education programs for advancement to these positions. Baccalaureate graduates are also prepared for beginning positions in public health agencies. Nurses with BSN degrees are the only nursing graduates that may elect to do graduate work in nursing at the master's and doctoral levels. Graduates of associate degree nursing programs outnumber BSN graduates. Starting in the mid 1990s, entry level BSN enrollments dropped nationwide and continue to do so. The number of diploma graduates continues to decline. This education mix is expected to continue.

All RNs function under the nurse practice act of the state in which they are working. Registered nurses use the nursing process to identify client problems, formulate nursing diagnoses, and plan and evaluate care. **Standards of care** are used instead of care plans in many acute care agencies. These standards include the priority nursing diagnosis for each client, with appropriate assessments, nursing interventions, and expected outcomes (goals). Standards provide minimum guidelines for a consistent approach to delivering client care. Standards are used as a reference by the RN in individualizing client care.

Registered nurses assign routine care and the care of stable clients to assistive personnel. This allows RNs to carry out the roles of

1. planning care,
2. coordinating all the activities of care,
3. providing care that requires more specialized knowledge and judgment,
4. teaching clients, families, and other members of the health care team, and
5. acting as client advocate.

Registered nurses function **independently** in nursing, initiating and carrying out nursing activities. For example, to prevent complications in the respiratory and circulatory systems, RNs assess the client on bed rest. They identify the need for a turning routine, deep breathing, leg exercises, and range-of-motion exercises. Registered nurses add these nursing interventions to planned care. Because of their level of education, RNs can identify which clients can and cannot receive these nursing interventions. In the community, RNs will initiate dietician and social worker orders.

When RNs carry out the legal orders of another health professional, for example, the physician or physical therapist, they are functioning in an **inter-** **dependent** role. Frequently, RNs function interdependently (collaboratively) when decisions about client care are made jointly by members of the health care team. It is the independent role in decision making that distinguishes RNs from LP/VNs. Registered nurses have the ultimate responsibility for care given to clients.

Education Beyond the Basic Nursing Programs for Registered Nurses

CERTIFICATION. After graduating from a nursing program and gaining work experience, RNs can receive certification from various professional nursing groups. The certificate that is awarded after passing a comprehensive examination indicates that the nurse has demonstrated competence in a select area of practice. As of February 2000, the Open Door 2000 policy of the credentialing center of the American Nurses Association (ANCC) makes certification available to all RNs. Those with a BSN and higher preparation will take examinations leading to "board certification." RNs with a diploma or associate degree will take examinations leading to "certification."

ADVANCED PRACTICE. With additional degrees, RNs can pursue expanded roles, called advanced practice. **Clinical nurse specialists (CNSs)** have a master's degree in a specialty area (for example, medical-surgical nursing). When employed by acute care organizations, the CNS serves as a mentor, role model, and resource person for staff by setting standards for nursing care. The CNS also is employed by clinics and nursing homes and in other community settings. In all sites of employment, the CNS also serves as an educator, consultant, researcher, and administrator.

Nurse practitioners (NPs) are found in the same settings as the CNS. Some NPs have their own offices. They are involved in providing primary and preventive health services. NPs diagnose and treat common minor illnesses and injuries. An MSN is the basic requirement for advanced practice as a nurse practitioner.

Certified nurse midwives (CNMs) provide preventive gynecologic care and low-risk prenatal and postpartum care to women at home and in hospitals and birthing centers.

Certified registered nurse anesthetists (CRNAs) are the primary providers of anesthetics in acute care facilities. They are found in every setting where anesthesia is given: operating rooms, clinics, and outpatient surgical centers.

Advanced practice nurses (APNs) may also prepare themselves to prescribe medications, and all states have given APNs the authority, with varying restrictions, to do so. Through advanced degrees or certificates, these nurses specialize in treating specific groups such as the family, adults, and children. All APNs have a minimum of a master's degree.

Practical/Vocational Nurses

Practical/vocational nurses are the second largest group of health care workers in the United States. The educational program for practical/vocational nurses varies in length from 9 to 12 months. The practical/vocational nursing program is found in trade, technical, and vocational schools as well as community colleges. These institutions are usually public, tax-supported institutions. Practical/vocational nursing programs are also found in private schools. Courses in the biologic and behavioral sciences as well as nursing theory are offered. Clinical experience in acute care facilities, extended care facilities, and the community is included. Upon graduation, the practical/vocational nurse receives a diploma in practical nursing and is eligible to take the NCLEX-PN examination to become an LP/VN.

Role of the Practical/Vocational Nurse

Practical/vocational nurses must be aware of the content of the nurse practice act of the state in which they are employed. The practical/vocational nurse's role is found in this law, and the law differs from state to state. Regardless of the site of employment, practical/voctional nurses provide care in basic and complex client situations under the general supervision of an RN, physician, podiatrist, or dentist. In acute care facilities, the increasing number of clients requiring more complex care reflects the practice of discharging clients from hospitals for continued recuperation in extended care units and nursing homes—excellent places of employment for practical/vocational nurses.

Every three years a job analysis is performed by the National Council of State Boards of Nursing, Inc. to determine the content areas for the NCLEX-PN. The findings of the latest job analysis (1997) (Yocum, 1998) indicate that newly licensed LP/VNs are continuing to provide care in all types of settings, with the majority continuing to be employed in long-term care settings. No statistically significant changes have occurred in work settings since the last job analysis in 1994 (Chornick et al, 1995).

Practical/vocational nurses function interdependently when they offer input to the RN about the effectiveness of care or offer suggestions to improve the client's care. Because practical/vocational nurses provide actual care at the bedside in acute care situations, their collection of data while engaged in giving care is valuable in determining whether progress is being made to meet client goals. A major criterion in differentiating between the roles of the registered and practical/vocational nurse is that the practical/vocational nurse never functions independently. Practical/vocational nurses must function safely and are accountable for their actions. They should assume responsibility only for nursing actions that are within their legal role and that they feel safe in carrying out. Table 2–1 helps identify differences between the LP/VN and the RN.

Regionally, the demand for LP/VNs in acute care settings has increased, but nursing homes and long-term care units continue to be the major source of employment. The employment of practical/vocational nurses is expected to increase faster than the

TABLE 2–1: Differences Between the RN and the LP/VN, Using the Five Roles of the Professional Nurse (RN) as a Guide

Five Roles of RN	RN	LPN
Professional	Belongs to and is actively involved in ANA at state and local levels	Belongs to and is involved in NFLPN/ NAPNES at state and local levels
Provider of care	Independent role Initiates all phases of nursing process; formulates nursing diagnoses	Dependent role Assists with all phases of the nursing process; works with established nursing diagnoses; identifies nursing problems
Manager of care	Controls decisions regarding staff and care of clients	First-line manager in nursing home/extended care. Responsible to nurse manager
Teacher	Initiates all health teaching	Initiates health teaching for health habits (nutrition, cleanliness, health habits, etc.). Reinforces health teaching of RN in all other areas
Researcher	Theory included in four-year program. All levels interpret and implement research findings. Participates in the research process	Theory not included in one-year program. Assists in implementing research findings

average for all occupations through 2006 ("Bright job future," 1999, p. 11). Practical/vocational nurses are also employed in the community. Sites of employment include physician's offices, weight loss clinics, freestanding clinics, ambulatory care centers, home health care agencies, and industry. Sites of job placement for the practical/vocational nurse in the community increase each year. These include clinics, dialysis centers, group homes, home health agencies, adult day care centers, Red Cross (as a phlebotomist), Alzheimer's disease units, companion centers, and various entrepreneurship opportunities.

Expanded Role of the Practical/ Vocational Nurse

In all settings, practical/vocational nurses are being used in their expanded role. Because practical/vocational nurses work under another professional's di-

rection, their role is called an interdependent one. Employers expect practical/vocational nurses to think critically and solve problems in client care situations. During implementation of care by the LP/VN, the RN is available to help in decision making when questions arise, either on site (direct supervision) or by phone (general supervision). See Chapters 13 and 14 for further discussion of the expanded role of the practical/vocational nurse.

   Critical Thinking Exercise

Refer to your state's nurse practice act to determine the circumstances under which you may function with the direct or general supervision of an RN and in your expanded role.

Student Nurses

Student professional and practical/vocational nurses come to the clinical area under the supervision of clinical instructors. The clinical area is an extension of the classroom. It provides an opportunity to apply theory to practice. When assigned to clients, students have a responsibility to give safe care and function responsibly under the supervision of the instructor. Students are in the clinical area to learn, not to give service. It is possible that a clinical instructor can remove them from the assigned clinical site at any time for additional learning experiences.

Students are members of the health care team. They are expected to assist other team members in addition to performing their client assignment. Examples of such assistance include passing trays, answering call lights in acute care situations, and assisting clients and staff in the community. These activities help students learn how to get along in a team situation. *Student practical/vocational nurses are responsible for giving the same safe nursing care that LP/VNs provide.* This is a legal matter. Therefore, the student role demands preparation and supervision.

Nursing Assistants

Nursing assistants are trained for their positions by combining federally mandated classroom instruction with close supervision by RNs while in the clinical area. Vocational schools offer programs that last a *minimum* of 75 hours. These programs combine classroom or autotutorial instruction with clinical practice. During the course, testing for competence occurs to meet federal Omnibus Budget Reconciliation Act (OBRA) requirements. When test results are satisfactory, the names of NAs are placed in a directory.

Nursing assistants function under the direction of registered or practical/vocational nurses. NAs who work in hospitals, nursing homes, extended care units, or psychiatric hospitals assist in providing personal and comfort needs for stable clients. They are assigned routine tasks, sometimes involving housekeeping chores. A large number of NAs are employed by nursing homes. At the beginning of the twenty-first century, the supply of NAs is not meeting the high demands of employers. People in some areas of the country refer to male NAs as orderlies.

Some states offer an advanced NA course. More complex skills are taught in these courses. These skills include many of the skills performed by the practical/vocational nurse. The demand for home health care workers continues to increase. NAs are allowed to perform a wider variety of skills in the home as home health care workers. Some states offer a postgraduate course for NAs to prepare them for the transition to home care. The comprehensive home care program is also available to individuals without NA experience.

Unlicensed Assistive Personnel

In an effort to use health care workers more efficiently and effectively, health care organizations have added a new level of worker to the health care team. **Unlicensed assistive personnel** are trained by health care organizations to function in an assistive role to RNs and practical/vocational nurses. Some health care organizations require applicants for UAP positions to be registered as NAs. These workers learn selected skills, sometimes by the autotutorial method or module method combined with some clinical teaching. Actual skills learned depend on which skills are needed in specific client care units. Unlicensed assistive personnel are also known by the terms patient care technician (PCT), patient care associate, care pair, nurse extender, multiskilled worker, and so on. See Chapter 16 for a discussion of UAPs under Changes in Health Care Facilities and Chapter 14 under Assigning Tasks in the Extended Care Unit.

Clerk Receptionists (Ward Clerks, Health Unit Clerks, Health Unit Coordinators)

The job of the **clerk receptionist** is mainly secretarial in nature, but the duties vary from site to site. With the clerk performing this job, nurses are freed from much of the paperwork involved in client care. Clerk receptionists are trained on the job or in programs of several months' duration in technical schools. Clerks prepare, compile, and maintain client records on a nursing unit. Duties include transcribing physician's orders; scheduling lab tests, x-ray procedures, and surgery; scheduling other appointments for services; routing charts on client transfer or discharge; compiling the client census; answering the phone; maintaining established inventories of supplies; distributing mail to clients; and generally ensuring that the unit functions smoothly.

Unit Managers

Some large health care organizations have **unit managers** to supervise and coordinate management functions for client units. Some college background and supervisory experience are desirable for this position. This job is combined with on-the-job training for specific duties. Responsibilities include budgeting, supervision of ward clerks, assignment and evaluation of clerical personnel, inventory of client's valuables, coordination with housekeeping and maintenance, and clarification of hospital compliance with Medicare requirements. If a health care organization does not have unit managers, these duties are assumed by the clerk receptionist and the nurse manager.

Delivery of Client Care Services in Acute Care Settings

With the goal of providing optimal care, the health care team uses different methods to assign clients to staff. The methods evolved as a response to changing needs in staffing. Each of the methods is discussed in its general form as it was intended to function. Keep in mind that health care organizations modify these methods to fit their individual needs.

Case Method

At the turn of the century, families hired nurses to meet a client's special needs in the home. By the 1920s, private duty nursing was popular. This **case method** of client care continued in various degrees into the 1960s. Vestiges of the case method, or a one-to-one relationship with a client, are found today in acute care situations as total care nursing (comprehensive care). In the case method, one nurse is assigned to one or two clients and is responsible for the total care of these clients. Today, total care nursing occurs in intensive care or special care units, as Mrs. Brown experienced in the ICU after she left the PACU. Nursing instructors frequently use the total client care method when assigning students to the acute care clinical area.

Functional Method

In the 1950s, the **functional method** was a popular method of client assignment. Registered and practical/vocational nurses were in scarce supply. The functional method of client care is task oriented. The tasks that have to be done for clients are divided among the staff. For example, one person might measure all vital signs, another might do all treatments, and still another might make all the beds. This method's emphasis on efficiency and division of labor is based on the assembly line production concept found in industry.

The nursing home nearest Mrs. Brown's home schedules resident assignments by the functional method. An NA helped Mrs. Brown with her physical care. A practical/vocational nurse gave her medications and did her treatments. In addition to assuming responsibility for all care given to residents, the charge nurse, a practical/vocational nurse, would be kept busy with managerial and non-nursing duties.

Functional nursing can easily overlook holistic care, especially in the area of psychological needs. This results in fragmentation of care. Although this method is efficient and appears to be less costly to implement, it can discourage client and staff satisfaction. The functional method, however, may work well in times of critical shortages of personnel.

Team Method

After World War II, the **team method** of client care was introduced because of the increasing numbers of practical/vocational nurses and NAs. The team method is more a philosophy than a method. It is based on the belief that goals can be achieved through group action. The clients on a unit are divided into small groups. Small teams are assigned to care for the clients in each group. Assignments are based on the needs of each client and the skills of the team members. The team is led by the team leader, the RN. The RN continues to have the final responsibility of planning, coordinating, and evaluating the implementation of care for each client and supervising the personnel giving the care.

In this method, the capabilities of each team member are used effectively. This increases the quality of care for the client and the satisfaction of the team member. An integral part of the team method is the team conference. During this conference, which is intended to be held daily, information is shared by team members about specific clients, problems are identified and solved, and plans of care are developed and revised. The team method is rarely carried out in this manner. When busy, the team leader may administer medications and perform treatments. Team conferences are often postponed. The team method then becomes a functional method of assigning care. Several years ago, the nurses on the medical floor where Mrs. Brown was a client used the team method, but frequently the team leader functioned as the medication nurse.

Primary Method (Primary Care)

The hospital in which Mrs. Brown was a client adopted the **primary care method** several years ago to replace the team method of assigning care. The intention was to increase the quality of care for clients. This method was instituted in the late 1960s as a result of the dissatisfaction of professional nurses with their lack of direct client contact and the fragmentation of care that resulted from functional and team nursing. In primary nursing, RNs individualize client care and accept responsibility and accountability for total client care. Ideally, staffing for this method requires a nursing staff composed entirely of RNs. Each nurse is assigned a maximum of six clients. There are no team leaders in this method. Each primary nurse is a bedside nurse, who has received the assignment from and in turn reports to the nurse manager.

The major characteristic of this method is the responsibility and accountability of the primary nurse. The primary nurse is assigned to a client on admission, develops the nursing diagnoses after the admission interview, and is responsible for the care of that client 24 hours a day until discharge. When the primary nurse is off duty, an associate RN continues care as planned by the primary nurse. If any changes are contemplated in client care, the primary nurse must be contacted.

Primary nursing facilitates continuity of care. Positive aspects of the primary method include shorter hospital stays for clients, improved communication among staff, and a more holistic focus of care. Negative aspects included the difficulty of recruiting a sufficient number of RNs when this method was first introduced. But the greatest negative aspect of this method is the cost of a staff composed entirely of RNs. Practical/vocational nurses are used as assistive nurses in primary care situations and have performed safely and effectively.

Case Management Method

The **case management method** of delivering client care is evolving over time and need. This method became popular in the 1980s in response to the increasing complexity of client care, the need to utilize scarce nursing resources, and meeting client needs in a cost-effective manner in acute care. Depending on client needs, this method uses baccalaureate registered nurses, diploma and associate degree registered nurses, licensed practical/vocational nurses, nursing assistants, and unlicensed assistive personnel in varying ratios to deliver nursing service. Care pathways or critical paths are used to coordinate care with this interdisciplinary staff. The case manager keeps an eye on timely discharge and continuity of care in the community by planning, directing, and evaluating care throughout the client's stay in acute care. The strength of this method of delivering nursing services is its focus of delivering cost-effective, quality care to clients with complex needs. Quality, service, and cost—timely considerations for the beginning of the twenty-first century.

Supply and Demand

The fact of a nursing shortage has again surfaced. Around 1989, nursing journals began talking about **differentiated practice** as a system of assigning clients for care. This system recognizes that persons on the health care team with less education than RNs are important in reorganizing the delivery of client care in a more cost-effective manner. Starting in the 1990s, the **skill mix** on the health care team changed. Acute care agencies began decreasing the percentage of RNs on staff and increasing the number of practical/vocational nurses and unlicensed personnel. Registered nurses are being used as coordinators of the health care team in these situations.

These changes are regional and are continuing. As we begin the twenty-first century, there is an increased demand for RNs in specialty areas in acute care, especially neonatal, operating room, and intensive care units. There is a decrease in RN to BSN enrollments as well as entry-level BSN enrollments. Currently, the average age of RNs in acute care is the forties and for nursing faculty is the midfifties. Generally, the average age of RNs is the

midforties. Because of the future retirement of these nurses and their leaving the workforce for various other reasons, a shortage of RNs is projected well into the future.

Critical Thinking Exercise

Investigate the skill mix of staff in acute care agencies and other health care agencies in your community.

Patient-Focused Care: Another System for Delivering Client Care

Have you ever experienced the following situation in an acute care setting? Rhonda, an LP/VN, tried to find out when her nauseated, elderly client was scheduled to have his chest x-ray, physical therapy session, and special lab studies. The radiology department, physical therapy department, and laboratory were unable to give even a ballpark time frame when Rhonda called. Instead, they answered, "We'll come when we can." So Rhonda started the bath. After she finished washing the client's face, a transport aide appeared at the door to take the client to the radiology department. Rhonda cautioned the transport aide that the client was nauseated, but the aide said she was not trained to take care of things like that.

After 40 minutes, the client returned to his room. Fortunately, he did not have to vomit while he was in the x-ray department. After Rhonda started the bath again, lab personnel came to take the client to the laboratory for the special blood test that had to be done in that department. The lab personnel looked shocked when Rhonda included the emesis basin with the client with instructions that they might need to assist him. Forty-five minutes later, the patient returned to his room.

Rhonda continued the client's bath from where she thought she left off. Then the physical therapy transport aide came to take the client to his physical therapy session. Thirty-five minutes later the client was back, but he had not had his physical therapy session. The client was waiting in line for his turn for therapy when he had to go to the bathroom, but nobody was available to help him get to the bathroom. The client could not have his physical therapy because he had been incontinent.

Critical Thinking Exercise

Identify two ways of doing things differently in this acute care situation that could help make the situation more patient-focused and efficient and would make more sense.
The client would benefit if:

1. _____

_____

2. _____

_____

The following are innovations created by management people to apply to acute care situations similar to the one just described:

1. Relocate small departmental units to the nursing area instead of making the client go to them.
2. Cross-train health care workers so that each has the skills and can perform the tasks of other health care workers.

What Is Patient-Focused Care?

Patient-focused care is an attempt to improve the quality of care by using hospital resources more efficiently to better meet the needs of clients. It is a consolidation and change of inpatient services that affects all departments found in hospitals. The major change in patient-focused care is **"decentralizing"** centralized service departments within hospitals and locating them in each client unit. For example, in this system of delivering care, the radiology department would cease to be a department of its own. Each client care area would have its own radiology suite, and an x-ray technician would be assigned to this area. Each unit could also have its own pharmacy and lab areas and even an admitting desk.

These health care workers would also be cross-trained to perform specific skills on the unit when needed by clients. Examples of **cross-trained** skills would be drawing blood, giving baths, feeding clients, taking x-rays, assisting patients with basic needs, providing health teaching about medications, and so on. As coordinator of the team, the RN would assign care duties to this team of health care workers. Patient-focused care can build a stronger team delivering higher quality care because the resources of the health care organization are focused on the client.

Patient-Focused Care

One of the authors recently had an outpatient mammogram at a hospital she has been using for years. The hospital recently went through a major renovation and restructuring. In the past, the author had to fight for a parking space, walk one block to the outpatient admission desk, walk one block to an elevator, another one-half block to the x-ray department, and then retrace her steps to find her car. After the restructuring, the author walked a total of 70 steps from valet parking to the registration desk and then to the mammogram room and back to the valet for her car.

Summary

☐ Health care organizations include a large number of specialized services and health care workers to provide these services. As a result, clients in the United States have some of the best and most expensive health care services in the world. Each member of the health care team provides a valuable service to the client. All members of the health care team are equal in importance to each other. Nurses on the health care team include registered nurses, practical/vocational nurses, student nurses, and cross-trained staff. Unlicensed assistive personnel, clerk receptionists, and managerial personnel round out the nursing team.

☐ To understand where you as a practical/vocational nurse fit into the picture, it is important for you to be aware of the educational background, role, responsibilities, and possible licensing requirements of all levels of personnel on the health care team. To understand your position on the health care team, it is necessary for you to keep up to date about new levels of health care workers and the different methods of delivering client care. As we enter the twenty-first century, practical/vocational nurses are recognized as important members of the health care team in acute care facilities and the community.

Review Questions

1. What is the difference between a diploma, ADN, and BSN registered nurse?
   A. There is no difference because the graduates of these programs take the same licensing examination to become a registered nurse.
   B. ADN and diploma registered nurses find jobs only in the acute care setting.
   C. Only the BSN registered nurse is prepared to work in public health at the time of graduation.
   D. Only the ADN and BSN registered nurse is capable of assuming a leadership position at the time of graduation.
2. What is the difference between a practical/vocational nurse and a registered nurse?
   A. Practical/vocational nurses are never hired for management positions.
   B. Practical/vocational nurses are hired only in nursing homes and extended care units.
   C. The practical/vocational nurse functions independently in all client situations.

D. Practical/vocational nurses function in a dependent role and under at least the general supervision of a registered nurse.
3. Select the statement that best describes the practical/vocational nurse's role in primary care nursing.
   A. Nursing care is very task-oriented.
   B. Client goals are achieved through group action.
   C. Each nurse is assigned to one client for total care.
   D. Personal responsibility and accountability for total client care is stressed.
4. Select the statement that best describes a clinical nurse specialist.
   A. This registered nurse works only in a hospital.
   B. This registered nurse has had additional training.
   C. This registered nurse has a minimum of a PhD.
   D. This registered nurse has a master's degree in nursing.

5. Select the statement that best describes to-
   day's demand for nurses.
   A. There is a surplus of LP/VNS
   B. Practical/vocational nurses are in de-
      mand.

C. here is a decreased demand for registered nurses.
D. There are adequate numbers of nurses
   at all levels.

References

American Nurses Association. *Nursing—A Social Policy Statement.* Kansas City: American Nurses Association, 1995, pp. 9–13.

"Bright job future." Practical Nursing Today 2(1):10–13, 1999.

Chornick N, Yocum C, Jacobsen J. *Job Analysis of Newly Licensed Practical/Vocational Nurses 1994.* Chicago: National Council of State Boards of Nursing, 1995.

Henderson V. *The Nature of Nursing: A Definition and Its Implications for Practice, Research and Education.* New York: Macmillan, 1966.

Yocum C. *Job Analysis of Newly Licensed Practical/Vocational Nurse 1997.* Chicago: National Council of State Boards of Nursing, 1998.

Bibliography

Chornick N. How it all began . . . . Journal of Practical Nursing 47(2), June 1997.

Fralic M. Nursing leadership for the new millennium: Essential knowledge and skills. Nursing and Healthcare Perspectives 20(1):260–265, 1999.

Mason D, Leavitt J. *Policy and Politics for Nurses.* Philadelphia: W.B. Saunders, 1998.

McBride A. Breakthroughs in nursing education: Looking back, looking forward. Nursing Outlook 47(3):114–119, 1999.

Nursing Data Source; 1994. Focus on Practical/Vocational Nursing. Vol. 3. New York: National League for Nursing, 1994. (Most recent on back order. Expected in the year 2000.)

Occupational Outlook Handbook. Bureau of Labor Statistics. Home page http://stats.bls.gov/ocohome.htm 1998.

Poliafico J. Nursing's gender gap. RN 61(10):39–42, 1998.

Shindul-Rothschild J, Berry D, Long-Middleton E. Where have all the nurses gone? Am J Nurs 96(11), 1996.

Smith C, Maurer F. *Community Health Nursing: Theory and Practice,* 2nd ed. Philadelphia: W.B. Saunders, 1999.

Swanson J, Nies M. *Community Health Nursing: Promoting the Health of Aggregates.* Philadelphia: W.B. Saunders, 1997.

Chapter 3

The Adult Learner

Outline

The Adult Learner Defined
Formal and Informal Educational Experiences
Geared for Success
Liabilities, Pitfalls, and Hidden Dangers
    Hidden Danger Shared by All Adult Learners

Dangers for the Traditional Adult Learner
Dangers for the Returning Adult Learner
Dangers for the Recycled Adult Learner
Special Challenges for Practical/Vocational Nursing Students

Learners Have Rights
Responsibilities of Learners
    Teaching Versus Learning
    The Role of Evaluation
    Dealing with Referrals
    Other Responsibilities of Learners

Key Terms

active learning
constructive evaluation
facilitator
First Amendment
formal education
generalization

informal education
passive learning
performance evaluation
positive mental attitude
recycled adult learner
referral

returning adult learner
self-directed learner
self-evaluation
teaching
traditional adult learner

Objectives

Upon completing this chapter you will be able to:

1. Identify yourself as a traditional adult learner, returning adult learner, or recycled adult learner.
2. Identify personal areas of strength that will help you ensure success in the practical/vocational nursing program.
3. Identify personal areas that could interfere with your success in the practical/vocational nursing program.
4. Explain in your own words three rights of learners.
5. Discuss personal responsibility for learning and active participation in the learning process as learner responsibilities.
6. Identify the purpose of evaluation in the practical/vocational nursing program.
7. Discuss ten learner responsibilities.

Welcome! You are one of thousands of adult learners in the United States who have decided to pursue a formal program in education this year. Every year adults enroll full-time and part-time in educational activities and programs. These programs and activities help them achieve job skills, increase self-esteem, and generally improve their quality of life. You are not alone.

You are entering school at an excellent time. Schools have put full effort into attracting and keeping adult learners in their programs. The adult learner is a very serious and capable learner. These learners help raise standards in our schools. Schools have looked seriously at the special needs of adult learners. To enable the adult learner to succeed, schools have taken these needs into consideration

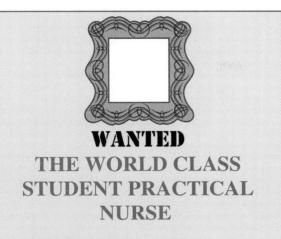

WANTED
THE WORLD CLASS STUDENT PRACTICAL NURSE

Age: Late teens up to the sixties and beyond.

Gender: Male and female

Personal characteristics:

- Married, single, looking, not looking.
- Has had work experience in a variety of settings and/or may have been through another program of study.
- Needs more knowledge and skills.
- Has clear, specific goals.
- Motivated and responsible.
- Serious about education.
- Seeking to have mind opened to the world of practical nursing.
- Would like to change practical nursing for the better.
- Willing to make considerable sacrifice of time, money, family, and personal pleasures.
- Wants to master practical nursing skills for the twenty-first century.

The **traditional adult learner** comes to an educational program directly from high school or from another program of study. Many traditional adult students are in their late teens and early twenties. Traditional adult learners are in transition from late adolescence to young adulthood. In addition to their own developmental tasks, these students are being propelled into situations of responsibility for others.

The **returning adult learner** has been out of school for several years. Many have not taken any courses since high school. Although returning adult learners can be any age, most are in their mid to late twenties. Returning adult students are experiencing many different life transitions. Because of life experiences, returning adult learners have built a strong foundation for the personal commitment and transitions needed in nursing school and practical/vocational nursing.

Another type of adult learner has emerged on the scene in practical/vocational nursing. Adult learners with prior education beyond high school are also an important part of practical/vocational nursing. This student shares some of the characteristics of both the traditional and the returning adult learner. But this adult learner might have technical school or college experience or an undergraduate or a graduate degree in a discipline other than nursing. Because these adult learners are starting a new cycle in their lives, we call them **recycled learners.** Reasons for choosing to enroll in the practical/vocational nursing program include:

1. Desire to change careers.
2. An attraction to nursing.
3. Desire to acquire new job skills.
4. The outlook for a full-time job with benefits may be more promising in practical/vocational nursing.
5. Possible lack of jobs in area for which person has a degree.

Regardless of the reason for enrolling in the one-year practical/vocational nursing program, recycled learners find that this program meets their needs in both time and cost. In addition to characteristics of returning adult learners, the recycled learner brings experience in tackling a challenging educa-

when setting up educational programs. And to think, over the years you might have been saying, "I was born too soon," or "I was born too late." It turns out you were born at just the right time.

The Adult Learner Defined

Who is the adult learner? Adult learners perceive themselves as adults and have adult responsibilities.

tional program and valued life and work experience. Just as recycling is good for America, recycled learners are good for practical/vocational nursing programs. Nursing in general and practical/vocational nursing in particular are benefiting from the maturity and experience of this new type of nursing student.

Which type of adult learner are you? Survey your classmates. Determine who consider themselves to be traditional, returning, or recycled adult learners.

Formal and Informal Educational Experiences

Generalizations can be made about each type of learner. Keep in mind that generalizations are broad, sweeping statements. The characteristics of each type of adult learner are not found in every individual. The traditional adult learner is accustomed to planned, organized learning. This type of learning is called **formal education.** The practical/vocational nursing program in a vocational-technical school or junior college is an example of a program of formal education. Frequently, returning adult learners say they are rusty and have not been to school since high school. Only the latter part of this statement is true. They might not have been in a classroom for some time. But they have been learning. They have had informal educational experiences every day of their lives. Some examples of their **informal educational experiences** are learning to make a new recipe, using a digital camera, programming the VCR, filling out a new income tax form, driving a new car, and handling a new family problem.

Returning adult learners tend to put more emphasis on formal educational experiences. They underemphasize the value of informal learning experiences. As you read your nursing texts, you will find that these experiences can be helpful when you are learning new material. Recycled learners may have recently graduated from college. Some may have entered practical/vocational nursing after a career in

**Learning Exercise:
Educational Experiences**

List at least five informal educational experiences you have had since high school.

_____

_____

_____

_____

_____

another field of work. Recycled learners have many formal and informal educational experiences that help them in a practical/vocational nursing program.

Geared for Success

All adult learners have things going for them that allow them to succeed in school. Traditional adult learners are generally experts at educational routine. They know how to get through registration as painlessly as possible (even on-line), find the fastest way to get from one class to another, find the best time to get through the cafeteria line, and know how to take a test using a computerized answer sheet. In comparison, some returning adult learners may feel they have used up the last bit of their energy in trying to find a parking space, and once they do, they may be puzzled about how to find their way to their assigned classroom.

Traditional adult learners have been given the opportunity to develop reading, writing, studying, and test-taking skills. They are at their prime physically, are filled with energy and stamina, and often have fewer out-of-school responsibilities to distract them from their studies. The returning adult learner is a serious learner who is ready to work. Returning adult learners have had many responsibilities and life experiences that help them relate well to new learning, make sense out of it, and get the point quickly. They are mature, motivated, and self-directed and have set a goal for themselves. Many have made economic, personal, and family sacrifices to go back to school.

Recycled learners are also experts in educational routine, and they too have had the opportunity to develop reading, writing, studying, and test-taking skills. They are serious, motivated, and self-directed students. All adult learners are geared for success, and each group has its own strong points. But each group also has some liabilities—things that could stand in the way of success.

Liabilities, Pitfalls, and Hidden Dangers

Hidden Danger Shared by All Adult Learners

One of the greatest liabilities shared by all adult learners is the fear of failure. Fear of anything is a very strong motivator but in a negative sense. Fear of failure in school is a feeling that usually develops as a result of past negative experiences with learning situations. Perhaps you did not do well in some high school or college classes. Maybe you did not study, studied the wrong way, or allowed yourself to be put down by teachers or professors in the past. Maybe you allowed yourself to underachieve because of peer pressure. Regardless of the cause, you may look at school in a negative, threatening way.

A surprise is in store for you. Your past is history. You have a clean slate ahead of you! Many adult learners with the same history and fears as you may experience have succeeded in their educational programs. You are not a child in grade school. You are an adult in an adult educational experience. You will do yourself a favor if you

begin to picture in your mind the rewards of succeeding in the practical/vocational nursing program. Forget the failures and setbacks you may have suffered in high school and other educational experiences. Replace your fear of failure with the desire for success. Keep your thoughts positive. Practice these positive thoughts continuously. Watch the content and tone of your thoughts and words. Negative thoughts and words can play like a tape. As surely as you learned this negative script, you can learn a positive script. But it takes time. Replace all your "I can'ts" and "I never coulds" with "I want to," "I can," "I will," and "I'm going to." Do not dwell on the past but look to the future. Dominate your thoughts with positive ones. You know, go all the way with PMA—**positive mental attitude.** If you consistently expect to succeed and combine this expectation with hard work in your studies, you will succeed. Did you know that your brain believes anything you tell it? Well, if it believes you can fail, it can learn to believe you can succeed. Start today to engage in positive self-talk.

Sometimes students who have not succeeded in other nursing programs enroll during midterm in the practical/vocational nursing program. Reasons for not making it in prior nursing programs are varied, personal, and confidential. These students may feel the need to be on their guard. They may behave in a defensive manner, especially if there were teacher-student conflicts in the prior nursing program. It is good for these students to remember that the past is history. All that counts is their performance in the present. For them, it is possible to start over with a clean slate.

Dangers for the Traditional Adult Learner

Although traditional adult learners often have fewer outside responsibilities to distract them from their studies, they may allow social events to compete with school and study time. A serious interference with school responsibilities is a party mentality. Parties and "hanging out" used to be special occasions for celebrating and getting together. They were a well-earned and much-needed break from work and everyday routine responsibilities. Today, sometimes work and everyday responsibilities in life and at school get in the way of the traditional adult learner's party habit. Another interference is the amount of time occupied by employment outside of school hours. Ask yourself, "How much of the time I am employed outside of school is necessary for food, shelter, and other realistic expenses?" Many explanations can be given for these behaviors. Some traditional adult learners may still be working at developing an awareness of who they are and what life is all about for them. They may lack a sense of direction and have no clear goal or idea of what they really want to do in life. These examples of pitfalls for traditional adult learners are good examples of **generalizations.** They may or may not apply to the traditional adult learners you know.

Dangers for the Returning Adult Learner

Returning adult learners may experience difficulties with academic behavior. Their reading, writing, test-taking, and study skills may be rusty. Physical changes occur as adults age and can affect learning. The senses of vision and hearing are at their peak in the adolescent years and decline very gradually through the adult years. As the decades go by, these adults may notice the need for more illumination when they read. They also may experience problems with reading small print. Some returning adults note that they are not as energetic as they once were. Socially, returning adult learners have many roles to play outside of school. They may be husbands, wives, daughters, sons, grandparents, employees, or volunteers, and generally they are very busy people. Returning to school may result in feelings of guilt because they know it will affect their relationships and routines outside of school.

Because of their many roles, more demands are placed on returning adult learners. Some families may not support mom's or dad's choice to continue

their formal education. Spouses may object to the extra demands placed on them. In many cases, the returning adult learner must struggle with learning how to juggle the worlds of learner and head of the family.

Despite these demands, returning adult learners, like traditional and recycled adult learners, need to learn how to manage their time. They need to learn how to concentrate when time for concentration is made available. Sometimes returning adult learners set unrealistic goals for themselves and have to re-adjust their game plan. Although past experience can be an asset, returning adult learners may have to rethink and possibly unlearn some things they have learned in the past. They might have allowed some of these things to become habits.

■ When faced with obstacles, some adults may decide to throw in the towel and write off school as a bad idea. This book can help you avoid this negative way of thinking and go on to succeed. ■

Dangers for the Recycled Adult Learner

The recycled adult learner shares the same pitfalls as do the traditional and returning adult learners. Depending on their age and personal responsibilities, recycled adult learners may feel an energy crisis as they pursue their academic life. An additional danger for recycled adult learners may be an attitude that because they have earned a degree or have some college experience, the practical/vocational nursing program will be a breeze to get through. It is good to remember the difference between obtaining a college degree and obtaining a technical college education. In college, a student might have no practical experience with his or her major subject until junior or senior year or after graduation when hired for the first job in the chosen field. In the practical/vocational nursing program in a technical college, application of current learning is stressed continuously. Students need to apply theory continuously to the clinical area. What you learn on Monday will be used on a clinical basis on Tuesday. And you will be expected to apply learning from past nursing classes consistently. Cramming for examinations will be useless with this consistent expectation of application of theory to the clinical area.

Special Challenges for Practical/Vocational Nursing Students

No matter what type of adult learner they are, some students have special challenges to success in practical/vocational nursing. Students with a spouse at home may be extremely busy with school and family affairs. Single parents may feel overwhelmed when the student role is assumed in addition to all their other roles. It may be good for students with spouses to imagine what it would be like to be a student without a spouse to offer support.

Occasionally, practical/vocational nursing students with English as their first language complain about the difficulty of schoolwork and the amount of time it takes to complete assignments. It may be good for these students to imagine being responsible for the same amount of schoolwork when English is the second language. Students who speak English as a second language need to strive continually to understand content presented in a language different from their native tongue. This is comparable to presenting English-speaking students with textbooks written in Spanish or Russian.

We have met many students facing such challenges and commend them for the good job they have done, against great odds, in the practical/vocational nursing program. They are a testimonial that success is within your reach even if you are faced with these special challenges.

Learners Have Rights

You must start thinking about some fundamental rights that you have been granted as an American

citizen through the U.S. Constitution that will affect you as a learner. The **First Amendment** gives you freedom of expression as long as what you want to express does not disrupt class or infringe on the rights of your peers. So, when your instructor asks you to join in a discussion, do not be afraid to do so. Instructors want your input in a class session. They have no intention of holding your comments against you. The Fourteenth Amendment assures you due process. Due process means that if you are charged with a violation of policies or rules, you will be presented with evidence of your misconduct and will be entitled to state your position. So relax. The institution in which you are enrolled cannot terminate you at whim, nor do they want to. They exist to help you succeed. A more detailed account of these two rights can probably be found in your school's student handbook. You did not get one? You lost yours? Hurry to Student Services and get a copy today.

An important learner's right is the right to have an organized curriculum and a responsible instructor who is prepared to teach it. Although your tuition and fees do not pay for all the services you receive at school, you are the most important person on campus. You are the reason the instructor was hired. You do not interfere with the instructor's work—you are the focus of it. You have the right to know the requirements of each course and how you will be graded for each course.

Responsibilities of Learners

The first responsibility of learners is to learn. The authors want you to test your knowledge about the process of learning before you read any further. Read the following four statements and answer "true" or "false" to them. As the chapter continues, these statements will be discussed. You will be expected to check the accuracy of your responses. *Remember, your answers are for your eyes only.*

Learning Exercise: Responsibilities of Learners

_____ 1. The instructor has the responsibility for my learning.
_____ 2. If I fail, it is the responsibility of the instructor.
_____ 3. If I succeed, the credit for my success should go to the instructor.
_____ 4. My instructor has the responsibility to pass on to me all the information I will need to know in my career as a practical/vocational nurse.

Teaching Versus Learning

Years ago, a wonderful thing happened in the area of adult education. Teachers were exposed to the difference between **teaching** and learning. Great emphasis was placed on the role of the learner. Changing emphasis from *teaching* to *learning* is called a paradigm (a way of thinking) shift. We think learners need to be aware of the exciting world of learning and the roles of teaching and learning in that process. In doing so you will know what is expected of you as an adult learner.

Many of you (and this includes us and some of your instructors) have had educational experiences in the past that encouraged dependency and passivity on the part of the learner. Think back to the educational experiences you have had. Did they involve sitting in classes in which the teacher did most of the talking and you just took notes? Did you view the teacher as someone who possessed knowledge and somehow was going to pass it on to you? And if you did not pass, did you say, "The teacher flunked me"? When you think about it, these situations are characterized by the adjectives dependent and **passive.**

The last time you were dependent from necessity was when you were an infant. Even then you were far from passive. When you became a toddler, you became very independent and began to learn about the world in earnest. You very actively pursued your learning—that is, the acquiring of new knowledge and skills. And you did it with gusto! Now, here you are an adult learner. How unfair of an instructor to expect you to become dependent and passive in your learning. This is especially true because studies have proved that people learn best when they are actively involved in their own learning and have an interdependent relationship with the instructor. Today, instructors are viewed as **facilitators** of learning.

You have already learned that it is the instructor's responsibility to set up a curriculum. Your state's board of nursing dictates the content of the curriculum in a school of nursing. It is then up to the faculty of your school to decide how that content will be included in the nursing program. Instructors have the responsibility to create a learning environment in which learning can take place. They do this by arranging for a variety of activities and experiences. Part of that learning environment involves being available to learners when they encounter questions and problems they cannot solve themselves. Instructors also have the responsibility to evaluate learning. They do so by testing and observing learners.

To learn is to acquire knowledge and skills. The verb *acquire* means to obtain or gain by one's own effort. Learners must open themselves up, reach out, and stretch to gain their knowledge and skills. They are agents of their own knowledge and skill acquisition. **Learning** is a very **active** activity, not a passive one. Learners have the personal responsibility to acquire knowledge and skills. It is impossible for instructors to pour knowledge and skills into the heads of learners. Learners must become **self-directed** in their learning. Instructors will not hover over you and guide your every step. Instructors are there to help you along when needed.

Do not expect the teacher to assume your skill for you, be your medical dictionary, or replace Chapter 2 in *Body Structure* because you did not have time to study. Instead, expect your instructor to observe you while you are trying to work through a difficult skill. The instructor will make suggestions and demonstrate a point here and there to help you along. If you are having trouble, expect your instructor to help you put a definition of a medical term in your own words. Expect the instructor to answer specific questions you may have about Chapter 2 in *Body Structure*. These are the roles of teacher and learner and examples of their interdependency.

If you are to learn and succeed, you must become actively involved in your own learning. You say you are too old to learn? You say you cannot teach an old dog new tricks? Much study has been done in this area. To date, studies of adult learning clearly indicate that the basic ability to learn remains essentially unimpaired throughout the life-span. Now review the answers to your true/false questions on page 46. Are there any answers you want to change before looking at the key?

1. *False.* You have the responsibility for your own learning. You must become actively involved in the learning process.
2. *False.* If you fail, it is your own fault. Adult educational programs are geared for success. You are geared for success. Although you could list many reasons why you might not succeed, the teacher's flunking you is not one of them. Learners sometimes allow themselves to flunk.
3. *False.* When you succeed (and you are perfectly capable of doing so), only you can take credit for the success. You were the person who assumed responsibility for your own learning. You became actively involved in the learning process.
4. *False.* Instructors have had much experience in nursing. They do not know all the experiences you will have in your career as a practical/vocational nurse. Even if they did, there would be no time or way to transfer this knowledge to you. Instructors help learners learn how to learn. This is important in an ever-changing field like nursing. Your instruc-

tors will encourage you to develop critical thinking and problem-solving skills. These skills will enable you to handle new situations as they arise in your nursing career.

If you had no wrong answers, you should be an expert on learning. Now put your expertise to work for you. If you had one wrong answer or more, the authors suggest you reread the section Teaching Versus Learning.

The Role of Evaluation

The second responsibility of learners is to receive and participate in **self-evaluation**. Evaluation plays an important role in your education in the practical/vocational nursing program and throughout your career. You have set a goal to become a practical/vocational nurse. As the year goes on you will be evaluated by your instructors in several different ways as a means of determining whether or not you are progressing in the achievement of that goal. When you graduate, you will be evaluated periodically while on the job, sometimes as a means of determining whether you are to receive a salary increase. At other times you will be evaluated to see if you are functioning well enough to keep your job. Evaluation generally occurs in two areas: written tests that measure your knowledge of theory and performance evaluations that measure your progress in the clinical area. Evaluation in these areas is a learning experience in itself.

Theory Tests

Learners and instructors look at test results very differently. Learners focus on the number of items they answered correctly. Learners need to identify what they did right on a test so they can apply the process of getting the right answer to future tests and using this information in the clinical area. Instructors focus on the specific items the learner had wrong. Wrong items indicate critical knowledge the learner does not have. Do not just ask for your grades. Try to arrange time with your instructors to review your tests. It is impossible to say grades do not count. You must earn the minimum grade established by your nursing program. But consider this. If you got 80% on a test, that means you failed to answer 20% of the questions correctly. Now place yourself in the client's slippers. What about the 20% your nurse got wrong? Was it something the nurse should have known to care for you safely? For this reason, try to look at tests as learning experiences. Be as interested in your wrong answers as you are in your correct answers. Take time to look at your test with the goal of understanding why the correct answers are correct and why the wrong answers you gave are wrong.

Clinical Performance Evaluations

The most meaningful evaluations you will receive during the year will be the **performance evaluations** given while you are in the clinical area. Because these evaluations give you an opportunity for career and personal growth, it is important to understand this form of evaluation and the responsibilities you have with regard to it. Clinical performance evaluations provide an example of how to evaluate others in your expanded role.

In the clinical area, instructors will be observing you as you go about caring for clients. They are observing you to discover the positive things you are doing to reach your goal of becoming a practical/vocational nurse. These behaviors are to be encouraged. They indicate that learning has taken place and you are growing and progressing toward your goal. Instructors are also observing you to discover behaviors that stand in the way of reaching your goal. These behaviors are to be discouraged. Your instructor will update you daily on your progress in a verbal or written manner. At the end of a clinical rotation, you will receive a written performance evaluation during a conference with your clinical instructor.

From the start, you need to look at performance evaluations as a two-sided coin. The instructor is on one side and you are on the other. As part of their job, instructors have the responsibility of evaluating your performance. As a learner, you have the responsibility of being aware of your clinical behaviors. You are responsible for self-evaluation. The National League for Nursing has indicated that practical/vocational nursing students, at the time of graduation, should be able to look at their nursing actions and be aware of their strong behaviors and behaviors that need improvement. Development of the ability to be aware of one's behaviors begins with day one in the practical/vocational nursing program, including the skills laboratory. Objective awareness of one's own behaviors is an important skill to have as an employee. A learner does not automatically have this skill. Learners must consistently work at viewing themselves objectively. Instructors will help in this area. For example, when learning how to make a bed, ask yourself, "Is the finished product as good as I had intended it to be when I started?" *Do not wait for the instructor to identify areas of success or areas of needed improvement.*

Think back to when you received comments from your teachers and parents about your behavior in grade school and high school. How did you feel when you received these comments? Many people grow up with bad feelings about these episodes of criticism and even about the word itself. Criticism means evaluation. Many persons attach a negative meaning to criticism and view it as a put-down.

The phrase "constructive criticism" may evoke negative feelings. The phrase "constructive evaluation" is frequently used instead. This choice of words may help you look at evaluation of your behaviors in a positive way. It is important to distinguish what is being evaluated. You must separate your behaviors or actions from yourself, the person.

Constructive evaluation directed toward your behaviors has no bearing on your value as a person. Look at your behaviors as being either positive and helping you reach your goal or as needing improvement. Behaviors needing improvement must be modified so that you can reach your goal.

As you progress in the nursing program, you will learn about a systematic way of conducting client care called the nursing process (see Chapter 12). An important part of the nursing process is evaluation of client goals while giving client care. If your actions are not helping clients reach their goals, they must be modified. Knowledge of the nursing process will help you develop your ability to look at your actions and evaluate them. Comments from instructors will help your self-awareness. Remain open with yourself. The comments you receive are directed toward your behaviors and not you as a person.

A good way to start learning self-evaluation is to look at yourself in everyday life. Ask yourself how you look through the eyes of others:

How would you like to be your own spouse?
How would you like to have yourself as a learner?
How would you like to be your own mother or father?
How would you like to be your own nurse?

If you would not like to be any of these people, identify the reasons why. Another good exercise is to make two lists. On one list note your assets or strong points. On the other list note your liabilities or areas that need improvement. When asked to evaluate themselves, learners traditionally rate themselves more negatively. They tend to neglect their strong points. Identifying strong points is not proud or vain behavior. It is dealing with yourself honestly and openly. After you have identified assets and liabilities, review your assets periodically. Make an effort to continue these strong points while modifying your liabilities. Pick one liability at a time to work on. If you do so, your assets list will grow and your liabilities list will shrink.

A good place to start self-evaluation in nursing is in the skills lab of your basic nursing course. Practice becoming very observant of the results of your actions. Are the top sheets centered when you are making an unoccupied bed? Are you using the bath blanket as a drape to avoid chilling and invading the client's privacy? Are you aware of the effect of the tone of your voice on your instructors and peers?

Evaluation is an ever-present reality in any career. Getting into the practice of self-evaluation early in your program of study will help you develop a skill you will use daily in your career and personal life.

Learning Exercise: Self-Evaluation

List one of your strong areas that you have identified as a new practical/vocational nursing student.

_____

_____

List one area needing improvement that you have identified as a practical/vocational nursing student.

_____

_____

_____

Dealing with Referrals

If you are assessed by your instructor as having areas that need improvement, the instructor will refer you to a counselor at school. Examples of areas that require **referral** are a grade below passing in a major test and frequent absences from class. Counselors at technical colleges and junior colleges are academic counselors who have expertise in helping students identify reasons for academic problem areas. A referral to a counselor is an attempt to help you succeed. These counselors can help students set up a plan of action to remedy the problem. We have seen some students resist "going to the counselor." Some students think this is a waste of time.

Critical Thinking Exercise: The Counselor

What could be one reason for thinking that an appointment with the counselor is a waste of time?

Other Responsibilities of Learners

In addition to assuming responsibility for your own learning, becoming actively involved in the learning process, and receiving and participating in evaluation, it is necessary to be aware of some other responsibilities you have as a learner.

1. Be aware of the rules and policies of your school and the practical/vocational nursing program. Abide by them.
2. When problems do develop, follow the recognized channels of communication both at school and in the clinical area. The rule is, go to the source. Avoid "saving up" gripes. Pursue them as they come up.
3. Be prepared in advance for classes and clinical experiences. You expect teachers to be prepared. They expect the same of you. When you are unprepared for classes, you waste the time of the instructor and your peers. When you are unprepared for clinical experiences, you are violating an important safety factor in client care. When you are scheduled for the clinical area, your state board of nursing expects you to function as a licensed practical/vocational nurse would function under your state's nurse practice act.
4. Prepare your own assignments. Use your peers and the experiences and knowledge they have and learn from each other.
5. Seek out learning experiences at school and in the clinical area. Set your goals higher than the minimum.
6. Seek out resources beyond the required readings. Examples of these resources can be the library, information from past classes, and the Internet.
7. Assume responsibility for your own thoughts, communication, and behavior. Avoid giving in to pressure from your peers. BYOB: Be Your Own Boss.
8. Be present and on time for classes and clinical experiences. Follow school and program policies for reporting absences. Getting into this habit will prepare you to be a favored employee.
9. Enter into discussion when asked to do so in class.
10. Treat those with whom you come into daily contact with respect. Be mindful of their rights as individuals.
11. *Seek out your instructor when you are having difficulties in class or in the clinical area.* Often instructors can tell when students are having problems. More important are the times when they cannot tell and only the student knows a problem exists. Do not be afraid to approach your instructors. They are there to help you.
12. Keep a record of your grades as a course proceeds. At the beginning of a course, the instructor will explain the method of calculating your final grade. You are responsible for knowing how you stand gradewise in a course at any point in time.

Summary

☐ Adult learners are numerous today on campuses throughout the United States. Adult learners can be classified as traditional adult learners, returning adult learners, and recycled adult learners. Each category of learner possesses characteristics that can help the learner succeed in the practical/vocational nursing program. Each group also possesses characteristics that can prevent success. Liabilities occur in areas where learners have control over their solutions. They are not concrete barriers to success. Although learners have rights, they also have responsibilities. The most important of their responsibilities are the personal responsibility for learning, taking an active part in the process, and participating in the evaluation of their learning and growth.

Review Questions

1. Which of the following statements best explains the role of learning in the practical/vocational nursing program?
   A. Instructors will teach students everything they need to learn about practical/vocational nursing.
   B. Students will be responsible for their learning and will need to get actively involved in the learning process.
   C. Credit for students' anticipated success in the practical/vocational nursing program will go to the faculty of this program.
   D. Learner responsibilities include showing up on time and having the correct notebooks and pens.
2. If a student with a poor previous school record expresses fear of failing the nursing program, the best response is:
   A. "You should not feel that way."
   B. "Underachievers from the past never succeed in this program."
   C. "Instructors are very tuned in to your past achievements."
   D. "Focus on success. Your past is history in this program."
3. If you are informed during a daily clinical evaluation that several areas of your basic nursing skills need improvement, you should:
   A. Immediately go to the counselor.
   B. Drop the course before you fail.
   C. Focus on improving the behaviors that need improvement.

D. Make an appointment for the study skills center and spend more time on developing your care plans.
4. Students who love finding out their score on theory tests but hate having to review the tests should focus on:
   A. Developing a concern for the items they get wrong on tests.
   B. Reviewing tests so they can find instructor error in grading.
   C. Always striving for a minimum grade as decided by their program's grading system.
   D. Stop being concerned about theory tests and focus on learning, as the theory tests are not important to progress in the practical/vocational nursing program.
5. Students who are embarrassed about identifying strong areas in their own clinical performance need to understand that:
   A. This is the instructor's responsibility and students need not be concerned with it.
   B. Identifying strong areas is necessary to meet course expectations and will not have to be done after nursing school.
   C. Identifying strong areas is not a good expectation of instructors because identifying positive things about oneself is egotistical.
   D. Identifying strong areas involves looking at yourself honestly and objectively and is a skill practical/vocational nurses will use throughout their careers.

Bibliography

Brookfield S. *Discussion as a Way of Teaching: Tools and Techniques for Democratic Classrooms.* San Francisco: Jossey-Bass, 1999.

Chenevert M. *Mosby's Tour Guide to Nursing School.* St. Louis: Mosby–Year Book, 1995.

Galbraith M. *Adult Learning Methods: A Guide for Effective Instruction.* Melbourne, FL: Krieger Publishing Co, 1998.

Knowles M. *The Adult Learner: The Definitive Classic in Adult Education and Human Resource.* Houston: Gulf Publishers, 1998.

Patterson B. Partnership in nursing education: A vision or a fantasy? Nursing Outlook 46(6):284–289, 1998.

Siebert A, Gilpin B (contributor). *The Adult Student's Guide to Survival and Success.* Portland, OR: Practical Psychology Press, 1997.

Wilson J. Generation X: Who are they? What do they want? NEA Higher Education Journal 14(2):9–18, Fall 1998.

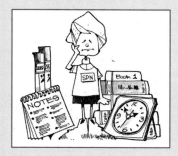

PART **TWO**
Developing Your Learning Skills

Chapter 4

For the Organizationally Challenged

Outline

Self-Test of Time Management
Benefits of Time Management
Review of Personal Goals
Getting Organized with the Nursing
   Process
      Data Collection (Assessment)

Before You Continue
Planning
Arguments Against Planning
Scheduling Time
Setting Priorities
Delegating Activities

Implementation
   General Hints
   Procrastination
   Hints for Handling the Home or
      Apartment
Evaluation

Key Terms

assessment
delegating
effectiveness
efficiency
evaluation

habits
implementation
long-term goal
minitask
planning

priorities
procrastination
schedule
short-term goal
support system

Objectives

After reading this chapter you will be able to:
1. Discuss three benefits of time management for an adult student.
2. List the activities of the various roles you fill in daily life.
3. Arrange the list of various roles in two columns according to whether they are high priority or low priority items.

4. Keep at least a one-day activity log to determine the present use of your time.
5. Devise a semester schedule and a weekly schedule to reflect present time commitments.
6. Make a daily "to do" list.

7. Carry out weekly and daily schedules for two weeks.
8. Evaluate the effectiveness of a personal time management plan and modify it if necessary.
9. Identify right-brain techniques to use in time management.

■ Becky, a fulltime student in the practical/vocational nursing program, consistently scores As and Bs on her tests and quizzes. She always hands assignments in on time. She is always prepared to demonstrate nursing procedures in the skills lab. On Thursday evenings, she bowls with her husband in a couples' league. It is hard to believe she is the mother of six children, aged 3 to 17. ■

Have you noticed at school and in your personal life that some people seem to get more done than others? Worse yet, some of the busiest people are the ones getting the most done. To add insult to injury, all of us are given the same amount of time, 168 hours a week, in which to get the job done. How can some individuals get the job done and some not? The answer does not lie in the fact that some people have fewer responsibilities and less to do in a week's time. The answer lies in their ability to manage their own time.

There are several explanations for being disorganized and managing time poorly. These traits can be related to a trauma in your personal life. Organizing may be the last thing on the mind of a person who has been through a divorce or a death in the family. A state of disorganization may be the result of a disorganized upbringing. Disorganization can be the style you grew up with. You might continue this style as a source of comfort. Other disorganized persons may not have committed themselves to something they really want to do. They may use disorganization as a symptom of their discontent. Regardless of the reason for disorganization, millions of dollars are spent annually to hire time management experts to help people get organized. This chapter contains information and tips that can help you get organized and manage your time more efficiently and effectively. If you follow the suggestions, they will help make a challenging year more tolerable for you.

Self-Test of Time Management

Time management is a major skill that contributes to learner success. It is also a necessary skill for

practical/vocational nurses so they can better manage their time in the clinical area to meet client goals. To start this chapter, it is necessary for you to take a self-test of time management so you will know how you stand with regard to this important skill. If you are going to be responsible for managing clinical time, you must be able to manage personal time. Answer yes or no as you read each of the statements in the following Self-Test of Time Management and apply them to your personal use of time.

The answers to the self-test are the ones suggested by time management experts. Although different time management techniques work for different people, these suggested answers reflect basic time management techniques that could help you succeed in the practical/vocational nursing program.

Benefits of Time Management

Time management is a technique designed to help you do not only the things you have to get done but also the things you want to finish in a definite time period. Time management can put you in control of your life rather than making you a slave to it. You will have to give up some of the things you were accustomed to doing before you became a practical/vocational nursing student. Time management techniques can help you gain some personal time for your family and yourself so you will not feel that there is time only for school. Time management can help you work smarter, not harder. It will not give you more hours in the week but will help you use what hours you do have more efficiently and effectively. **Efficiency** will help you get things done as quickly as possible. Time management does not deal solely with efficiency, as did the efficiency experts of the 1950s. The efficiency of the 1950s can bring images of robot-like individuals working to get *every* task done in the shortest time possible in a machine-like manner. Efficiency needs to be balanced with effectiveness. **Effectiveness** involves setting priorities among the tasks

Self-Test of Time Management

————— 1. I keep a semester or course calendar to reflect requirements and due dates of work for all my classes.

————— 2. I keep a written weekly schedule of everything that must be done at school and in my personal life.

————— 3. I keep a written daily list of things I must do at school and in my personal life.

————— 4. Daily I list and rank in importance my priorities for using school and personal time.

————— 5. After listing and ranking my daily priorities for school and personal life, I stick to the list I have made.

————— 6. I use my best working time during the day for doing my high-priority work for school.

————— 7. I plan to do lower-priority schoolwork before higher-priority schoolwork.

————— 8. I start school tasks before thinking them through.

————— 9. I stop a school task before I have completed it.

————— 10. I spend the few minutes before class talking to my classmates about anything other than the class.

————— 11. I have trouble starting a major task for school.

————— 12. I become bored with the subject I am studying.

————— 13. I have a hard time getting started when I sit down to study.

————— 14. Sometimes I avoid important school tasks.

————— 15. I find myself easily distracted when I study.

————— 16. I always try to get everything done in my personal life that must be done.

————— 17. I frequently watch television instead of doing schoolwork.

————— 18. I manage to turn a short coffee break into a long coffee break.

————— 19. I study nightly for my classes.

————— 20. I frequently have to cram for exams.

Suggested Answers to Self-Test

1. Yes	11. No
2. Yes	12. No
3. Yes	13. No
4. Yes	14. No
5. Yes	15. No
6. Yes	16. No
7. No	17. No
8. No	18. No
9. No	19. Yes
10. No	20. No

Count the number of statements you disagree with and plug yourself into one of the following categories:

1–5 Disagree with	You deserve the *Alan Lakein** award.
5–10 Disagree with	Hang in there! With a little guidance you will get on the right track.
11–20 Disagree with	We know you must be exhausted, but keep on reading, fast!

———————

*Alan Lakein is a famous time management expert. In 1973 he first published a very readable book entitled *How to Get Control of Your Time and Your Life.* The key to using time wisely has not changed since his first edition was published.

that need to be done and doing them the best way possible. Efficiency involves doing things as quickly as possible. Effectiveness involves choosing the most important task to do and doing it the right way.

Review of Personal Goals

How did you score on the self-test? If you are a typical adult, you are probably reading quickly right now to find out what to do to improve. Take heart. Very few of us get the Alan Lakein award. Most of us could stand to learn how to use our time more efficiently and effectively. Ineffective use of personal time is learned behavior, better known as a habit. Any behavior that is learned can be unlearned if you work at it, and new habits can be acquired.

If you have set a goal to be a practical/vocational nurse, you are already on the right track in time management, no matter what you scored. This is your **long-term goal** and the bull's eye to which you will direct your efforts for the next year. It would be beneficial to write that goal on an index card and place it where you will see it frequently. Some suggestions are your car visor, the bathroom mirror, and the refrigerator door. Be specific when you write your goal. Be sure to include the date of your graduation. There will be some tough days in the months ahead, and the visibility of your long-term goal can keep you going. Use all your senses to experience what reaching your goal will be like (the weather, how you feel, celebrations that may be planned, and so on).

To realize this long-term goal, you must break it down into smaller, more manageable goals. These are called your **short-term goals.** Examples of short-term goals are passing each of the courses you must take to graduate from the practical/vocational nursing program. These short-term goals can be broken down even further to include the individual requirements for each of the courses you must take. For example, for your professional issues course you might have to meet the following requirements to pass the course:

1. Earn a minimum grade on each of a certain number of major tests.
2. Give two oral reports.
3. Write a four-page paper on a selected topic.

Fulfilling each of the requirements will eventually lead to passing the course. When each of the courses you are required to take is passed, you will graduate from the program. While keeping your eye on your long-term goal, you will fulfill requirement after requirement until that goal is reached.

Now, let us start learning how to manage your time.

Getting Organized with the Nursing Process

At all levels, nursing has a special way of getting organized called the nursing process. Chapter 12 discusses the nursing process and your role as a practical/vocational nurse in using it. The nursing process and its four components, data collection (assessment), planning, implementation, and evaluation, will be used to help you get organized as a student and in your personal life.

Data Collection (Assessment)

According to *Webster's Dictionary,* assessment is the act of placing a value on something. To do this, the element of judgment must be brought into the picture. Data collection **(assessment)** in time management involves two important areas: (1) collecting data on how you actually spend your time and (2) discovering what roles you fill in your daily life.

Enrollment in a vocational-technical program, whether you are single, divorced, widowed, or married, requires some degree of change in the activities in which you were involved before entering the program. Regardless of your state in life, all the roles you fill can be classified in any of five general categories: school, job, family, community, and recreation.

The activities involved in going to school are very structured. You must get there, attend classes and clinical programs, and get home. When you are enrolled in a vocational-technical program such as practical/vocational nursing, your school day is chock-full. Seldom do you even have the choice of when you will take a specific course. The same structure is not evident in the other four roles. In your other roles, you might be involved in activities that you either did not plan to do, do not enjoy doing, do not have time to do, or feel do not need to be done.

You are encouraged to complete the activity on page 374 of Appendix E in order to collect data about your *personal roles and activities* for the data collection (assessment) portion of time management. A sample exercise and explanation are on page 373 of Appendix E. You are now ready to document how you actually use your personal time. Ideally, a time log should be kept for about one week to document how you use your personal time. Because time is marching on, a one-day time log can give you a general idea of how you use your time at present. Page 375 of Appendix E explains the exercise entitled Use of Personal Time. On page 376 of the Appendix you will find a blank page on which to record your Personal Time and Activity Log.

Now, supply only one more piece of information and your assessment will be complete. Following this paragraph, list one activity you wish you had time for. The activity could have been listed under your roles, but maybe it was not listed at all. Remember, the sky's the limit as long as your wish is something that is really important to you.

My special wish is

_____

_____

Before You Continue

How students use their time is partly due to which side of the brain is dominant. Chapter 5, Discovering Your Learning Style, discusses the difference between right and left brain dominance and gives you an opportunity to assess your specific dominance on page 73. Time management systems generally reflect the left brain thinking style. This style is linear (prefers a step-by-step approach) compared with right brain thinkers who are nonlinear (prefer to jump around). Traditional tools of time management are directed to left brain thinkers because of their ability to process information in sequence. Right brain thinkers look at the picture as a whole. Right brain thinkers prefer their own tools/ideas for time management and are good at making them. Neither system of thinking is good or bad. Both sides of the brain work together and complement each other.

The challenge of time management for practical/vocational nursing students is to find on which side your brain dominance lies. Use the strengths of this side. But, strive to use the resources of both sides of your brain. We will provide some right brain strategies in this planning stage. But we are sure right brain thinkers will be able to develop tools with which they are more comfortable.

Planning

When you have completed the assessment (data collection) exercises in Appendix E, you will be ready to proceed to the planning stage. The planning phase of time management will result in a blueprint for action. In this phase you will learn how to plan use of your precious 168 hours a week. **Planning** involves thinking about setting priorities (most important tasks), but to be successful, these thoughts need to be written down. You need to devise written **schedules** for yourself so that you can program your time on a monthly, weekly, and daily basis. The schedules should include the activities that are part of all the roles you fill and not just your role as a student. Your schedules should reflect the total of your activities.

Schedules help keep you honest. They reflect the classes you must attend and the studying you must do to reach your long-term goal. With a schedule you will avoid the roller coaster phenomenon all too familiar to students—falling behind in school and then trying to catch up. Schedules help you include time for friends and family. Schedules help you avoid overlooking an important part of your well-being: recreation. And schedules help you avoid the pitfall of allowing extracurricular activities to come before schoolwork. Allowing extracurricular activities to come before schoolwork is the major reason for failure in postsecondary educational programs.

Arguments Against Planning

At this point some individuals will say they do not have time to plan and will pass off the suggestion about scheduling. Individuals who are too busy to plan are the very persons who should be planning. They cannot afford not to plan. If you do not plan, you will overlook priorities and possibly miss some available free time. For the small amount of time planning takes, the benefits are great. Some persons who say they do not have time to plan really do not want to find time to get priority work done. They may use lack of time as an excuse. Some individuals look at planning and scheduling as leading to inflexibility and loss of freedom. They want to "hang loose" and go in different directions as the opportunity arises. Flexibility of this sort can result in disorganization and the accomplishment of few, if any, important tasks. As imposed deadlines near, guilt, frustration, and anxiety appear. These individuals wind up being a slave to time instead of being its master. A schedule written in accordance with the principles of time management will help you be a master of time and not a slave to it. The schedule will be written with flexibility in mind, and you will be able to trade time with yourself when unexpected events come up.

Unlearning old **habits** and learning new **habits** is not an easy task. It takes work in the form of self-discipline and determination to drop old, comfortable ways. But it is possible. Be sure to practice the new habit whenever the opportunity to do so

presents itself. In doing this, the new habit will eventually become a part of you. Ah! You say you slipped up and reverted to old habits. Do not give up! Start from where you left off and try again.

Scheduling Time

The only special equipment you need for scheduling is some form of calendar. Ideally, you need a device that has blank space for each date so that you can list activities. These calendars should be available at the bookstore. Some school bookstores provide a semester calendar for students. You can also make your own monthly calendar by copying a current calendar. Examples of other methods used for planning include:

1. On-line day planners; for example, when.com and anyday.com contain calendars.
2. Some students prefer to use index cards or Post-it notes for each activity. One color card or note can be used for roles and another color for activities. The cards can be piled or notes stuck on a wall. This method also helps put activities in appropriate categories or roles.
3. Some students prefer to use a timeline for planning instead of a calendar.

Setting Priorities

To schedule your time, you should be able to set **priorities** and delegate activities. In Appendix E, there is an exercise entitled Setting Personal Priorities to help you decide which of your activities are most important or which activities need to come first.

To have a successful year in the practical/vocational nursing program, teamwork is important. Identify the persons in your life who make up your team. This is your **support system.** Inform them of the goals and priorities you have set for yourself for this school year.

Critical Thinking Exercise

List the persons in your personal support system. Use the lines below, or a piece of paper, index cards, or Post-it notes.

_____   _____

_____   _____

_____   _____

Delegating Activities

Some of your activities can be **delegated** to specific persons on your team. On page 60 is a chart of activities with examples of tasks that can be delegated in this manner. Taking growth and development into consideration, the tasks listed for children are excellent ways for them to learn responsibility.

As in the study of growth and development, these suggested activities apply to the typical child of each age group. The suggestions may or may not apply to your children. But do not underestimate your children. You will be able to come up with some ideas that do fit your children and add to the list. At first it may take some time to instruct your children, but in the long run it will be worthwhile. Have you ever heard of the saying "You have to spend money to make money"? Well, in time management, sometimes it takes time initially to teach the people near you what is expected of them. In the long run it will pay off handsomely in time saved. Plus you get the added bonus of encouraging independence.

The same principle will be used in client care. It may take time to teach clients how to master a skill for themselves. In the long run it will save you time once they learn, and as a bonus the clients gain independence. These suggestions are a wonderful

way to help a child become independent and develop lifelong skills.

Are you having trouble getting your spouse to cooperate? Avoid interpreting stubbornness as lack of love or laziness. Chances are that your spouse grew up in an environment in which household chores were divided by sex. The spouse may feel that assuming new tasks jeopardizes his masculinity or her femininity. Gather your thoughts and decide on the areas in which you think your spouse could be most helpful during this. hectic time of your life. The answer lies in communication. Talk to your spouse (and only you know the best time and situation for this). Hopefully, you both agree that you should be going to school and have identified the positive features of this endeavor for both of you. Review these positive features. If you have not identified them, do so together. Then collaborate on solutions to ease your lack of time. While you are at it, establish some precious "spouse only" time to be honored during your hectic year at school. You do not want to create in your spouse the feeling of being left out during this whole experience.

Page 377 in Appendix E has an exercise entitled Delegating Activities to help you decide which personal roles and activities can be delegated, which you can indicate on your paper, index cards, or Post-it notes.

Implementation

Implementation is the part of your time management program in which your plans become action. The only value of a plan lies in its being used. Thanks to the planning you have done, you now have an incentive to get started because you already know exactly where you have to be and what you have to do. Now for some hints on how to follow that plan.

General Hints

As you begin to follow your personal plan, you may notice that some of your peers at school are

Text continued on page 63

Chart of Shared Tasks That May Be Delegated

Significant Other	Preschool and Early School Age (4–8 years)	School Age (9–12 years)
Pay bills	Fold laundry	Cook simple meals
Help clean	Make laundry piles	Wash dishes
Take charge of car maintenance	Deliver laundry to correct room	Dry dishes
Mow the lawn	Clear dishes from table (not best china)	Put dishes away
Paint		Start laundry
Do small repairs		Shop for a few food items as indicated on list
Sort laundry		Dust
Transfer laundry to dryer		Run vacuum
Shovel snow		Sew patches on own shirts
		Plant garden
		Weed
		Shovel snow
		Make own bed

Rationale for activities chosen for:

Preschool and early school age. Children in these age groups are experiencing muscle development and notice their psychomotor development; they want to try new things. Make-believe rides high with these kids and they love to play house. Capitalize on this.

School age. These children are adults-in-training. Muscles continue to develop and psychomotor skills are increasing. They need tasks of the real world to engage in and should be encouraged to carry them through to completion.

Adolescents (13–18 Years)	Friends	Relatives
Run errands with family car if they have a license; use bike if no license	Replace you at bowling the night before a big exam	Substitute for mom or dad at Scout meetings, PTA meetings, or school activities
Plan menus	Feed you occasionally	Spend time with children
Prepare grocery list within budget		Holiday baking or shopping
Mow the lawn		
Paint		
Make own bed		

Rationale for activities chosen for:

Adolescents. Sometime during adolescence, the ability to think as an adult will develop, allowing this age group to budget, apply principles of basic nutrition, to everyday life. One of the tasks of adolescence is to become independent. Help its development by delegating meaningful activity to this age group.

School-age children and adolescents can also do activities in the column preceding their column but would probably prefer the specific activities listed for their age group.

Learning Exercise

Scheduling for the Semester

TIME INVOLVED: Approximately 10 minutes

On your planning calendar/system, list the things that must be done during this time frame. Examples of activities to include here are

- Your class schedule
- Dates of major examinations
- Dates papers are due
- Dates of doctors' appointments
- Dates of club meetings
- Dates for haircuts, and so on

Include activities that are delegated. Indicate them by circling the activity on your calendar/planning system. Write the name of the person who is responsible for it. Post these sheets, one month at a time, on your refrigerator for you, your family, or your roommate or significant other to see. The semester schedule is done only once, in pencil. Additions or corrections are made as needed. This is also a way of communicating your new life to those with whom you live. Keep in mind, if you do live with other people, that your new schedule is something to which they must get accustomed.

Weekly Scheduling

TIME INVOLVED: Approximately 10 minutes

The weekly schedule is for your peace of mind. A blank form can be found on page 378 of Appendix E. You can copy this sheet on looseleaf paper or use index cards or Post-it notes. Fill in all your classes and other fixed activities for the week or paste/tape your cards or Post-it notes here. Photocopy as many sheets as there are weeks in the semester or time period of your current classes. Use some time each weekend to plan your week. Be sure to include in your planning the time you spend before and after classes. As assignments are made, add them to your weekly schedule. Your weekly schedule not only will reflect study time but also will specify what should be studied when. The following are some suggestions to keep in mind when planning your week.

1. Schedule studying for your prime time. Prime time is the time at which you are most effective in doing a task. High-priority courses need to be studied during personal prime time.
2. Schedule blocks of time for studying by identifying your personal attention span for various school activities. For example, when reading, note the time you start reading and when you begin to lose your concentration. Note the amount of time that has passed. Do this for several sessions of studying. You will begin to see patterns in your attention span. Take a three- to five-minute break at this point in your studying. Vary your activity.
3. Some people may find they have a 20-minute attention span. Others may have an attention span of one hour. The important thing is not to let your break extend beyond a few minutes. Condition yourself to get right back to work, without the need for start-up time.
4. It is impossible to tell you exactly how much time you will need for studying for each of your classes. This will vary from student to student and from class to class. Does the class meet daily? If so, you will have a daily assignment. The old suggestion of two hours of study for each hour of class will be just right for some classes, too much for others, and not enough for the rest.

Box continued on following page

Learning Exercise *Continued*

5. Identify small blocks of time. Make them work for you. They are important sources of time. These minutes can add up quickly to large time losses. These small blocks of time usually occur between classes. During these small blocks of time:

a. Get up.   b. Stretch.   c. Take deep breaths if staying in the same classroom.   d. Walk briskly while taking deep breaths to get to your next class.   e. Review in your mind the class you just attended.

These activities will force more oxygen into your bloodstream and help it circulate to your brain. This results in better thinking and a fresher state of mind. One of the worst things to do is to grab a soda or a cigarette. The soda, if nondiet, will quickly elevate your blood sugar level and encourage insulin to be deposited in the blood. The insulin will quickly lower the sugar content of your blood, leaving you with a tired, dragged-out feeling. Smoking constricts your blood vessels and decreases the amount of oxygen carried to your brain. Your brain needs oxygen to help you think and to keep you alert.

6. While waiting for your next class, select one of the following activities:

a. Review your notes from the class you just finished. This will allow you to fill in any gaps you may have in your notes. You will aid your retention and understanding of the material by reviewing it in this way.

b. Mentally prepare for your next class. If it is a lecture or discussion class, review your assignment. If it is an autotutorial class, review your plan of activities for the class.

c. Discuss an assignment with a peer. School is a social activity, but do not waste time by fooling around during all of your small blocks of free time. The more you get done at school, the less you will have to do at home.

7. Include only what is essential on your schedule. Details take too much time to write down and are a real turn-off.

8. Plan for three meals a day with appropriate snacks, based on the food pyramid. Eating properly will help avoid tiredness and irritability. With a busy schedule, you need to avoid being tired and irritable at all costs.

9. Plan for adequate sleep. Individuals have personal sleep patterns. Try to get in tune with yours. Do you ever wake up before your alarm? Next time you do, calculate how many hours of sleep you have had. Odds are your hours of sleep are some multiple of 1.5 hours. Brain research has shown that you will function better if you get up after 6 hours or after 7.5 hours of sleep rather than after 7 or 8 hours. Apparently, we repeat a sleep cycle every 1½ hours. If you get up one-half hour into your next cycle, you could be very sluggish. Think of this when you set your alarm. And when the alarm goes off, resist the temptation to reset the alarm on snooze.

10. Remember, although some sacrifices must be made, your life is more than just school. Review your "sky's the limit" wish on page 57 of this chapter and include it on your weekly schedule.

Daily Scheduling

TIME INVOLVED: Approximately 5 minutes.

This schedule could prove to be the most important one as far as getting things done. Alan Lakein, the time management expert, calls the daily schedule a "to do" list. He states that both successful and

Learning Exercise *Continued*

unsuccessful persons know about "to do" lists. Successful persons use such a list every day to make better use of their time. Unsuccessful people do not (Lakein, 1989, p. 64). This is the simplest schedule to make.

1. Use a 3 by 5 inch card and head it *To Do.* List the items you plan to accomplish directly on the card or on Post-it notes that you attach to the card. Be sure to include the high-priority activities for school and your personal life that you identified on pages 374 and 377 of Appendix E. Refer to your weekly calendar/planning system to refresh your memory about your assignments and their due dates. Rank (prioritize) your activities so that you can handle first things first. Use numbers, Highlighters, or colored Post-it notes to indicate priority.
2. Mind-mapping a "to do" list. See Chapter 6, Learning How to Learn and Retain Information, for an explanation of mind-mapping.

Decide for yourself the best time of day for preparing your "to do" list. Some persons like to prepare this list while eating breakfast as a way to get into the activities of the day. Some people like to prepare the list right before they go to bed. These persons may be getting an extra benefit that they are not aware of. Their subconscious will be able to go over the to do list while they peacefully sleep and renew themselves. Carry your list with you. Stick to the activities and priorities you have listed. Cross off/tear off the activities when you have completed them. Ah, what a feeling!

Planning takes so little time. It can be fun and not a chore. Just think of all the benefits that come out of taking 10 minutes to plan each month, 10 minutes to plan each week, and 5 minutes to plan each day. What great returns for so little effort! And, by writing your schedules and lists, you have freed your brain from one more source of clutter and saved it for all the learning you need to do.

not planning their time. They may even give you static for attempting to plan yours. Even if it means leaving some peers in the shuffle, have the intestinal fortitude to follow your schedule. You paid your tuition and have your own personal time problems to contend with to get full mileage out of that tuition. There may be some students who put their efforts into games instead of scholastic pursuits. They think they will look better if others do not succeed. You will recognize these students when they tell you straight out that your efforts will make them look bad. Whose problem is that, anyhow? Make sure you never miss a class, regardless of peer pressure or any reason other than an emergency. When you miss a class, you spend more time than the class would have taken trying to obtain the information from the class. You may never capture all of it.

In actually carrying out your schedule, be aware of a pitfall that can happen when you assign a spe-cific time to a task. Sometimes the time it takes to do a task, whether for home or school, can stretch out to fill whatever time you have assigned to it. So practice setting realistic time limits in which to complete tasks so you do not fall into this trap.

Procrastination

You know what you have to do and when it must be done, but do you ever find yourself putting off high-priority tasks to some time in the future? Take time now and list one task that you have put off this week.

_____

_____

_____

How did you feel about postponing this task? Such action usually leads to tension. What is causing your reluctance? Reevaluate the task you have been avoiding. Is it really a high-priority task? Remember, your planning should be flexible. The priority status of tasks can realistically change. But be careful if you find yourself using this explanation too frequently. Other causes for putting off what is important are ill health (you do not have the energy), laziness (you do not have the motivation), and past successful episodes of procrastination (if you did not do it, someone else did or nobody cared). Regardless of the cause, we all **procrastinate** to some degree. Some persons make more of a habit of it than others do.

If you look truthfully at the tasks you keep postponing, odds are they are unpleasant, difficult, or time consuming. It seems we never postpone things that are fun or simple to do. In fact, sometimes we avoid high-priority tasks and do a bunch of low-priority ones. This action gives us an immediate yet false feeling of accomplishment. For others, fear of failure causes them to put off things to the last minute. This provides the individual with an excuse for not doing well.

A sure way to finish those unpleasant, difficult, and time-consuming tasks you have been putting off is to reduce the entire task to a series of **minitasks.** There are two rules for doing this. First, the minitask must be simple to do and take no more than five minutes of your time. Second, for best results, the minitasks should be written and carried in your pocket for quick reference. Many students fear upcoming major tests and put off studying for them. Some examples of minitasks for this situation could be:

1. Before and after each class, review your current notes and related material covered previously.
2. Write the more difficult information you must know for the test on index cards. For example, write a term on one side of the card and its definition on the other. List causes of, consequences of, prevention of, and differences between items of class content and have these cards handy for quick reference whenever you have a spare minute. One of us studied vocabulary for a German final in this way while undergoing a root canal procedure.

3. Follow the same procedure as in minitask 2 for items you got wrong on quizzes.
4. Talk to a peer about course content.

Refer to Chapter 5 for information on identifying your personal learning styles.

Now, write some minitasks for the high-priority task you identified as having put off.

1. _____
2. _____
3. _____

These minitasks will get you involved in starting the task in a less painful way. Just starting a task, even in a minimal way, is a positive force. Getting started takes more effort than keeping going.

Whatever the cause of your procrastination, to be behind in work is to be behind in success. Most times it takes more time and energy to escape the task than to do it in the first place. Start today to keep life in the present. Avoid deferring life and all its opportunities to the future.

Hints for Handling the Home or Apartment

No matter how much you delegate, if you are a spouse and parent, a single parent, or a single adult, you must realize that your house or apartment is not going to be as spic and span as usual while you are a student. A few hints may help ease the transition. Some of these hints are also helpful for spouses who are helping out while the other goes to school and for single adults who are living on their own for the first time.

■ Grandma always said tidy up to make it look like you really cleaned. Pick up papers and magazines as you pass through a room. If you don't have time to wash dishes, rinse and stack them to be done later rather than just collecting them on the counter in the kitchen. If you have a dishwasher, rinse briefly and stack. Make your bed each morning when you first get up. It only takes a minute and improves the appearance of the bedroom dramatically. In fact, you can teach yourself to smooth out the top covers before you get out of bed and then slither out. Place dirty clothes in a laundry basket in your bedroom or bathroom instead of just heaping them on the floor. Hang up other clothing instead of just draping it over furniture. Clean the tub after using it by soaping up your washcloth and washing the sides of the tub while it is still warm. The soap and dirt ring will not have to be scoured. (Be sure to put your washcloth in the laundry and get out a clean one.) Put hair dryer, cool curling iron, and so on away after use or collect them in a basket to reduce clutter. These suggestions take hardly any time and really help things look straightened up.

- If you live in a two-story home, put a box at the top of the stairs and another one at the bottom for objects that need to go upstairs or come down. There is always something coming or going, and this will save extra trips.
- Having trouble with the family remembering their assigned chores? Draw the shape of a house on cardboard, draw 31 windows on the house and number them in sequence. Cut three of the four sides of each window so that it opens up. Place the cardboard over a piece of shelf paper and write in names and chores for each day on the paper. Paste this chore sheet in place and tape up the windows. The first month takes the most time, but the chore list is a snap after that. Be sure to include a surprise or treat occasionally.
- A fun and fast way for an adult or child to dust is to wear a washed garden glove. Briefly spray the glove with furniture polish and go to it.

The sky's the limit as far as creative ideas for saving time at school and in your personal life. You will come up with some ideas out of sheer necessity as the year goes by. When you do, be sure to share them with your peers and authors (care of W.B. Saunders Company).

Evaluation

Evaluation of your time management program will take place continuously from the minute you start implementing your plan. Evaluation involves determining how well your plan is working and how you are progressing toward meeting your long-term goal. It is a crucial part of time management. Why continue with a plan if it is not helping you reach your goal?

If the plan is not working, modify it. Ask yourself, "What changes should I make in my plan so that it will help me reach my long-term goal?" The best gauge you have for evaluating your plan is your test grades. They will tell you if you are devoting as much time as you need to make the grade in a course.

And how is your daily participation in class? Do you have assignments completed when they are due? Are you even aware that you had an assignment? Did you forget the test was on Thursday because you didn't mark it on your weekly calendar/planning system? Are you lapsing into the habit of procrastination? Not only will evaluation help you see how well you are progressing toward your goal, it will also help you develop the evaluation and modification skills you will need as a practical/vocational nurse.

Summary

☐ Time management is the efficient and effective use of personal time to meet long-term goals. Techniques of time management can help you gain control over your life rather than being a slave to it and can help you work smarter, not harder. Most systems of time management are geared to the left-brain style of thinking. Students with a right-brain thinking style need to adapt time management systems to styles that reflect their interest and strength. By using elements of the nursing process, you can set up time management techniques to fit your personal life. Assessment includes collecting data about present personal time use and the activities included in the various roles you fill. Planning involves composing semester, weekly, and daily schedules to include high-priority activities. Implementation involves carrying out your plan. Evaluation involves deciding whether your plan is helping you meet your long-term goal and modifying it accordingly.

Review Questions

1. Select the strategy best suited to the long-term goals of graduating from a practical/vocational nursing program and getting a job in an area nursing home:
   A. Pay your graduation fees now, including the fee for a cap and gown.
   B. Begin to search help wanted ads in the newspaper for nursing home jobs.
   C. Make sure you get plenty of sleep each night and eat a well-balanced diet.
   D. Set a small-term goal to pass the courses you are currently taking and do the same throughout the school year.
2. Select the statement that best describes the planning stage of time management.
   A. Planning is not a necessary step in time management to reach goals.
   B. Brain dominance will determine each student's approach to planning.
   C. All students will approach the planning stage in the same manner.
   D. Planning can be very time consuming when students already have full schedules.
3. When you have a few minutes between classes, select the activity that would *not* be good preparation for the next class.

   A. Stretching.
   B. Deep breathing.
   C. Taking a soda break.
   D. Review of the class just finished.
4. Which statement applies to when you forget an appointment because of a busy schedule?
   A. You are too busy with school to remember an appointment.
   B. You need to redo the implementation phase of time management.
   C. Missing the appointment is a definite indication that time management does not work.
   D. You need to evaluate your daily scheduling system and modify how you indicate daily "have to"s.
5. If you put off studying for the next *Body Structure* major examination, you are practicing
   A. Prioritizing.
   B. Procrastinating.
   C. Implementation.
   D. Educational negligence.

Reference

Lakein A. *How to Get Control of Your Time and Your Life.* New York: New American Library–Dutton, 1996.

Bibliography

Chenevert M. *Mosby's Tour Guide to Nursing School.* St. Louis: Mosby–Year Book, 1995.

Mayer J. *Time Management for Dummies.* Foster City, CA: IDG Books, 1995.

Pauk W. *How to Study in College,* 6th ed. Boston: Houghton Mifflin, 1997.

Shepherd J. *College Study Skills.* Boston: Houghton Mifflin, 1998.

Silber L. *Time Management for the Creative Person.* New York: Three Rivers Press, 1998.

Chapter 5

Discovering Your Learning Style

Outline

Key Terms

adult ADD
auditory learner
bodily/kinesthetic learner
critical thinking
hard wiring

interpersonal learner
intrapersonal learner
left brain
linguistic learner
logical learner

musical learner
right brain
spatial learner
tactual learner
visual learner

Objectives

Upon completing this chapter you will be able to:

1. Define critical thinking in your own words.
2. List two differences in the development of the male and female brain.
3. Explain what is meant by learning style.
4. Discuss three major learning styles.
5. Describe four secondary learning categories.
6. Identify your personal learning styles.
7. Describe five characteristics of an undependable memory and learning system.

Introduction to Critical Thinking

Critical thinking is an advanced way of thinking. It is the problem-solving method plus more. Critical thinking is used to resolve problems and to find ways to improve even when no problems exist. For example, the critical thinker will routinely ask himself or herself questions such as these about the subject of the thinking task at hand:

What is the **purpose** of my thinking?
What precise **question** am I trying to answer?
Within what **point of view** am I thinking?
What **information** am I using?

How am I **interpreting** that information?

What **concepts** or ideas are central to my thinking?

What **conclusions** am I coming to?

What am I taking for granted, what **assumptions** am I making?

If I accept the conclusions, what are the **implications?**

What would the **consequences** be, if I put my thought into action?*

For each element, the thinker must be able to reflect on the standards that will shed light on the effectiveness of her or his thinking.

Critical thinking is an essential part of nursing. The overall purpose of nursing is to assist people to (1) stay well or (2) regain their maximum state of health as quickly as possible, in a cost-effective manner, and in a way that fits with their belief system. Decisions nurses make affect both. Nursing decisions must be accurate and must be based on sound thinking and data. As a nurse, your critical thinking skill will vary according to your education and clinical experience. Challenge yourself critically by:

1. Anticipating questions that the client or instructor might ask.
2. Asking for clarification of what you do not understand.
3. Asking yourself if there is more you can do.
4. Rewording what you have read or been told in your own words (for example, stating the nursing diagnosis as a nursing problem).
5. Making comparisons with something similar to help you understand.
6. Organizing information in more than one way to see if you have missed anything im-

portant. This is to avoid being impressed when the "facts" fall into place but you have missed the obvious.
7. Asking your instructor to check out your conclusions.
8. Striving for objectivity. Keep an open mind and avoid drawing conclusions in advance.
9. Reviewing all your data again, especially after a period of time. It may look different.
10. Getting used to saying "I do not know but I will find out."
11. Learning from mistakes. Fix them if you can, and for goodness' sake, do not hide an error. Someone's life may be at stake, plus others can learn from your error.
12. Thinking about what you are reading about while you are reading it. Ask your instructor to challenge you to think critically while you are on the clinical unit.

Discovering Your Learning Style

Most individuals have wondered why one classmate takes voluminous notes while another just listens, and another equally successful student says, "I'll understand this better when I practice it." Everyone learns differently. Some of you may have attempted to emulate a classmate's learning style because of his or her success. Perhaps you continue to practice a learning method that has never been as successful for you as you would like it to be. We are here to say that if a learning style is not working for you, change it. After completing this chapter, you are encouraged to review what you have learned about learning styles and to support or change your present learning styles accordingly. Before reading any further, take time to complete the self-evaluation quiz given here.

After you have identified your major learning style(s), find out how the information can be helpful in your studying.

*From Paul, R. *Critical Thinking: What Every Person Needs to Survive in a Rapidly Changing World*, 3/e. Dillon Beach, CA: Foundation for Critical Thinking, 1993, p. 22 (www.criticalthinking.org).

Self-Evaluation of Major Personal Learning Style(s)

Identify Your Major Learning Style(s)

Directions: Underline the answer that is most accurate for each statement.

	Yes	Sometimes	No
Prefers to talk rather than read.	○	△	□
Likes to touch, hug, shake hands.	△	□	○
Prefers verbal directions.	○	△	□
Uses finger spelling as a way of learning words.	△	□	○
Likes written directions better than verbal directions.	□	○	△
Reads to self by moving lips.	○	△	□
Likes to take notes for studying.	□	○	△
Remembers best by doing.	△	□	○
Likes or makes charts and graphs.	□	○	△
Learns from listening to lectures and tapes.	○	△	□
Likes to work with tools.	△	□	○
Might say, "I don't see what you mean."	□	○	△
Good at jigsaw puzzles.	□	○	△
Has good listening skills.	○	△	□
Presses pencil down hard when writing.	△	□	○
Learns theory best by reading the textbook.	□	○	△
Asks to have printed directions explained.	○	△	□
Chews gum or smokes almost continuously.	△	□	○

Scoring

Count all of the ○ △ □. The highest number indicates the major learning style(s).

Key

□ = visual; ○ = auditory; △ = tactual.

Adapted from and used with the permission of Jeffrey Barsch, Ed.D. Complete copies of the test may be obtained by writing directly to Jeffrey Barsch, Ed.D., Ventura College, 4667 Telegraph Rd., Ventura, CA 93003.

Major Learning Styles

Different people think differently. They think in the system corresponding to the sense of vision, hearing, or touch. Those who think in terms of vision (**visual learners**) generate visual images—that is, they think primarily in pictures. People who think in terms of hearing (**auditory learners**) talk to themselves or hear sounds. Individuals who think in terms of touch (kinesthetic or **tactual learners**) experience feelings in regard to what is being thought about. This does not mean that a learner thinks exclusively in any one of these overall systems. What it does mean is that most people think more in one system than another. There are ways to enhance learning by supporting the overall system.

No learning style is better than another. It is usually easier to feel connected to someone who shares a similar learning style: "We think in the same language." It is easy to label a peer with a different learning style as either smart or dumb. A similar implication is there for an instructor.

A learning style just is. There are ways to make it work for you.

Visual Learner

If you are a visual learner, you learn best by watching a demonstration first. You learn something by seeing it. Make this style work for you by:

1. Sitting in front of the class.
2. Staying focused on the teacher's facial expression and body language.
3. Making notes in class and highlighting important points.
4. Rewriting notes in your own words as a form of studying. Writing notes in the margin of your book.
5. Using index cards for review or memorization.
6. Reviewing films or video tapes.
7. Looking for reference books with pictures, graphs, or charts or drawing your own.
8. Requesting demonstrations and observational experiences prior to demonstrating a new skill.
9. "Picturing" a procedure rather than memorizing steps.

Auditory Learner

If you are an auditory learner you learn best by hearing. Make this style work for you by:

1. Reading aloud or mouthing the words. Concentrate on hearing the words, especially when reading test questions.
2. Reading important information into a tape recorder and then playing it back.
3. Listening to the teacher's words instead of taking notes during class. Tape presentations and discussions if permission is granted by the instructor and students. Play the tapes back several times.

4. Finding a "study buddy" with whom to discuss class content. Verbalizing the information aids in learning the material.
5. Requesting permission to make audio tapes or oral reports for credit instead of written reports.
6. Making up rhymes or songs to remember key points.
7. Requesting verbal explanations of illustrations, graphs, or diagrams.

Tactual Learner

If you are a tactual learner you learn best by doing. You have difficulty in processing both visual and auditory input. You follow directions best by watching and doing. Make this style work for you by:

1. Handling the equipment before you practice a nursing procedure.
2. Moving while reading or reciting facts; rocking, pacing, using a Stairmaster or stationary bike, and so on.
3. Changing study positions often.
4. Using background music: your choice.
5. Taking short breaks and doing something active during that time.
6. Offering to do a project as a way of enhancing a required classroom presentation. For example, you have been asked to explain how oxygen gets out of the capillary and carbon dioxide gets in. You develop a project to use as the basis of your explanation.

Specific Categories of Learning Styles

Gardner (1990) described what he termed "multiple intelligences" as being more accurate than the single measure of intelligence quotient (I.Q.) that most are familiar with. The seven identified styles include linguistic, musical, logical/mathematical, spatial, bodily/kinesthetic, interpersonal, and intrapersonal intelligences. This knowledge translates into information that will further assist you in determining your learning style(s).

Linguistic Learner (The Word Player)

If you are a **linguistic learner,** you learn best by saying, hearing, and seeing words. You like to read, write, and tell stories. You are good at memorizing names, places, dates, and trivia. Make this style work for you by:

1. Taking notes when you read this text and reducing the number of words you have included in the notes. Use those notes as your study source. Your love of words and vocabulary may cause you to become distracted from the key points.
2. Reviewing all written work before handing it in. Delete extra words and phrases that are not directly related to the topic.

Logical/Mathematical Learner (The Questioner)

If you are a **logical learner** as well, you learn best by using an organized method involving categorizing, classifying, and working with abstract patterns and relationships. You are good at reasoning, math, and problem solving. Make this style work for you by:

1. Taking the time to organize a method of study that fits you personally.
2. Redoing your notes to fit your study method; categorizing the material under titles.
3. Studying in an area that is orderly.

Spatial Learner (The Visualizer)

If you are a **spatial learner,** you learn best by visualizing, dreaming, working with colors and pictures, and studying diagrams, boxes, and special lists in the text. You are good at imagining things, sensing changes, puzzles, and charts. Make this learning style work for you by:

1. Making your own diagrams, boxes, or lists when they are not available in the book.
2. Redoing your notes using key concepts only.
3. Boxing key information in the text.

Musical Learner (The Music Lover)

If you are a **musical learner,** you learn best by humming, singing, or playing an instrument. You are good at remembering melodies, rhythms, and keeping time. Make this style work for you by:

1. Playing your favorite music or humming when studying. Remind yourself what music relates to the content you are studying.
2. Playing an instrument while reviewing information in your head.

Bodily/Kinesthetic Learner (The Mover)

If you are a **bodily/kinesthetic learner,** you learn best by touching, moving, and processing knowledge through bodily sensations. You are good at physical activities and crafts. Make this style work for you by:

1. Moving around when studying. If you work out on a treadmill, stationary bike, or Stairmaster, it becomes a good time to read or review notes.
2. Dance or act out concepts you are studying to experience the sensations involved.

Interpersonal Learner (The Socializer)

If you are an **interpersonal learner,** you learn best by sharing, comparing, cooperating, and interviewing. You are good at understanding people, leading others, organizing, communicating, and mediating. Make this style work for you by:

b. Organizing and/or participating in a study group.

2. Comparing your understanding of material with that of other students.

Intrapersonal Learner (The Individual)

If you are an **intrapersonal learner,** you learn best by working alone, self-paced instruction, and having your own space. You are good at pursuing interests and goals, following instincts, understanding yourself, and being original. Make this learning style work for you by:

1. Working on individualized projects.
2. Trusting your instincts in regard to study needs.

Choose ideas from those suggested to fit the combination of learning styles that defines you; add or subtract as needed (Gardner and Hatch, 1990; Miller and Babcock, 1996).

Our Incredible Brain

The battle of biology (**hard wiring**) versus socialization in brain development is finally backed by sound scientific evidence. Originally biology alone was credited for male/female differences in areas such as learning (and behavior). For a number of years until the late 1980s, the importance of socialization became the focus. It was thought that men and women became what they are based on their specific socialization. Looking back, it has not worked out this way and both boys and girls have paid dearly for this singular emphasis.

The Right and Left Hemispheres of the Cerebrum

It is accepted that the **left** hemisphere of the brain is verbal; the **right** is not. The left hemisphere processes in sequence; the right, spatially (how parts fit together). Confining the activity of creativity to the right hemisphere lacks scientific evidence (Springer and Deutsch, 1997, pp. 292 and 297).

The two sides of the brain are designed to form a partnership. Musicians process music in their left hemisphere, not the right as a beginner would. Among left handers, almost half use their right hemisphere for language. Higher-level mathematicians, problem solvers, and chess players have more right hemisphere activation during these tasks, whereas beginners in those activities usually are left hemisphere-active. The right hemisphere recognizes negative emotions faster; the left hemisphere is more active while experiencing positive emotions (Jensen, 1998, p. 8). In the activity of speech, for example, the left side of the brain, being very verbal and fluent, would cause us to talk in computer-like patterns if the right side were not available to add tone and inflection to our voice. The right side of the brain helps us recognize a face in the crowd quickly, even if the person has shaved off his beard, whereas the left side would puzzle over this missing part. In school, the left side helps us break down new information into bits and pieces so we can master it. The right side gives us the total picture of our learning. Unfortunately, we usually limit ourselves to using about *1% of 1%* of the brain's projected processing capacity.

Developmental Differences

This brief review of brain development will be limited to developmental issues that affect learning in the classroom and clinical area.

 Critical Thinking Exercise

What is your belief at this time about biological (hard-wired) influences versus environmental (socialization) factors in male/female learning differences?

The male brain is about 10% to 15% larger than the female brain. The reason for and use of the additional space has not been clearly identified. Size alone is not intelligence in humans any more than it is in other animals.

In utero (fetal life), the female brain develops earlier than the male brain. The left half of the brain, which controls thinking, develops somewhat later than the right brain, which is related to spatial relationships. Brain development is even slower for the male. When the right side of the male brain is ready to connect with the left side by sending over connecting fibers (corpus callosum), the proper cells for the connection do not exist. Consequently, the fibers go back and form connections within the right side. This is why the male brain ends up with enriched connections within the right hemisphere (spatial capability). The ability often shows up early in the male child, such as moving blocks to see how they use up space.

The female brain develops faster and is able to develop a larger system of connecting fibers (corpus callosum) between the left and right hemispheres of the brain. There is more communication between both sides of the brain. Being able to draw on both hemispheres benefits the female in reading skills, for example (Gurian, 1997, pp. 13–19).

Practical Application of Information

In the following chart, we will look at specific characteristics related to brain development. Individual differences can always apply in nature. Socialization also enters into expanding the original work of both hemispheres of the brain. Personalize the chart as it applies to you. Mark the characteristics that apply to you in the boxes provided.

How We Learn

Scientists are not exactly sure how the brain can rewire itself with each new stimulation, experience, or behavior and cause learning. Their idea is that a stimulus occurs and is processed by the brain on several different levels. Neural pathways (traces) become more and more efficient when a learning

Brain Characteristics

Check all that apply:

☐ Better at sensory data (hear, smell, touch, taste, and see minute detail).

☐ Hear better from one ear. Visual is best sense: I interpret best from left eye.

☐ Differentiate background sounds readily.

☐ Do less well in picking up background noises: may not "hear" someone speaking to me.

☐ Satisfied with limited space. Process data in sequence.

☐ Increased focus on spatial relationships and activities. Tend to use more space. Like video and computer games and participate in activities that fill more space, such as football, baseball, and so on.

☐ Easy to express myself verbally.

☐ Not so easy to express myself verbally.

☐ Do less well with abstraction skills.

☐ Good abstraction skills. Test out better at math (abstract spatial construction of right hemisphere).

☐ Reading is easy.

☐ Reading takes more time.

☐ Multitask: I can work on several tasks at one time.

☐ Focus on one task at a time. Irritated by interruptions.

☐ Handle issues involving emotions readily.

☐ Difficulty in identifying and expressing emotions.

☐ Detect emotions easily.

☐ Have difficulty detecting emotions in another's face.

☐ Process information or think about things all the time.

☐ Brain shuts down with overload or fatigue.

☐ Rarely aggressive.

☐ Tend to be aggressive.

exercise, like reviewing notes, is repeated. This is done through myelination (coating) of the neurons. Stimulation occurs when you learn something new. The mental or motor stimulation lights up the brain in several areas, producing even greater beneficial electrical energy. Example: A new assignment or clinical experience.

The brain gets its energy for learning primarily from blood—about eight gallons per hour. Remember to keep up the water intake—8 to 12 glasses per day. "Dehydration is a common problem in school classrooms, leading to lethargy and impaired learning" (Jensen, 1998, pp. 10 and 12).

Undependable Memory and Learning System

There are average and above average individuals with potential and talent who embrace failure messages and low self-worth. Some of these individuals are part of a population who continue to live with an untreated attention deficit disorder (ADD) as adults. Among the characteristics of **adult ADD** is an undependable memory and learning system.

Some Suggestions for the Student with Adult ADD

1. Identify your learning style from the categories presented in this chapter. Practice the suggestions offered.
2. Use relaxation exercises to quiet your mind and reduce anxiety.
3. Use background music (not TV) to shut off background noises.
4. Schedule study time for when you feel most alert and fresh.
5. Use color to help focus your attention. A colored transparency over the page you are reading or a large colored poster board on the desk where you work help draw your attention.
6. Use physical activity to enhance study: play study tapes while walking, or ride a stationary bike while reviewing notes.
7. Invent your own comfortable ways of studying.

Signs of Possible Adult ADD

Check the statements that apply.

_____ 1. Trouble hanging on to a steady job.

_____ 2. Difficulty getting assignments in on time; late in filing taxes or renewing driver's license.

_____ 3. Supervisor or instructor complains that you do not do your share of the work.

_____ 4. Feel others are responsible for what happens to you.

_____ 5. Impulse buyer: I need, I want, I must have. Credit cards frequently maxed out.

_____ 6. Thrill-seeking impulsive behavior: live for the moment without considering consequences.

_____ 7. Use alcohol, tobacco, and caffeine to pick you up or calm you down.

_____ 8. Overreact to everyday situations: very happy, very sad, very angry or irritable, grumpy, pessimistic.

_____ 9. Short attention span: easily distracted.

_____ 10. Superfocused: difficulty detaching from task at hand.

_____ 11. Normal noise, sight, or sound causes feelings of intense anxiety or irritation.

_____ 12. Protective of own physical space but will invade others' space without forethought.

_____ 13. Experiences shame after unexplained explosive outbursts.

_____ 14. Fatigued: seen as a night person but often stays up until exhausted because of nightmares and disturbed sleep patterns.

_____ 15. Problems with organizing activities of daily living.

_____ 16. Uses charm and humor to manipulate.

_____ 17. More comfortable with monologue than with dialogue.

If you recognize several of these traits, check with your school counselor for further information. We also recommend the book *You Mean I'm Not Lazy, Stupid or Crazy?!* (Kelly and Ramundo, 1993).

Putting It Together

It is not unusual to read information but then say, "But of course this doesn't apply to me." This information does apply. Quality education encourages you to explore and apply alternative thinking, multiple answers, and creative insights. You become a self-directed learner by:

1. Practicing critical thinking with the goal of developing noncritical thinking most of the time.
2. Identifying your major and specific learning styles. Studying becomes easier.
3. Understanding basic right and left brain functions and how they work together. It helps you appreciate your capacity for learning.
4. Doing your part to prevent dehydration when studying and participating in classes. Water is a major ingredient of the blood, which motivates the brain.
5. Behaving in a successful manner. Successes reinforce this attitude.
6. Setting realistic goals and evaluating the results to see whether these goals are being met. **It is an obstacle to learning to think that learning can take place without effort.**
7. Not letting established styles harden into such fixed beliefs that new styles cannot be tolerated; at that point, education ends.
8. Tying in new learning to previous lessons and experiences. This gives the material meaning and makes it easier to remember.
9. Seeking help when needed. Sometimes being alone is best; sometimes it is best to study with others. Beginning studies, problems with studies, and the need to be with someone are reasons for seeking out others.
10. Learning beyond the point necessary for doing or performing the skill. Keep reviewing and practicing the skills learned. Practice, practice, practice.
11. Fitting your new information into what you already know.
12. Remembering that whatever your learning style is, the best memory aid is **writing it down.** According to a Chinese proverb, the weakest ink lasts longer than the strongest memory!

Summary

☐ Critical thinking is an advanced form of thinking. It is used to solve problems and to find ways to improve even when no problems exist. It is an essential part of nursing.

☐ People think in different representational systems; the way they think determines their major learning style. Some think in pictures (visual learners). Some hear sounds or talk to themselves (auditory learners). Some experience a feeling in regard to what they are thinking about and learn best by doing (tactual learners). Each learning style can be enhanced through specific techniques.

☐ There are secondary learning categories as well. Identifying whether you are a linguistic learner (love words and new vocabulary), a logical learner (organized, consistent), a spatial learner (likes boxes and diagrams rather than words), a musical learner (likes to hum, sing, or play instruments), a bodily/kinesthetic learner (likes touching and moving), an interpersonal learner (likes sharing, comparing, cooperating), or an intrapersonal learner (likes working alone, self-paced instruction) further enhances your learning ability.

☐ Each side of the brain processes things separately. Based on experimental evidence, it is accepted that the left hemisphere is more verbal and processes things in parts or sequentially. The right hemisphere is nonverbal and sees the total picture. A connection between the right brain and music is established.

☐ Male and female brains develop differently, which therefore accounts for some different characteristics.

☐ One's personal attitude toward learning also influences the learning process. Attitude is closely related to whether you are a reactive learner who expects to be taught or an active learner who takes charge of his or her own education.

Review Questions

1. Which of the following is a partial definition of critical thinking?
   A. A 5- to 6-step process used to find a solution to a problem.
   B. Intuition used as the basis for finding a solution.
   C. Open to possibilities with focus on accuracy and truth.
   D. Trial-and-error method that assists in building character.
2. Which difference(s) in how the right and left hemisphere process information is/are based on scientific evidence?
   A. Right brain is creative.
   B. Left brain combines parts of a whole.
   C. Right brain is verbal.
   D. Left brain processes in sequence.
3. Which major learning style is needed to grasp information accurately during a lecture?
   A. Visual
   B. Tactual
   C. Auditory
   D. Kinesthetic
4. What major learning style is used during demonstration/return demonstration?
   A. Auditory
   B. Tactual
   C. Visual/tactual
   D. Visual
5. How would you assist a classmate with an interpersonal learning style in her or his learning?
   A. Encourage participation in a study group.
   B. Suggest having music on while studying.
   C. Encourage studying alone at own pace.
   D. Suggest using charts, diagrams, or lists.

References

Barsch J. *Understanding Your Learning Style.* Ventura, CA: Ventura College Learning Disability Clinic.

Gardner H, Hatch T. Multiple Intelligences Go to School: Educational Implications of the Theory of Multiple Intelligences (Technical Report No. 4). New York Center for Technology in Education, March, 1990.

Gurian M. *The Wonder of Boys.* New York: Jeremy P. Tarcher/Putnam, 1997.

Jensen E. The learning brain. In *Teaching with the Brain in Mind.* Alexandria, VA: Association for Supervision and Curriculum Development, 1998.

Kelly K, Ramundo P. *You Mean I'm Not Lazy, Stupid or Crazy?!* New York: Scribner, 1993.

Miller M, Babcock D. *Critical Thinking Applied to Nursing.* St. Louis: C. V. Mosby, 1996.

Paul R. *Critical Thinking: What Every Person Needs To Survive in A Rapidly Changing World,* 3rd ed. Santa Rosa, CA: Foundation for Critical Thinking, 1993.

Springer S, Deutsch G. Attempts at applying asymmetry: Hemisphericity, education, and culture. in *Left Brain Right Brain; A Perspective on Cognitive Neuroscience,* 5th ed. New York: W. H. Freeman & Co., 1997.

Bibliography

Alfaro-LeFevre R. *Critical Thinking in Nursing: A Practical Approach,* 2nd ed. Philadelphia: W. B. Saunders, 1999.

Griggs D, Griggs S, Dunn R, Ingham J. Accommodating nursing students' diverse learning styles. Nurse Educator 19(6), 1994.

Iyer P, Taptich B, Bernocchi-Losey D. *Nursing Process and Nursing Diagnosis,* 3rd ed. Philadelphia: W. B. Saunders, 1995.

Marcus D, Mulrine A, Wong K. How Kids Learn. In US News & World Report 127(10), September 13, 1999.

Chapter 6

Learning How to Learn and Retain Information

Outline

General Hints for Learners
    Concentration
    Listening
    Notemaking

Remembering and Forgetting
How to Understand (Comprehend)
    Information

Visual Strategies to Enhance
    Understanding
Other Methods of Increasing
    Understanding
    Study Groups
    Tutoring

Memory Aids

Reading
    Hints to Increase Reading Effi-
       ciency

Hints for Successful Test Taking
    Preparation for the Test
    Taking the Test
    Hints for Specific Tests

Key Terms

active listener
analysis
application
external distractions
idea sketches
internal distractions

knowledge
mapping
mental imagery
mnemonic devices
outlining method

passive listener
study groups
tutoring
understanding
vocalization

Objectives

Upon completion of this chapter you will be able to:
1. Identify techniques that increase your degree of concentration in learning situations.
2. Identify techniques that improve your listening skills in learning situations.

3. Utilize techniques that enhance understanding of information needed to be a practical/vocational nurse.
4. Evaluate your personal need for help with reading skills to increase

speed of reading and degree of comprehension.
5. Utilize hints for successful test taking when taking tests in the practical/vocational nursing program.

Of all the reasons for not succeeding in school, lack of study skills is high on the list of causes. From our teaching experience, we have seen students fail because of lack of study skills more often than because of lack of time to devote to school. In fact, when failure is attributed to "I don't have the time," it often is really due to lack of knowledge about how to study and how to use time to advan-

tage. Many vocational schools and junior colleges offer courses in how to study before the student enters a program and have departments that offer study skill services after a student is enrolled. Not everyone who needs these services is aware that he or she needs them. Many learners think they will succeed because they have succeeded in high school or college courses. Learners cannot assume they have the study skills necessary to succeed in the practical/vocational nursing program because they have attended high school or college. Students who have developed study skills will be surprised at how much more effectively they can learn after reviewing their study habits.

Before going on, you must be aware of two things. First, you must get yourself organized into a study habit. Some people dislike the thought of being organized. Many times this feeling arises out of habit. The feeling can be overcome by keeping your educational goals in front of you and developing some organizational skills for studying. Second, you must realize that it is hard work to acquire the knowledge and skills needed for your chosen career. We cannot say it will be easy. Learning is hard work. It takes time and effort. Study skills are like any other skill. They are developed by practice and hard work.

General Hints for Learners

Concentration

Concentration is the ability to keep your mind completely on the task at hand. The major enemy of concentration is distraction. Many distractions in a learner's life compete with the need to buckle down to school assignments. These distractions can be summarized as two types: (1) those that come from outside yourself (external distractions) and (2) those that come from inside yourself (internal distractions).

External Distractions

External distractions occur in your physical and social environment.

PERSONAL STUDY AREA. Your physical environment is a potential enemy of concentration. Locate one or two realistic areas for studying. The chosen areas should be associated with learning and not with daydreaming or napping. If your school has a learning resource center, it can be used between classes and after school. Another area can be a place in your home or apartment. This could be

the kitchen, a corner of your bedroom, or part of the basement. The place you choose needs to be away from family or roommates. A writing surface, a lamp, and a chair are necessary. Have on hand a supply of pens, sharpened pencils, highlighter, felt marker, loose-leaf paper, scrap paper, index cards, calendar, English dictionary, thesaurus, and medical or nursing dictionary and add additional tools you identify that help you learn. Keep these items organized and readily available. You will save time and aggravation by not having to look for your study tools each time you sit down to study. Choose a chair you feel comfortable in but not one that you associate with snoozing. Avoid studying in bed.

LIGHTING. The light you choose for studying is almost more important than your chair. Many students have a table lamp. This is fine as long as the bulb is shaded and your writing surface is light colored to reflect light. It is important to eliminate glare. The shade and light surface will help in this matter. Try using a "soft white" light bulb to reduce glare further. Be sure that the bulb is screwed into its socket to ensure a tight connection to reduce flicker. If a ceiling light is also available, turn this on in addition to your table lamp to reduce shadows.

Eyestrain can occur if lighting allows glare, shadows, or flicker to exist in your study area. If you have tried to eliminate these three unwanted lighting conditions and you still experience symptoms of eyestrain, such as headaches, dizziness, tiredness, or blurred vision while reading, it is time to have an eye examination to rule out the need for corrective lenses. Some students discover that they need glasses only after they enroll in an educational program demanding much reading, such as the practical/vocational nursing program.

BACKGROUND SOUNDS. Keep in mind that research studies on learning styles show that some students concentrate better with background sounds (music, voices). Other students require quiet surroundings. Honestly identify the type of environment that allows you to get the most out of your study time. Your grades will be the criteria by which you can judge whether your environment is helping or hurting. Strive for a study environment that meets your learning style preference (see Chapter 5). If you require a quiet environment, sometimes home does not provide this. Past students have told us they were successful in disciplining themselves to ignore noise and concentrate on studying. Television, stereos, radios, and CD players are considered background noise. Frequently, despite learning style preferences, students state that they study best in the presence of these external distractions. If these habits are a carryover from high school and are interfering with your concentration, establish new habits to help you with your more difficult subjects. High school and college study habits do not automatically guarantee success in the practical/vocational nursing program.

YOUR PEERS. Are the persons you associate with at school encouraging your progress in the practical/vocational nursing program? Do you support and encourage each other? Do you pick a special person to sit with in class so you can privately chat while others are talking? Do you seek out other students who have negative attitudes? If so, what are the conversations you engage in during a supposedly relaxing coffee break? Do the persons you associate with love to belittle, complain, and tear down the instructor, the course, and various students in your group? Does your anxiety level increase when you carpool with certain students on test days? The energy devoted to any of these activities can seriously deplete the energy needed to achieve success with less stress and frustration.

 Learning Exercise: Personal Distractions

List any external distractions that are affecting your concentration.

_____

_____

What can you do to eliminate these distractions?

_____

_____

_____

THE INTERNET. The Internet offers a vast amount of resources for all your classes. You may have assignments that need to be completed by using the Internet. Much can be learned and discovered by getting "sidetracked" on the World Wide Web. However, watch your time when you are online. Hours can slip by before you know it.

Learning Exercise: Peers

Answer the questions asked in "Your Peers" above.

_____

_____

_____

_____

_____

_____

_____

_____

_____

Internal Distractions

You can have the perfect desk, lighting, chair, noise level, equipment, and peers for studying but still not be able to keep your mind on the task at hand. The culprit may be distractions arising from inside yourself. Here are some common examples of **internal distractions** and suggestions for overcoming them.

COMPLAINTS OF MENTAL FATIGUE. Most students confuse boredom with fatigue. In setting up a study schedule, make sure you do not study one subject so long that you get bored with it (see Chapter 4). Keep up your physical self with proper food, sleep, and exercise. At the first sign of "getting tired," take a short break (not a snooze) and come back to new material so that you can get your mental second wind.

DAYDREAMING. Daydreaming can be a creative adventure or wasted time. Every time you find your mind wandering from the topic at hand, put a checkmark on a piece of paper that you keep at your side. This will remind you that you are drifting off and need to get back to work. Students who use this technique find that the number of check marks decreases dramatically as the days go on.

Learning Exercise: Daydreaming

List four topics that you daydream about when studying.

_____

_____

_____

_____

List internal and external distractions that encourage you to daydream.

_____

_____

_____

_____

List suggestions for reducing or eliminating these distractions.

_____

_____

_____

_____

Another Technique for Improving Concentration

The following technique has been used successfully by students to improve their concentration. Try it out to see whether it can help you.

Using simple tools such as a pencil or highlighter will keep you active in your learning. Underlining or highlighting *main* ideas, writing in the margins, and so on will keep you active and your concentration at its peak. Remember the hints related to your personal learning style (see Chapter 5).

Listening

The human voice takes up much of class time. Whether you are involved in a minilecture class or discussion or activity, or are viewing videotapes as part of a course, you are going to miss a lot if your mind wanders. Listening is much more than the mechanical process of hearing. There are two kinds of listeners. Which type are you?

- The **passive listener** receives sounds with little recognition or personal involvement. This "listener" may be doodling, staring out the window, or even staring at the instructor but thinking about having to change the oil in the car or deciding what to cook for dinner.

■ The **active listener** listens with full attention and is open-minded and curious. This listener is searching for relevant information and strives to understand it. Active listeners realize that listening is an important method of gathering information and work at developing this skill. The active listener looks for ways in which the speaker's words can be put to practical use regardless of the student's level of interest in or degree of fondness for the instructor or the instructor's dress or mannerisms.

■ Are you an active or a passive listener? Hints for effective listening include:
1. Be well rested for class.
2. Have assignments, including extra readings, completed.
3. Ask questions before, during, and after class.
4. Listen for key information and central ideas, not specific facts.
5. Make eye contact with the speaker.
6. Listen when other students are speaking.
7. Seek help when a difficult concept is not understood.

Notemaking

An important part of listening is remembering what you have listened to. Some students say that taking notes interferes with their listening skills. They are correct if they are in the business of *taking* notes. Research has shown that a student remembers only 50% of a 10-minute lecture when tested immediately afterward and only 25% of that lecture when tested two days later. The secret to improving those percentages to as much as 80% to 90% is to engage in *notemaking* whenever you are listening. Because teachers derive test questions from minilectures, discussions, activities, videotapes, and readings, that 80% to 90% could translate into a comparable test score. Notemaking will help you to pay attention, concentrate, and organize your ideas.

Hints for Notemaking

Never try to capture every word the speaker says. This is *notetaking* and is impossible. A speaker can put out about 100 to 125 words or more per minute. Time yourself to find how many words you can write per minute. Have a peer time one minute and another peer read for the same time while you try to write everything down. The number will shock you. Besides not being able to get every word down, you will also not be able to capture the meaning of what was said. Instead, strive for *notemaking,* formulating condensations of what is said in a telegram-like manner. Actively listen for the main ideas. Capture them in a way that reflects your personal learning style or styles. You are recording ideas or key concepts that you will later add to, correct, and study.

HAVE ONE 8.5 × 11-INCH LOOSE-LEAF NOTEBOOK WITH DIVIDERS FOR EACH CLASS. Spiral notebooks have the disadvantage of not allowing handouts to be included easily with daily notes. With the loose-leaf system, the notebook can be left at home and a supply of paper taken to school daily. Make sure your name, address, and telephone number are in the notebook in case you misplace it.

DO NOT TAKE NOTES IN SHORTHAND. Shorthand notes have to be transcribed after class, another poor time-management technique. Develop your own personal symbols, abbreviations, and shorthand of sorts to help you capture the main ideas yet retain readability without having to transcribe the notes. Use your medical abbreviations as presented in your charting classes. Make your notes in pen so that they don't smudge. When a mistake is made, cross out the error, but do so neatly. Erasing is time consuming. Avoid typing or rewriting your class notes word for word. Instead, use this time to think about what is important in the notes and condense them as you rewrite. This is especially helpful for visual learners. At first your notes may seem to be a disaster, but remember that you are not competing for a penmanship award. With practice, they will improve. Your goal is a set of notes you can use today, next week, and at the end of the program for review for the NCLEX-PN.

Two Methods for Making and Reviewing Notes

OUTLINING METHOD. The first method is the **outlining method,** which has been used for ages. Outlining is especially popular with left-brain dominant individuals. It involves adapting normal loose-leaf paper so that you have room to take notes and summarize content and can test yourself on your notes. This method can be used to prepare you continuously for testing of the material. This method is useful for taking notes when reading textbooks. Figure 6–1 is an example of traditional *notemaking,* used to summarize this chapter so far. The actual form used can be adapted to your preference. Suggestion:

1. Use the margin at the top of the page to write the date and course number and any assignments that are given.
2. Extend the left margin another inch. Take your notes in your personal learning style to the right of this line.
3. After class, in the area at the left of the page, record key words or phrases that serve as cues for the lecture notes on the right. Also, use this area as a space for questions or comments. These will be useful in testing yourself.
4. The bottom inch of each page should be left blank. A summary of the content of the notes on that page can be made in this section. This summary forces you to think about and come to grips with the ideas in your notes.

Some students think that writing material in note form alone will help them retain the material. Active and frequent review of your notes is an important step in retention of material.

MAPPING. Brain researchers have suggested an alternative to the linear method of notemaking. It encourages using the right side of the brain with its emphasis on images. Color and drawings are processed by the right side of the brain and are important components in mapping. Information presented in a linear manner, as in traditional notemaking, is not as easily understood as information presented by key concepts. The use of key concepts is the primary way in which the brain processes information. The brain takes these key concepts and integrates them in relationships. So, if the brain does not work in lines or lists, the method of notemaking called **mapping** can enhance your ability to understand, review, and recall this information. Mapping is a method in which information is organized graphically so that it is seen in a visual pattern of relationships. Mapping is like drawing a road map. Figure 6–2 summarizes the information presented in this chapter so far in an unstructured mapping form called clustering. Suggestions for mapping include:

1. Start with your notepaper in a horizontal position.
2. Draw a small circle in the middle of the paper.
3. Put the main topic of the class in the circle.
4. Add branches off the circle for important ideas or subtopics. Arrange these branches like spokes of a wheel. Use a different-colored pen for each of the branches. Draw more branches off branches as needed for each topic.
5. Draw a picture to go with each key topic or idea. Artistic ability does not count here. What is important is that the picture gives meaning to you.

Regardless of the side of your brain dominance, you can benefit by using each of the above methods of notemaking.

Remembering and Forgetting

We all can recall things from the past, indicating that our brains have the ability to store information. But how many times have you said "I forgot," or "I can't remember"? Possible causes of forgetting include:

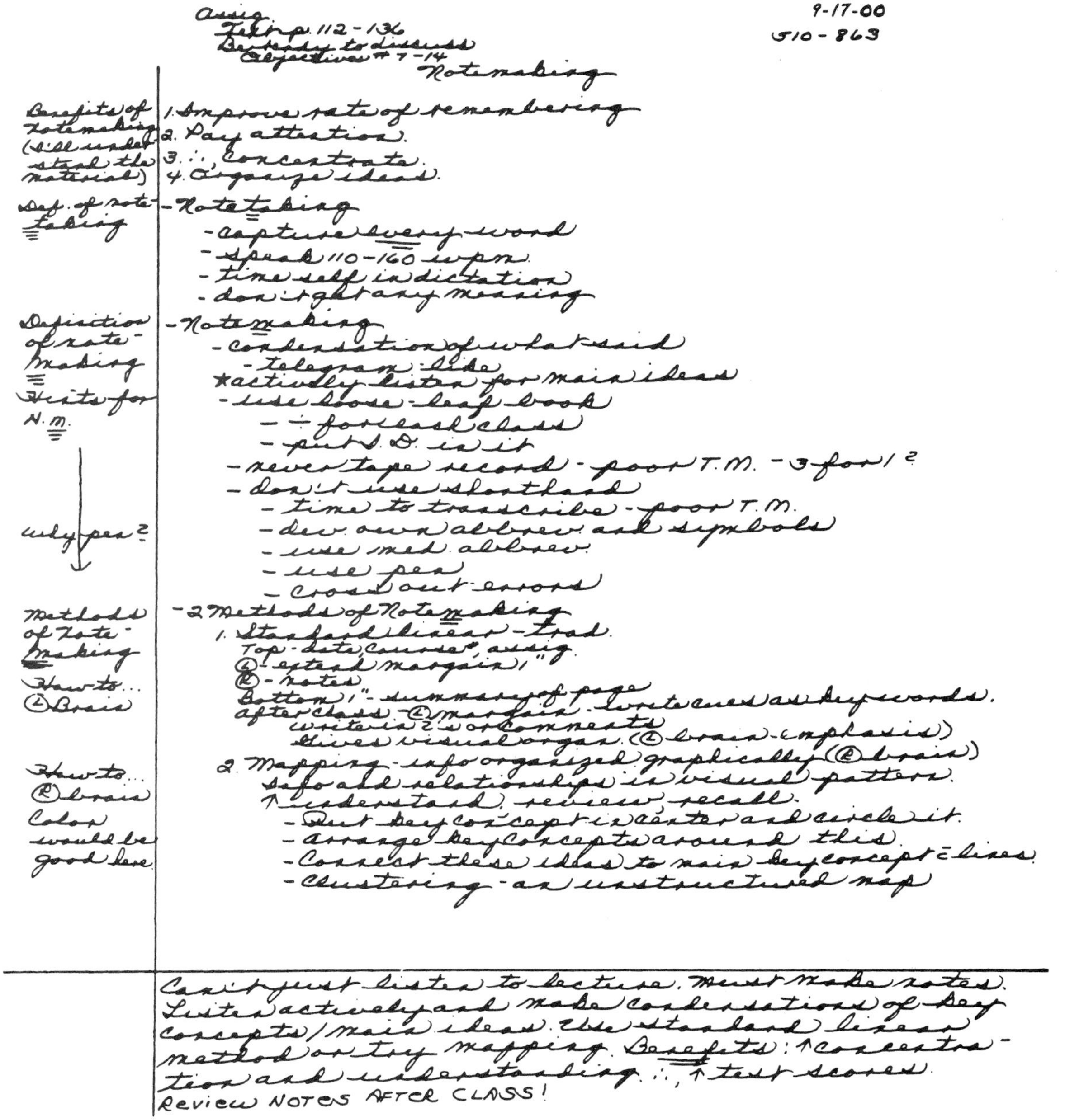

Handwritten notes:

Assign.
Text p. 112-136
Be ready to discuss
Objectives #7-14

9-17-00
JO-863

Notemaking

Benefits of Notemaking (I'll understand the material)
1. Improve rate of remembering
2. Pay attention
3. " Concentrate
4. Organize ideas

Def. of note taking — Notetaking
- capture every word
- speak 110-160 wpm
- time self in dictation
- don't get any missing

Definition of note-making — Notemaking
- condensation of what said
  - telegram style
★ actively listen for main ideas
- use loose-leaf book
  - - for each class
  - put S.D. in it
- never tape record - poor T.M. - 3 for 1?
- don't use shorthand
  - time to transcribe - poor T.M.
- dev own abbrev and symbols
- use med abbrev
- use pen
- cross out errors

Methods of Note-making — 2 Methods of Notemaking
How to... (1) Brain
1. Standard linear - Trad.
   Top - date, course, assig.
   (a) extend margin 1"
   (b) - notes
   Bottom 1" summary of page - write own as keywords.
   after class (a) margin (b) brain (emphasis)
   criteria 2 or 3 or comments
   Gives visual organ

How to... (2) Brain   Color would be good here
2. Mapping - info organized graphically (2 brain)
   info and relationships in visual pattern.
   ↑ understand, review, recall.
   - Put key concept in center and circle it.
   - arrange key concepts around this.
   - Connect these ideas to main key concept c̄ lines.
   - Clustering - an unstructured map

Can't just listen to lecture, must make notes. Listen actively and make condensations of key concepts/main ideas. Use standard linear method or try mapping. Benefits: ↑ concentration and understanding ∴ ↑ test scores.
REVIEW NOTES AFTER CLASS!

FIGURE 6–1. Traditional notemaking.

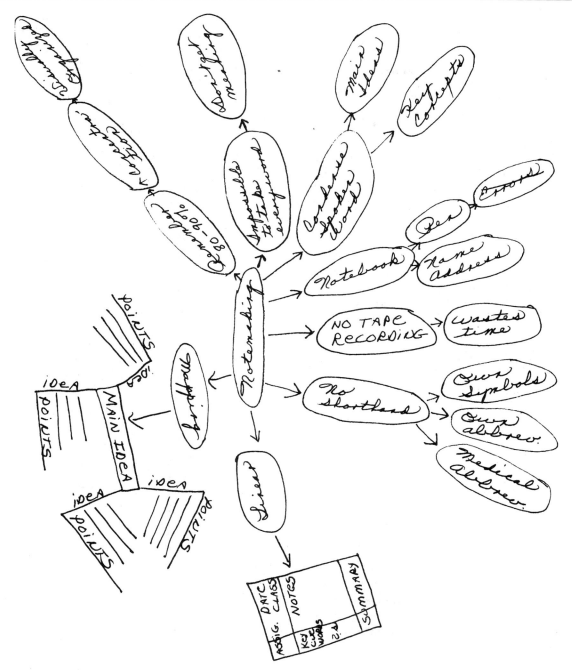

FIGURE 6–2. Clustering.

1. A *negative attitude* toward the subject, which interferes with the motivation to remember.
2. *New knowledge,* which interferes with the recall of old learning.
3. *Old knowledge,* which interferes with the recall of new learning.

Valid as these causes of forgetting may be, perhaps the most common reason why students cannot remember is that *they never grasped the information in the first place.* They really did not internalize the information and understand it to begin with. Perhaps they did not listen actively, or they just read words and created a mental blur.

To store information in your long-term memory, a neural trace or a record of the information must be laid down. Psychologists have found that it takes four to five seconds for information to move from the temporary, or short-term, memory to the permanent, or long-term, memory. To form a long-term memory of information, you must strive to understand that information. In doing so, you will give your brain the chance to lay down a neural trace. Presto! You have created a memory of that information. Short but frequent study periods will help you understand information and store it in your long-term memory.

How to Understand (Comprehend) Information

You will be exposed to much new knowledge during your year in the practical/vocational nursing program. You will gain knowledge as stated in the course objectives. Your real test as a practical/vocational nurse will be your ability to understand that information and use it as the basis for critical thinking in the clinical area. The national licensing examination for practical/vocational nurses tests the level of knowledge, understanding, application, and analysis. The following definitions will help you comprehend the meaning of the words knowledge (knowing), understanding, application, and analysis.

1. **Knowledge** means the ability to repeat information you have memorized. This is the lowest level of learning. Defining a concept as stated in a dictionary is an example of knowledge.
2. **Understanding** (comprehension) means to grasp the meaning of the material. This is the lowest level of understanding. Repeating information *in your own words* indicates that you understand the concept.
3. **Application** means being able to use learned material in new situations. For example, you apply what is learned in class to your clinical work. Application is a higher level of understanding that helps you retain what you are learning.
4. **Analysis** means to be able to break down information into its basic parts in order to understand its organizational structure (form/arrangement). An example of analysis is the ability to organize and prioritize (what is most important, most urgent) two or more pieces of information in a client situation in order to process a safe response. Analysis is a higher level of application.

Understanding, application, and analysis are what employers expect of a practical/vocational nurse on the job. Your instructors will also expect this level of competence in the clinical area as you continue to develop your critical thinking skills. Past students with college degrees have told us that the consistent need to apply and analyze both prior and newly learned information is the area about practical/vocational nursing that differs most from their college experience.

Visual Strategies to Enhance Understanding

Your scholastic world is bombarded with words, sentences, and paragraphs. One of the most beneficial techniques used to understand and remember all the new information is to balance this verbal mixture with visual strategies. Each of the following visual strategies will help you understand and ultimately remember information better. They deal with the right side of the brain. You will be tapping a

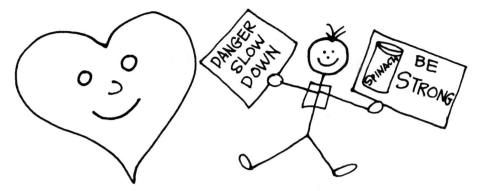

FIGURE 6–3. Idea sketch: Action of Lanoxin (digoxin).

resource that perhaps you have not used before. If you have right brain dominance, your understanding will be improved by adopting left brain strategies of organizing information, as discussed in Chapter 5. These strategies include improving the general organization of material and writing and restating new information in your own words.

Draw Idea Sketches

These drawings will probably be comprehensible only to you. The emphasis is not on the quality of the drawing but on the process you must go through to take a verbal concept and represent it graphically, without words. To go through this process you must understand the verbal concept. You can even set it up as a cartoon. Use stick figures and describe the concept verbally. Figure 6–3 is an **idea sketch** illustrating the function of the drug Lanoxin (digoxin), which is used to slow and strengthen the heartbeat.

 Critical Thinking Exercise: Idea Sketch

Choose a concept you are having trouble with in one of your classes. Draw an idea sketch to help you increase your understanding of that concept.

Use Color in Whatever Form of Notemaking You Use

Use highlighters, crayons, colored pencils, or felt-tip pens. Avoid merely underlining the sentences. Use the different colors to help capture and direct your attention to information that fits in different categories. The different colors will help your brain organize and retrieve information.

Make Your Own Diagrams as You Read

If you commit ideas to memory only by using words, you are using only half of your brain's resources, those of the left side. If you also produce a sketch of that idea, you will have brought the right side of your brain into use. The use of both sides of the brain is a powerful tool that encourages the storage and retrieval of information.

Engage in Mental Imagery

This technique will really help you remember because it demands that you understand the information. When you use **mental imagery,** you become the idea that you are having difficulty understanding. The right side of your brain generates pictures of the idea, and the left side supplies the script to explain what is going on in the pictures (and always in your own words).

The following is an example of a mental image developed by a practical nursing student to give herself a simple understanding of the function of insulin, a hypoglycemic agent that increases glucose transport across muscle and fat cell membranes. Notice how she uses the senses of hearing and feeling and also body movement to help achieve understanding. She also uses a metaphor, equating something she knows about with something she is trying to learn. The student recites this image to herself while she closes her eyes and visualizes it. At first, she had her roommate read the story while she visualized the scenario.

I AM INSULIN—A JOB DESCRIPTION. I am insulin and I am shaped like a canoe. In fact, I am a canoe, a green one. My job is to make the sugar or glucose in the blood available to most of the cells of the body for energy. I like my job. I like things that are sweet but not too sweet, so blood sugar is just my thing. Sometime after the person who owns the pancreas where I am stored in my canoe rack eats a meal, a whistle blows, and I know this is a signal for me to launch myself into the bloodstream. As I ride the currents of the blood, I rock gently back and forth and the sugar in the bloodstream jumps right in to be passengers. Blood sugar likes me. I think this is because I am green, but I might be wrong. When I am pretty full, but not full enough to swamp, I pass through the blood vessels, paddle through the sea of tissue fluid (boy, it smells salty) around the cells, pass through the cell membrane. Then I deposit the sugar by making these molecules jump out of the canoe and into the fluid inside the cell. I feel pretty important in my job. Without me, the blood sugar molecules would be unable to pass through the cell membranes. Because of this, I am given the official job title of hypoglycemic agent, because I lower the level of sugar in the blood. Excuse me, there goes the whistle!

Perhaps a physiologist would wince at this description. But it is nothing to be ashamed of if it helps you understand a concept. Plus, mental imagery can be fun!

Other Methods of Increasing Understanding

FORM A NEURAL TRACE. Positive mental attitude is a factor in allowing you to understand and remember. Remind yourself that all the basic courses in which you are now enrolled are essential. They are the building blocks for all the remaining courses you will take in the practical/vocational nursing program. You have already started your career. Most of the following techniques help increase understanding of your work by allowing neural traces to be recorded in your brain.

1. *As you listen or read, seek out key concepts, basic principles, and key ideas.* Be selective and learn to sift out and reject unnecessary details. You cannot memorize everything. If you could, you would not have an understanding of anything. The student who memorizes has difficulty in applying course information and solving problems in the clinical area. The activity of being selective helps you lay down neural traces. Emphasize accuracy, not speed. You want correct information to make a clear neural trace. It is difficult to unlearn wrong information and replace it with correct information.

2. *Short study periods followed by short rest periods are better than long study marathons.* This type of study will reenergize you and allow neural learning to continue during rest periods. Those seemingly wasted 10 minutes between classes or standing in the cafeteria line can be used to your advantage. It seems that cramming for examinations is treated like a rite of passage among students. Brain research has shown that short but frequent study periods help you to store information in long-term memory. This will make the information available for testing and later for application in the clinical area.

3. *Use as many body senses and as much body movement as possible when trying to learn new information.* Recite the information aloud

as you read, using your own words. If you can explain it, you must understand it and will know it. Hearing yourself say the information aloud is an additional channel that allows neural traces to be recorded. Write down the information in your own words. *Do not copy word by word from a book.* This muscle action will help you clarify ideas and improve thinking.

Vary your body position while studying. Lean against a wall. Sit on the floor. Pace. You will keep alert and awake. Using your muscles by gesturing can help improve memory of information by matching a gesture to information that needs to be remembered. When the gesture and word are associated in your mind, performing the gesture can retrieve the word. Physical motion can jog memory and promote recall. You should see some of the motions students go through during an examination! If it works, don't knock it.

These techniques of using body senses and body movement are all elements of tactual learning. They all help lay down the neural trace. Try them—they may work for you. Adopt the suggestions that help you understand the material in your classes. They will increase your long-term memory of that information.

Study Groups

Do you have a desire to achieve better grades? Do you need to study more efficiently? Do you need a little support? Joining a **study group** could be the strategy for you. Students usually form their own study groups out of need. Studies have shown that despite each person's preferred learning style, actively participating in a study group can improve academic performance. Notice we said *actively* participate. Sometimes students join a study group thinking that the group will help them pass, and they avoid active participation. Kind of like a freeloader. Study groups work when students use them to become actively involved in their own learning. The group provides an outlet for oral rehearsal of

material, which promotes retention. Active study group members usually develop questioning and reasoning skills on a higher level.

Tutoring

Tutoring is a very select study group. For best results, the student arranges tutoring through a special department by means of instructor referral or self-referral. The purpose of tutoring is to help a student understand the material better and pass the course. We guarantee one thing in tutoring. The person doing the tutoring will probably get an A. Students who need tutoring *sometimes* have learning disabilities. In these situations, because of an excellent attitude on the part of these students and their active participation in the tutoring process, tutoring can be beneficial. Students without learning disabilities who actively participate in the tutoring process also are successful in passing courses.

We are concerned about students at risk for failure who expect the tutor to "learn for them." These students do not actively participate in the tutoring process. We have also seen some privately arranged tutoring situations fail because the tutor felt that the student at risk needed to "be saved." Please note: Students cannot be saved. Nothing can replace active participation on the part of the learner. If you want to pass a course, you must become actively involved in your own learning. There are also students who need tutoring but say they do not have time for it. Comment on this response.

Memory Aids

Mnemonic devices are examples of memory aids. You know what they are. Some examples:

- *Rhymes*
  Thirty days hath September . . .
  I before *e* except after *c* . . .
  In fourteen hundred and ninety-two . . .
- *Acronyms*
  Every good boy does fine (to remember the line notes of the treble clef)

There are also devices in nursing that can help you remember information. For example,

- *CMTSP* (for assessment of the nerve and blood supply to an extremity)
  C = color
  M = motion
  T = temperature
  S = sensation
  P = pulse
- *PERL* (for assessment of the pupils)
  P = pupils
  E = equal
   and
  R = react
  L = to light

Memorizing these acronyms can help the practical/vocational nurse remember series of information. They do not take the place of understanding the information.

Reading

To think critically, you must have information. To acquire information you must be able to read with understanding. Because you are responsible for large amounts of reading in a practical/vocational nursing program, the ability to read with understanding (comprehension) is a necessary skill. Most of us are able to read the printed words on a page. But the reading demanded of a learner and future employee involves much more than this. Reading to learn and understand involves a rate of speed and a degree of understanding that are effective.

You probably had to take a reading test as part of your pre-entrance tests for the practical/vocational nursing program. Generally, these tests are brief. If you scored low, you were referred for help with this skill. Perhaps you are one of those who achieved an acceptable score on these short reading tests but could use some hints on how to increase your reading efficiency. Evaluate your reading habits by answering yes or no to the following questions.

1. Do you ever reread a sentence before you come to its end?
2. Do you ever have trouble figuring out the main point of an author?
3. Do you stop your reading every time you come across a word you cannot define and look up the word immediately?
4. Do you read novels, popular magazines, newspapers, and textbooks at the same speed?
5. Do you ever have trouble remembering what you read?
6. Do you ever have trouble understanding what you have read?
7. Do you ever think of other things while you read?
8. Do you ever read every word of a sentence individually?

If you answered yes to any of the above questions, you could benefit from some help with your reading efficiency. We suggest a visit to your school's study skill center for assistance with reading your textbooks with more organization and efficiency.

Hints to Increase Reading Efficiency

1. *Read in phrases, a few words at a time, rather than word by word.* Although the brain can view only one word at a time, it understands only when words are in phrases. For better understanding, you should read as you speak, in phrases.
2. *Move your lips while reading.* **Vocalization,** whether out loud or to yourself, is a tool used by the auditory learner to increase understanding. For some learners, reading aloud word by word can decrease speed and comprehension.
3. *Put expression into your reading.* You do not speak in a monotone, so why read that way? Musical learners can benefit by singing what they are reading. Try it. It may work for you.
4. *Be aware of your reading assignments that are technical or scientific in nature and vary*

your reading speed accordingly. The more recreational your reading material (novel, newspaper, and so on), the faster you can read. For more technical or scientific material, you must slow down. As you become accustomed to this type of reading, you will find yourself increasing your speed. Regardless of your learning style, when the going gets tough in a paragraph of assigned reading, reading the difficult material aloud may help clear up more challenging information.

5. *Underline unfamiliar words as you read.* When you are finished reading, copy the words on an index card and look them up in an appropriate dictionary. Most of the unfamiliar words you come across will be medical terms and can be found in your medical dictionary. At first you will think these words are Greek, and you are right. Quite a few of them are derived from the Greek language. The rest are derived from Latin.

Write the definition on the other side of the card. Break the word down with vertical slashes into its prefix (the word beginning), root (core word), and suffix (word ending), so that you can begin making associations with other words with the same prefix, root, or suffix. If your medical dictionary does not include this information with each word, the information can be found in medical terminology texts or as part of a computer program in your learning resource center.

Nursing involves learning a whole new language. If possible, include your own drawing to represent the definitions of these words with the verbal definition. This can help you recall the meaning of the word. Using index cards allows your language development to progress because you can take the cards with you wherever you go. Learning can occur whenever you have a few minutes to spare.

6. *Underline key phrases and write in the margin.* We assume you own your textbooks. Underlining will keep you active and result in the identification of key concepts for study and review.

Hints for Successful Test Taking

Focus on remaining an active learner in all your classes. Set a goal to *understand* the information you are learning with an eye to *application* of that learning. NCLEX-PN will be testing you at the level of understanding, application, and analysis, with very few straight knowledge questions. You can anticipate application and analysis–type questions on theory tests in the practical/vocational nursing program.

Test-taking skills are divided into two general areas: preparing for the test and actually taking the test. The following address these areas.

Preparation for the Test

1. Preparation for Test Taking Begins the First Day of Class

This includes (1) your system of notemaking for class and assignments and (2) your goal of understanding information as a preparation for tests and for clinical performance and their focus on application and analysis.

2. Clarify Content to Be Covered on the Test and the Form of the Test

Avoid asking *what* will be on the test. You already know what will be on the test. The instructor will be measuring your understanding and application of understanding of all the objectives that the test covers. Clarify the *types* of questions that will be asked on the tests. For example, will the test be multiple choice, short essays, and so on? Specific hints for taking multiple choice and short-answer tests are included in this chapter.

3. Periodically Review the Material You Have Already Studied

This is necessary to get the information into your long-term memory. Utilize the Test step of the PQRST method (see Chapter 7) frequently and the audible recitation suggested. Make index cards of the material you are having difficulty understanding. Cramming—last-minute studying of new material for a test—sometimes results in short-term memory of material that might help you pass a test. But since you did not engage in repetitions spaced over days, storage in long-term memory will not occur, and application of the material to the clinical area will be difficult. Cramming for an examination is like packing your suitcase for a vacation at the last minute. You will wind up with a suitcase filled with things you do not need and a whole list of things you forgot to bring.

4. Use Time-Management Techniques to Help You Organize Your Time Before the Test

Make a schedule to help identify study times to do a grand review for each test. Do not reread the textbook. Since you have studied the material periodically since the last test and used study-skill techniques, all you must do at this point is focus on your summaries, margin writings, underlinings, and index cards to check your understanding and retention of the information. The night before the test, do not be tempted to watch television or go to a movie. These activities will interfere with remembering. Instead, do your grand review as described above and get a good night's sleep.

Taking the Test

Arrive at the classroom in plenty of time to get your favorite seat and arrange your pencils and so on. Beware of peers who may try to get you nervous by saying "You didn't study *that,* did you?" or "You mean you didn't study *that?*" Keep a positive mental attitude. You organized your time and

systematically reviewed for this test after clarifying the content of the examination. Silently rehearse your facts to keep out distractions. Take slow deep breaths to reduce tension. It is almost test time and you are ready!

Would you believe that some people who have organized their notes and their time, systematically reviewed, and understood the material have nevertheless done poorly in tests? The main reason for this is that they probably did not follow the directions on the test. How well do you follow directions? Take out a blank sheet of paper and test yourself on the following directions.

 ## Learning Exercise: How Well Do You Follow Directions?

Directions: Read the following directions carefully. You will have one minute to do the exercise after reading the directions. Be sure to write legibly. When you have finished, check your answers against the directions before handing in the paper. *Be sure to read the entire exercise before beginning.*

1. On a sheet of paper, print your name in the upper left-hand corner, last name first.
2. Under your name, write your Social Security number.
3. In the upper right-hand corner, write the name and number of the course for which you are taking this exercise.
4. In the lower left-hand corner of the paper, write today's date.
5. In the lower right-hand corner, write your instructor's name, last name first.
6. Fold your paper in half lengthwise.
7. Number the left half of your paper 1 to 6, skipping three lines between each number.
8. Number the right half of your paper 7 to 12, skipping three lines between each number.
9. Now that you have read all the exercise, do only Number 1 of the exercise and hand your paper to the instructor.

How did you do? If you did not follow the directions, do you feel tricked? You were not. The directions were clear and you simply did not follow them. Listen meticulously to oral directions and read the written directions completely before each test. To those of you who did follow the directions for this exercise: keep up the good work! If directions are ever unclear, ask the instructor before proceeding. Clarify the time limit of the examination. Now you are ready to begin.

Quickly skim the entire examination to set up an overall picture of the types of questions on the test so you will be able to figure out the amount of time you can devote to each section. Then answer the questions you know well. This will boost your confidence level. Watch for absolutes such as always, never, all, and only. Avoid spending large amounts of time on difficult questions and do not get upset about them. Both these activities waste time and do not earn points. Go on to the next question and return to the skipped item later. However, be aware that on NCLEX-PN you will **not** be able to skip items and then go back to them. For NCLEX-PN, you need to answer each item as it comes up on the test.

Take the full time for the test. If you finish early, try to answer the questions you skipped. This brings up the point of guessing at answers. If you are not penalized for guessing, answer all the questions. But if the test will be graded by subtracting the number of wrong answers from the number of right, generally speaking, do not guess. Make sure you have not missed an item or group of items. Make sure your answers match up with the proper answer slot. The instructor cannot possibly know you put the answer to number 37 in the slot for number 36.

Should you change an answer? Although research has shown that test scores are generally improved by changing answers, we have seen many learners decrease their test scores by the same action. If you have given the item further thought and feel the item should be changed, change it. Test by test, keep tabs on your test scores to see whether changing answers is helping your final score and modify your behavior accordingly. If you are using a separate answer sheet that will be machine corrected, be sure you erase your first answer completely.

Chapter 3 discussed tests as a learning tool. When the examination is corrected and returned to you, do the following:

1. Read the items you missed. Why are they wrong? Did you make a careless mistake? Did you know the material? Can you correct the item without looking in your textbook or notes? If not, look up the answer.
2. Read the items you answered correctly. What did you do right to get credit for these items?
3. Decide which of your study skills and test-taking techniques are and are not working to your benefit. Modify your test-taking strategies accordingly.

Hints for Specific Tests

The types of tests you will be taking in the practical-vocational nursing program, including the NCLEX-PN, are achievement tests. They measure how much you have learned. Achievement tests are of two types: objective and subjective. Objective achievement tests include multiple-choice items. In objective achievement tests the answer is generally included in the test item. You must pick it out. The format of the NCLEX-PN is multiple-choice items that measure your understanding, application, and analysis of nursing knowledge. Subjective achievement tests include short-answer items. In subjective tests you must answer the item by formulating the answer. Samples of these two test forms are included here to help you understand them. Hints are provided for taking each type of test.

Multiple-Choice Items

Here are some hints for taking the short multiple-choice test that follows. Read over all the options given before making any decision. Eliminate the options you know are definitely wrong. When a number answer is involved, choose the number in the midrange. Remember the course subject matter for which you are being tested. Eliminate options that are not related to the subject matter.

Learning Exercise: Multiple Choice Statements

Choose the appropriate option for the following multiple-choice statements. There is only one answer to each multiple-choice statement.

1. Multiple-choice statements are examples of
   A. Sentences for which one-word answers are required.
   B. Incomplete statements with four options for answers.
   C. Two vertical columns that must be matched item by item.
   D. Statements that require a sentence to be written on the answer sheet.
2. When answering multiple-choice statements, it is not necessary to
   A. Read the directions.
   B. Match lists of items.
   C. Read each of the options.
   D. Watch out for negative words.

Answers to Multiple-Choice Statements

1B. A sentence or beginning of a sentence is given with four options. Usually only one option is correct. The rest of the options are distracters, that is, options that are there to test whether you really have learned the material and can apply it. Option A describes fill-in-the-blank items, option C describes matching tests, and option D describes short-answer terms.

2B. This multiple-choice statement contains a negative word in the stem that can complicate things. Read the stem without the negative word to get some meaning out of it and read the options. One option should not fit in with the others. Now reread the original

stem with the negative word and see whether the option you have already isolated fits in. Even though the test begins with directions, there may be additional directions before individual multiple-choice items. These directions may ask you to select one best answer or select what is most important of four correct answers. **Remember, do not stop reading when you think you have the correct answer.** There may be a better option yet to come. Incidentally, options A, C, and D are true.

Multiple-choice items are not "multiple-guess" questions. Think through each response thoroughly before choosing your answer. Should you ever guess? To be able to make a decision about guessing, you must know whether you will be penalized for wrong answers. Even if you are, figure out the odds. If you can eliminate one distracter for certain, you have a better chance of answering correctly. Can you eliminate two out of four distractors? Your chances are now even better. You make the decision. Remember, on the NCLEX-PN, you will have to answer every item as it comes.

Short-Answer Items

Learning Exercise: Short-Answer Items

1. Describe a short-answer item.
2. List five hints that the test taker should use in answering short-answer items to receive full credit for those items.

Answers to Short-Answer Items

1. In a short-answer item, you are given a simple command to carry out.
2. Five hints for answering short-answer items:

- Be sure to give the information that the statement asks for. Watch the verbs in these items, and do what they ask you to do.
- Give objective answers.
- Write in complete sentences.

- Concentrate on packing information into your answer.
- Think before you write.

Summary

☐ Learning how to learn is important because the theory and skills needed by the practical/vocational nurse can be understood and stored in long-term memory and used as the basis for critical thinking. When theory and skills are stored in long-term memory, they can be retrieved or recalled when needed. There is no easy way to learn information. Some techniques have been proved effective in increasing your level of concentration, improving your listening skills, and enhancing your ability to understand information. Perhaps your most important skill for success in the practical/vocational nursing program is your reading skill. Using the suggestions in this chapter, including hints for test taking, can help you succeed in the practical/vocational nursing program.

Review Questions

1. What is the most common explanation for lack of success in the practical/vocational program for students with college experience?
   A. College courses require a lot of memorizing.
   B. Because of the nature of college, college students have shown to be poor managers of their personal time.
   C. Party habits of college students do not allow them time to cram for an examination.
   D. A practical/vocational nursing program requires daily study and understanding of material so that theory can be applied to the clinical area.
2. Which most common explanation for forgetting information can help former college students find an intervention to help them be more successful on theory tests?
   A. They probably did not have the information in their long-term memory.
   B. They have a bad habit of mismanaging their study time.

C. They joined up with a study group and it made them feel intimidated.
   D. They did not apply themselves in college and need to learn how to be students.
3. Select the most common reason some practical/vocational students do not take advantage of study skills programs.
   A. Inability to afford the program.
   B. The attitude that they do not need it.
   C. Lack of time to devote to study skills.
   D. Past experience with study skills programs at the high school level.
4. Which of the following strategies will help you decide on the effectiveness of your study skills?
   A. Ask your instructors.
   B. Question your peers.
   C. Monitor your grades on tests.
   D. Compare your study habits with those of peers.
5. What is the most likely reason an instructor would refer a student with a failing grade to a counselor?

A. The student has a psychological problem.
B. The student has an emotional problem and needs counseling sessions.
C. Counselors at a technical/vocational school deal mainly with academic counseling.

D. Upon receiving a referral, technical/vocational school counselors are trained to counsel referred students to withdraw from the program in which they are enrolled.

Bibliography

Alfaro-LeFevre R. *Critical Thinking in Nursing: A Practical Approach,* 2nd ed. Philadelphia: W. B. Saunders, 1999.

Buzan T. *Use Both Sides of Your Brain.* New York: New American Library–Dutton, 1991.

Eison J. Challenging student passivity. *Advocate.* Washington, DC: NEA, 1(4); 5–7, 1999.

Hancock O. *Reading Skills for College Students.* Englewood Cliffs, NJ: Prentice-Hall, 1997.

Jensen E. B's and A's in 30 days: Strategies for better grades in college. Barron's Magazine, 1997.

Jensen E. *Teaching with the Brain in Mind.* Alexandria, VA: Association for Supervision and Curriculum Development, 1998.

Kay G. How to help students develop better notetaking skills. Teaching for Success 7(3):8, 1995.

Meltzer M, Palau S. *Learning Strategies in Nursing: Reading, Studying, and Test Taking.* Philadelphia: W. B. Saunders, 1997.

Pauk W. *How to Study in College,* 6th ed. Boston: Houghton-Mifflin, 1997.

Schacter D. How to remember what you cannot afford to forget. Bottom Line 19(16):1–2, August 15, 1998. Greenwich, CT: Boardroom, Inc.

Weil A. Ten steps to better memory. Self Healing, pp. 1, 6–7, January, 1999.

Chapter 7

Hints for Using Learning Resources

Outline

Textbooks
    The PQRST Method of Textbook
        Study
Professional Journals
    Articles
Magazines and Newspapers
Classroom Learning Strategies
    Lectures
    Lecture-Discussions
    Cooperative Learning
    Distance Learning

Other Learning Resources
    Syllabus and Course Outlines
    Nursing Skills Lab
    Study Skills Lab
    Audiovisual Materials
    The Internet
    Computer-Aided Instruction
Learning Resource Center
    Resources of the Library
    Locating Your Material

Staying Current in Practical/Vocational
    Nursing
    Periodicals
    Nursing Organizations
    Community Resources
    Guest Speakers

Key Terms

audiovisual (AV) materials
bucket theory
call number
CD-ROM
community resources
computer-aided instruction
computer simulation
cooperative learning
copyright laws
course outlines
database

discussion buddy
distance learning
guest speakers
interlibrary loan services
Internet
learning resource center
lecture-discussion strategy
librarian
microfiche
microfilm
nursing organizations

nursing skills lab
online catalog
periodical indexes
periodicals
PQRST method
reference materials
stacks
study skills lab
syllabus

Objectives

Upon completing this chapter you will be able to:

1. Describe each step in the PQRST method of textbook study.
2. Discuss the value of reading assigned periodicals.
3. Locate an article related to nursing by using:
   a. Cumulative Index to Nursing and Allied Health Literature
   b. one CD-ROM database (if available)
4. Discuss six hints used to gain full value from lectures.
5. Discuss your responsibilities for each of the following course learning strategies:
   a. mini lecture-discussion
   b. cooperative learning
   c. distance learning
6. Discuss the value of these learning resources to your personal learning:
   a. syllabus or course outline
   b. nursing skills lab
   c. study skills lab
   d. audiovisual materials
   e. the Internet
   f. computer-assisted instruction (CAI) and computer simulations
   g. learning resource center (LRC)
7. Describe how the following resources help you stay current in practical/vocational nursing:
   a. Internet
   b. periodical indexes
   c. CD-ROMs
   d. nursing organizations
   e. community resources
   f. guest speakers

There are three basic methods of obtaining theoretical information to prepare yourself to become a practical/vocational nurse: textbooks, professional journals, and course learning strategies. The purpose of this chapter is to provide suggestions to help you get full mileage out of these methods. In addition, other learning resources used by schools of practical/vocational nursing are discussed—also, how to stay up-to-date. Even if you have past experience in an educational program of study, you will find the information in this chapter helpful. The information will help you adjust to and succeed in the practical/vocational nursing program with less stress and frustration.

Textbooks

"I read the material four times and got a D. My friend read the material once and got an A. It isn't fair." The learner speaking is correct. It takes a lot of time to read material four times for a test. The missing ingredient is lack of understanding of information that is read. To think critically in nursing, you must have information. To acquire information, you must be able to read with understanding. Earning only a D is a poor return on your time investment.

The experts in study skills have come up with a variety of study systems for using textbooks and related reading materials. These systems are basically the same in that they present a method of reading that will increase comprehension by ensuring that the information is stored in long-term memory. We have chosen the **PQRST method** as described by Staton (1959) in *How to Study,* which was published in 1959 and is still available today. It is the method *we* used in nursing school, but do not ask which edition we used. Believe us, this method has stood the test of time.

The PQRST Method of Textbook Study

Each letter stands for a step in the study method. *Regardless of the length of time available for studying, studies have shown that learners who use each step of this method consistently scored higher on tests.* But each of the five steps in the method must be used. Learners have reported that the system is easier to use than they thought it would be. Each of the five steps will be discussed by identifying the meaning and benefits of each step and then describing how to carry it out and why it works.

P = Preview

WHAT IT MEANS. Preview is an overview or survey of what the material is all about. It gives you the general big picture of what the author wants to accomplish, not the fine details.

BENEFITS. Previewing helps you look for and recognize important points or main ideas of the reading material.

WHY IT WORKS. The Preview step makes you reflect or think about the material. It also increases your concentration level. These are important elements in the storage of information in long-term memory.

HOW TO DO IT

1. When you first buy your textbooks, look at the table of contents. This will give you a general sense of the organization of the book.
2. Read the Preface to find out the author's purpose for writing the book, the organization of the material, and suggestions for reading the book.
3. Preview the method of the author of each of your textbooks. Before reading each assignment,

   - Read each of the topics and headings.
   - Read the summary.
   - Read the first and last sentences of each paragraph.
   - Using the general hints listed for reading, read the assignment.

Q = Question

WHAT IT MEANS. As you preview the reading material, ask yourself **questions** that may be answered when you read.

BENEFITS. Formulating your own questions as well as using the author's questions will give you pointers about what details to look for in your reading. These questions will help you prepare for examinations.

WHY IT WORKS. By providing you with clues, this step points out what to look for in your reading. The Question step will also make you reflect on your reading and increase your concentration level.

HOW TO DO IT. Look at the chapter title and each heading. Turn them into questions. Some authors include questions at the end of a chapter. If so, read these before going on to the next step. Most authors include learning objectives at the beginning of each chapter. Use these to keep your mind inquisitive and to seek ends to these objectives.

R = Read

WHAT IT MEANS. In this stage you actually read the material. You are now gathering information to be stored. Look carefully at pictures and charts. They may contain new information or clarify what you have read.

BENEFITS. You will accumulate information and facts and be able to store them in long-term memory.

WHY IT WORKS. Being an active reader by seeking answers to the questions you have formulated will keep up your level of concentration. This allows you to store information in your brain.

HOW TO DO IT. Review the general hints under Reading in Chapter 6. Practice them so you can remain active during this step. You are seeking the answers to the questions you formulated. Remember to underline key phrases and to write notes in the margin.

S = State

WHAT IT MEANS. To state means to repeat in your own words what you have read.

BENEFITS. You will understand the organization of the material you are reading and the relationship of the facts to each other. By increasing understanding, you will be able to apply the information in the clinical area. *Rote memory fails when it comes time to apply information.* Stating will help you evaluate whether you did indeed store the information.

WHY IT WORKS. Stating something out loud involves another sense (hearing). This provides an additional channel for information to be stored. Stating facts in your own words indicates knowledge and understanding of the material.

HOW TO DO IT. At the end of each paragraph, look away from your book. Ask yourself the main ideas that were covered in the paragraph. State the ideas out loud and in your own words. This is the key to the success of this step. As you become more proficient in this step, you will find that you are able to read more than one paragraph and still state the main ideas and the answers to the questions you have formulated. Look at your marginal notes. Try to elaborate on them.

T = Test

WHAT IT MEANS. This final step occurs some time after your first study session and involves testing yourself on what you remember.

BENEFITS. Because the testing step is ongoing, it will indicate your weak areas. This gives you time to remedy them before an examination. Better grades are sure to follow.

WHY IT WORKS. This stage settles once and for all whether the information is in your long-term memory. It also indicates your comprehension of the material. When you identify your weak spots, you can review them and make sure they are retained in your long-term memory. You will be covering the information in small doses but more frequently. This activity is the best way to encourage the brain to remember.

HOW TO DO IT. This testing stage is really a review stage. Review your marginal notes. Restate the main ideas presented in the chapter. Review your class notes. Relate them to the information in the textbook. Write down the information you are having trouble with on index cards to be carried with you so you can test yourself while on the run.

To be effective, we suggest that about half of your study time be devoted to the Preview and Read steps. The other half should be devoted to Question, State, and Test. These steps require critical thinking (reflective thinking), use of your memory, and organization of ideas through your own efforts. The strength of this system lies in the State step. The reflective thinking required in this step takes work. Resist the temptation to skip over State.

An important part of any textbook is the index found in the back of the book. The subject index includes a list of topics that can be found in alphabetical order. Page numbers are included for information discussed. This index will help you locate information quickly.

Professional Journals

Practical/vocational nurses need to be aware of sources that will provide up-to-date information on nursing topics. Professional journal articles give you the opportunity to stay on top of the latest research in nursing and its application. In addition to articles that are assigned reading, practical/vocational nurses need to find and use articles that pertain to selected nursing topics and nursing problems in the clinical area. Student practical/vocational nurses need to be self-directed in looking up articles that apply to their current learning needs. Professional journals of interest to practical/vocational nurses include but are not limited to the following: *The Journal of Practical Nursing; Practical Nursing Today; RN; Nursing; and The American Journal of Nursing.*

 Learning Exercise: Nursing Journals

Identify these nursing journals in the learning resource center. Determine which of them help you keep up-to-date in nursing.

Articles

Learners are all looking for the perfect textbook, the one that is complete and self-contained. But it does not exist! Specific journal articles may be assigned to give you up-to-date information to supplement the readings in your textbooks. Use the PQRST method and hints for reading textbooks to read these articles.

Copyright laws prohibit the instructor from copying an article for each of you. For this reason, the required reading articles are available on a reserve basis in the learning resource center (library). You can make notes from these articles. Because copyright laws allow you to have one copy of an article, photocopy the article for your own use. Underline, highlight, and write in its margins. Remember, the instructor knows you are busy. Articles are not busy work but are a necessary part of any career education to keep current in your discipline.

Magazines and Newspapers

Include newspapers and popular magazines as sources of information on health-related topics. Magazine articles never replace professional journal reading, but they do provide information that your clients read. As one practical/vocational nursing student said, "I had better be up-to-date and understand what my clients are reading." Be aware of the author's expertise. This will help you evaluate the accuracy of the information on the topic.

 Learning Exercise: Popular Reading

List two newspapers or popular magazines that you read.

_____

_____

_____

Classroom Learning Strategies

Lectures

Some of your teachers may have been taught using the **"bucket theory"** of education. The bucket theory suggests that merely by lecturing, a teacher can transfer knowledge from the teacher's mind to the mind of the student. This teaching method evolved from the time of Aristotle. The teacher was considered the source and the vehicle of transmission of information. Kind of like a sage on the stage. Of course, the printing press had yet to be invented! Although traditional lecturing is an outmoded form of instruction, *brief lectures* (minilectures) can be valuable as a means of enhancing your assigned readings. However, they are passive learning experiences that do not actively involve you in the learning process.

Research has shown that students learn best from methods other than lecture. A minilecture situation needs to be a brief episode, taking no more than 30% of class time. Minilectures need to enhance your reading assignment, not replace it. A minilecture needs to reflect the fact that the teacher spent time searching, reading, selecting, and organizing information for your benefit. The instructor has done all the work and has become smarter in the process. You need to remain especially alert and actively involved during the minilecture to be able to benefit from this method of teaching.

The instructor may introduce various techniques to keep you actively involved during the minilectures.

1. You may be assigned to a **discussion buddy** before the class starts.
2. The two of you will be given a discussion task.
3. Focus carefully on the minilecture so you will be able to formulate an answer to the discussion task.
4. After the minilecture, discussion buddies share their answers with each other. A new answer is formulated from both your re-

sponses. The instructor will choose students at random to share their newly composed answers with the class.

What goes on in the classroom is just as important as what goes on in a reading assignment. There is, however, one great difference between the two. *You can repeat a reading assignment but you can never repeat a missed class.* Here are some hints to help you learn from a minilecture or any class situation.

1. *Never skip a class unless you are faced with an emergency.* Some students skip class to get another hour's sleep, use the time to prepare for another class or an examination, or get in their legal number of cuts. When an emergency does make it necessary for you to miss class, photocopying notes is not the answer to catch up on what you missed. Ask a peer to go over his or her notes and tell you about the class. Recall what you learned in Chapter 5 about personal learning styles.

2. *Come to class prepared.* By having the assignment completed, key terms and concepts will be familiar to you. You will be ready to participate in learning activities. You will save yourself embarrassment by avoiding questions that are answered easily by the readings. Come to class in time to get a seat close to the instructor and the blackboard. Heading for the last row is heading for distractions and lower grades. Have a pen and papers pertaining to the assignment ready to go.

3. *Listen for verbal cues that will inform you of key points during minilectures.* Some examples can be found in Table 7–1. Keep vigilant for nonverbal cues given by the instructor that will also inform you of key ideas. Examples are raising the hands, a long dramatic pause, raising or lowering the voice, and leaning toward the class. Be sure to copy everything that is written on the blackboard.

4. *The instructor speaks at a much slower rate than you are capable of thinking.* The fact that you can think faster than the instructor

TABLE 7–1 : Verbal Cues for Key Ideas in Minilectures and Discussion Activities
"The most important difference is . . ."
"The major principle in this situation is . . ."
"To sum up . . ."
"The main point is . . ."
"Finally . . ."
"In conclusion . . ."
"Moreover . . ."
"To repeat . . ."

can speak allows you to relate this new information to information you have learned in the past and formulate questions when you do not understand. Ask these questions in class or seek out the instructor after class. It is your responsibility to question what you do not understand.

5. *Look over your notes as soon after class as possible.* Use the hints given in Chapter 5 about personal learning styles. It is essential that you follow these techniques to place the information you learned in class into your long-term memory.

6. *Be present while in class.* Avoid using class time to work on other projects.

Lecture–Discussions

In the **lecture-discussion strategy,** the instructor shares several ideas with the class and then stops so that the class can discuss the ideas. Sometimes the instructor may say that the next class will be nothing but discussion of the assignment. The instructor then acts as a discussion leader. The instructor has developed several learning strategies to help keep your discussion focused on course objectives. Here are some hints for participating in discussions and related activities.

1. Be prepared to participate in the discussion by completing your assignment. This will allow you to be an active participant.
2. Be sure to have made a list of questions about the assignment. Discussions are the perfect time to clear up questions.
3. While other learners are speaking, listen to what they have to say. Some learners make the mistake of using other learners' speaking time to formulate their own comments.
4. You may disagree with others during a discussion. Do so assertively and firmly. Avoid yelling matches at all costs. It enriches your world to listen to another's point of view before responding.

Cooperative Learning

Cooperative learning is a technique that emphasizes individual accountability for learning a specific academic task while working in small groups. Cooperative learning encourages you to (1) be actively involved in your learning, (2) develop critical thinking skills, and (3) develop positive relationships with your peers. Besides helping you learn the course content, cooperative learning will help you encourage traits you will need in your future job. Cooperative learning encourages the development of teamwork. The ability to work in a team situation is what an employer is looking for in an employee. Use the suggestions listed under Lecture-Discussions to help you get full mileage out of this learning strategy.

Distance Learning

Perhaps some of the courses in your practical/vocational nursing program or parts of courses are available through **distance learning.** In this learning strategy, the student and teacher are separated by physical distance. The course could take part in "real time" in which all students in the course and the instructor participate simultaneously by means of interactive TV. A popular alternative is the type of instruction in which students can choose when and where they will attend class. This type of distance learning is carried out, for example, by videotapes, audiotapes, and World Wide Web based courses. The following hints will help you succeed in this type of distance learning.

1. Be sure you have the equipment needed *or access to* equipment needed to complete course assignments. Depending on the distance learning course, the equipment list could include any of the following:

   ■ word processor
   ■ fax machine
   ■ computer with adequate hard disk space
   ■ modem for e-mail
   ■ cable TV hook-up
   ■ VCR
   ■ telephone line

2. Time management skills, self-discipline, and motivation are important tools for success. The information in the chapter on time management (Chapter 4) will help you establish a weekly class and study schedule and stick to it. The nature of the course will not allow reminders from instructor and fellow students.
3. Good reading and study skills are a must. Chapter 6, Learning How to Learn and Retain Information, emphasizes the need for the proper study skills, including study environment. Since distance learning courses require much reading, this chapter and its stress on the PQRST method of study will be beneficial.
4. Since distance learning requires you to communicate by methods such as videotape, writing, e-mail, fax, etc., the contents of Chapter 8, Straightforward Communication Skills, will help you organize your thoughts so that you can present them in a concise manner and communicate your intended message.

Distance learning has proved to be at least as effective as traditional methods of instruction. Positive features include the fact that students become more active in personal learning and have more involvement in and control over the learning process.

Other Learning Resources

Syllabus and Course Outlines

A **syllabus** is an up-to-date course document given to you at the beginning of a course. It includes, at a minimum, a course description, course objectives, course requirements for a passing grade, required textbooks, grading scale, instructor information (office location, office phone number, office hours), course policies, and testing policies.

Some schools of practical/vocational nursing also use **course outlines** for each course. These outlines are a great help to an adult learner. They contain unit-by-unit course objectives and content areas, which indicate what the learner must know. Each objective begins with a verb. Watch the verb carefully. The verb tells you the level of understanding you must achieve to meet the objective. If an objective states you must *list* something, that task is quite different from having to *compare* and *contrast* the same information. Instructors develop their test questions from the course objectives and course content. The course outline will include a list of resources indicating where the information to answer the objectives is found. Supplementary material in the form of worksheets, charts, activities, and additional reading may be included to round out your learning.

Nursing Skills Lab

The **nursing skills lab** is a resource that will allow you to practice and develop your physical nursing skills. It is to be used throughout your program of study. This lab contains the physical items needed to make the practice area as similar to the workplace as possible. *Skills must be practiced.* Reading about them, watching a film, and watching other students practice are only the first steps in developing a physical skill. Practice until you are proficient in each skill, so that you will feel comfortable performing these tasks in the clinical area. Remember that you recall 10% of what you hear, 20% of what you see, 50% of what you read, and

90% of what you do, so *do* all you can. The Teton Lakota Indians have a proverb that summarizes how practical/vocational student nurses need to approach the skills component of their nursing program. "Tell me and I'll listen. Show me and I'll understand. Involve me and I'll learn."

You will be required to make appointments to give a return demonstration of skills. This routine will give you an opportunity to organize your time. This is what is expected of the practical/vocational nurse as part of client care. When you make an appointment with the skills lab, you are entering into an agreement with the lab personnel. Your responsibility is to practice the skill until you can perform it in the time frame of your appointment. If you are unable to keep your appointment, inform the lab personnel. This will allow them to schedule other students into lab time for skills testing.

Study Skills Lab

The **study skills lab** is available to help you with academic problem areas. Examples of areas in which help is available are study skills, time management, reading (including vocabulary and comprehension), listening skills, math skills, test-taking skills (especially situation tests), notemaking, writing, and any other academic problem you may have. You can go to the skills lab on your own or by referral of your instructor or the counselor.

 Critical Thinking Exercise

Some students who need the study skills center state they do not have time to go for help. Comment about this response.

Audiovisual Materials

In addition to lectures, discussion/activities, textbooks, and articles, the instructor may have included films and videotapes as part of your assignment. **Audiovisual (AV) materials** are not considered extra or additional assignments. They are a significant part of all areas of learning. These learning resources give faith to the saying, "One picture is worth a thousand words." AV materials provide an additional sensory channel for learning, compared with reading. In some nursing courses, especially autotutorial skills courses, the AV medium *is* the course. The student progresses independently, attending periodic lecture-discussion classes and seeking out the instructor when questions arise. Approach the AV material as you do a class. Realize that you have the option of repeating all or part of the presentation when you do not understand it. Remember, television, especially the cable network, can be a source of information for topics related to your coursework.

The Internet

The **Internet** offers an unlimited amount of information about any subject desired. The Internet is the physical infrastructure that allows the electronic circulation of vast amounts of information to computer users who have a connection to the Internet. A provider service charges a monthly fee and is a computer user's link to the Internet. When people are linked to the Internet, they are said to be online. An example of a provider service is America On Line. The World Wide Web (www) is the most effective means of providing access to the vast amount of information available on the Internet. Everything on the Internet has an address (called a URL) which helps in locating a specific site. All addresses begin with http://www followed by a dot. The next letters are specific to the site you are accessing, for example, nordstrum followed by a dot. This is followed by three letters denoting the site's type.

    com = commercial
    gov = federal government
    edu = education
    org = organization

Search engines and Web directories can help students zero in on the exact information they are looking for. Search engines periodically scan the web and index it. Therefore, search engines are like book indexes. Search engines are most effective in finding information when your subject is narrow, for example, Practical/vocational nursing. Examples of search engines are AltaVista and HotBot. Web directories are like tables of content and provide general categories of information. Web directories are most helpful when the information you are seeking is broad, for example, nursing. An example of a Web directory is Yahoo. Appendix F contains some suggestions of Internet sites that can be used by practical/vocational nursing students as learning resources, for client teaching resources, and just for fun.

Some guidelines for gathering Internet information follow:

1. The Internet is not regulated in any way. Everyone can publish anything they want to on the Internet. When searching the Internet, you can find the most recent and accurate information as well as the most inaccurate and out-of-date.
2. Let the user beware—people can spend a lot of time on the Internet. To save time, take a few minutes to read the section that gives hints for using the site. Stay focused on your purpose. Avoid getting sidetracked.
3. Check the professional credentials and qualifications of the author of the information.
4. Determine the organization, group, agency, company, and so on who created the site. This will help you evaluate the credibility of the information.
5. Check the date the information was created and last modified. This will ensure up-to-date material.
6. What are the objectives of the author of the material? Does the author express opinions? Does the author have a personal bias?
7. When conducting searches, supplying keywords helps the search tool narrow the documents you call up to the ones you really want to see. When using keywords for a search engine, use phrases or single words that are

pertinent to your topic and describe it objectively. Use nouns only and put the most important words that describe your topic first.

Computer-Aided Instruction

No segment of society has been left untouched by the computer. **Computer-aided instruction** (CAI) is an increasingly used teaching strategy in nursing education. It has the following benefits:

- It allows learners to be actively involved in their own learning.
- It encourages problem solving, a skill employers expect in practical/vocational nurses.
- It provides immediate feedback by quickly evaluating answers and decision-making strategies.
- It provides an opportunity to develop the ability to follow directions.

Learning by CAI is enhanced for students with right brain dominance. CAI can also be used effectively by any student to master new material. It simplifies concepts and reinforces skills that have been presented previously. If CAI is used in your practical/vocational nursing program, you will be taught the skills necessary to use the computer. The process is simple even if you do not have any computer experience. Many of you will also be using the computer in the clinical area to store and retrieve client information. And in less than one year, all of you will be taking the NCLEX-PN examination by computer.

Computer Simulation

Computer simulation is a learning activity that makes use of an imaginary client situation. The student is required to gather data, set priorities, plan, and evaluate care as in an actual clinical situation. The computer client simulation continually changes, as it would in the clinical area. This requires the student to evaluate the situation and plan new nursing interventions. Computer simulations may be used when the client census is inadequate for client assignments, when a desired client situation is unavailable, or when enhanced learning of specific concepts is desirable. A review of the available software reveals that few computer simulations are intended specifically for practical/vocational nursing students. Your instructors can suggest modifications of existing simulations for your use.

Learning Resource Center

If you are over 30 years of age, you know this resource as the library. Its name, often abbreviated LRC, merely reflects the increased scope of the library as we begin the twenty-first century. It consists of a lot more than books. How do you feel when you find out you must use the **learning resource center?** If you have some negative feelings, perhaps it is because you are unfamiliar with the sources of information contained in this resource, their location, and how to use them.

If you investigate your Learning Resource Center you will find that it contains a wealth of services that will help make your time in the practical/vocational nursing program much easier. Ask the librarian for a tour. Some Learning Resource Centers have self-guided tours on audiotape. An hour spent touring can save you many wasted hours and much frustration later in the school year. Ask for an informational brochure so that you have an idea of the Learning Resource Center's general hours of operation and its physical layout. Identify the special study areas available to you and groups of learners. Because the Learning Resource Center is a learning area, you need to keep it a quiet environment.

Resources of the Library

Librarian

This is perhaps the best resource in the whole school. The **librarian** is a college-educated specialist in what the library has to offer in the area of information and where that information can be found. Look at the librarian as a professional educator about information for learning and as a person who is always ready to assist you. When you do go for assistance, be sure to watch the process the librarian uses to obtain the information you need. Next time, you will be able to help yourself.

Interlibrary Loan Services

Interlibrary loan services allow your LRC to borrow materials you need that are not in your library's holdings. Books and audiovisual materials are available through this service. If your LRC does not have the periodical in which an article you need is located, a photocopy of the article, free of charge, can be obtained from a library that does have the periodical. Allow about one week to receive articles obtained in this manner.

Vertical File (Pamphlet File)

The *vertical file* contains pamphlets of various subjects arranged in alphabetical order by topic.

Circulation Desk

The *circulation desk* is the area where library materials are checked out and returned. Materials reserved by your instructor will probably be found here and can be checked out for short periods, along with audiovisual equipment to use with the material, if needed.

Online Catalog

You can obtain a lot of information in an LRC by yourself once you understand the cataloging system. Most LRCs have converted their card catalogs to an **online** (computerized) **catalog.** All books found in your LRC, but not magazines and newspapers, are indexed in this computerized system. Cataloged materials also include audiotapes and videotapes.

You can search for desired materials by subject, title, or author. Sometimes you know an author's name but not the title of the material you need. Select "author" on the initial computer screen. Type in the author's last name and first name. All the materials in the LRC by that author will appear on the screen with their call numbers (location in the LRC). If you know the title but not the author, information will appear on where to locate the material.

Sometimes you are investigating a topic but have no information about authors or titles of material on that topic. Type one or two words describing the topic you are investigating. Authors and titles relating to that topic will be displayed on the screen. Some systems will indicate whether the material is on the shelf or checked out. If the LRC does not have the material you are searching for but another LRC on the system does, this information might also be included.

At a moment's notice, students can determine the availability of a source miles away. In some systems, students are able to access the online catalog from home via computer. This system of cataloging can save students valuable time and energy.

Directions and brochures for how to use the online catalog are located next to the computer terminals. It is impossible to give you a step-by-step guide to using the online catalog because different LRCs use different computer systems to organize this information. However, a few hints might help you keep body and soul together at the computer terminal.

1. Read the directions on the screen, top to bottom.
2. Locate the keys with arrows up ↑, down ↓, left side ←, and right side →. Up and down arrows move the blinking cursor up a line or down a line. These arrows can also be used to scroll through lists quickly (the information appears on the screen and rolls by). The side-to-side arrows can move the blinking cursor left or right.
3. When you press the enter ↵ key, do so firmly

but do not hold it down. Press it and remove your finger quickly.

4. If your system tells you to press a letter and a number (for example, F1), look for keys that have the letter and the number on one key. These are located at the top of the keyboard. Do not type an F and then a separate 1.
5. If you are unsuccessful in finding information, ask an LRC staff member.
6. YOU WILL NOT CAUSE THE SYSTEM TO BREAK DOWN.

Locating Your Material

Now to locate your material in the LRC. Libraries may choose to use either of two systems to classify materials so they are easy to locate: (1) the Dewey decimal system, and (2) the Library of Congress classification system. Regardless of the system your library uses, the **call number** shown on the author, title, or subject screens is the same number as that on the material itself. Get in the habit of copying, in order, *all* the letters and numbers in the call number.

The Stacks

Armed with the call number, you can proceed to the **stacks**—the place where the majority of materials that can be checked out is located. When you do find the material you are looking for, note that materials covering the same subject are shelved in the same area. You might find additional useful material on the same shelf.

Reference Material

Reference materials include dictionaries, including medical and nursing dictionaries, encyclopedias, almanacs, yearbooks, atlases, handbooks, and other similar categories of books. You will find up-to-date information on any subject in this area. Reference material generally does not circulate. It cannot be checked out. Some libraries allow certain reference books to circulate for brief periods. Information from reference materials may be copied on a copy machine.

Staying Current in Practical/Vocational Nursing

Periodicals

Because magazines are published weekly, monthly, and quarterly, that is, periodically, they are often called **periodicals.** They are also referred to as journals—publications that contain news or material of current interest to a particular discipline. Professional journals contain articles that include the most recent information available on a specific subject and subjects that are too new to be included in books. This is the reason periodicals are important resources for a learner in a field changing as quickly as nursing and health care. The titles and authors of various articles cannot possibly be included in the online catalog. These can be found instead in two sources: bound books called periodical indexes and CD-ROM databases.

Periodical Indexes

Entries in **periodical indexes** are listed by author, title, and subject. Two periodical indexes are of special value to practical/vocational nursing students.

1. *Reader's Guide to Periodical Literature.* This comprehensive index to more than 160 popular American nontechnical magazines includes articles published between the dates printed on its cover. This guide is useful for recreational reading on specific topics, such as setting up a workshop, decorating with stenciling, and learning about the Internet. The *Reader's Guide,* or green book, is valuable for practical/vocational nursing students because technical data on health topics are presented in understandable language for the general public.

2. *Cumulative Index to Nursing and Allied Health Literature* (CINAHL). This comprehensive and authoritative periodical index contains current listings for nursing and allied health fields and for others interested in health care issues, including biomedicine, consumer health, and alternative medicine. Nearly 1200 nursing, allied health, and related journals are reviewed, indexed, and included in five bi-monthly issues and cumulative (arranged by year) bound volumes of past issues. Figure 7–1 illustrates the information found in a typical entry in the CINAHL.

Near the indexes is found a **periodical listing.** The listing includes the professional journals and magazines and the dates of the issues that are found in your library. If the article you need is in a journal or magazine that is not held in your library, see the librarian. The librarian will track down the article in another library and arrange for you to receive a photocopy by interlibrary loan. If your library has the date and issue you need, go to the section of the library that contains the periodicals. If the issue you need is not there, it may be on *microform.* To conserve space, back issues of magazines are microphotographically produced. Two commonly used microforms are **microfilm** and **microfiche** (mī-crō-fēesh).

1. Microfilm. Using microfilm, a whole year's issues of magazines can be reproduced on 16-mm or 35-mm film that threads on a wheel about 3 inches in diameter with room to spare.

2. Microfiche. Microfiche involves a 4 × 6-inch film card that carries reduced images placed on the card in rows. One microfiche can contain up to 98 pages of text.

Both these microforms must be read with a device that enlarges the very small image. Many libraries have reader-printers that will print the image seen on the screen on a sheet of paper you can take with you. See the librarian for help with microforms.

CD-ROM

Public and school libraries have these valuable sources of information. The audio CDs you use at home play music. The **CD-ROM** in the library plays "information." This information, via disk, may already be loaded into the computer so you do not have to insert a disk. CD-ROM systems differ in the subjects and the level of coverage they offer.

The CINAHL CD-ROM **database** is valuable to practical/vocational nursing students. This is the *Cumulative Guide to Nursing and Allied Health Literature* discussed under Periodical Indexes but in CD-ROM form and with some additional informa-

---

1–HYPERTENSION
  2- Managing hypertension **3-** (Woods AD) **4-** (tables/charts)
    5- Nursing 6- 1999 Mar; **7-** 29(3): **8-** 7–12 **9-** (4 ref)

Key: 1. Subject. 2. Title of the article. 3. Author of the article. 4. Additional information found in article. 5. Periodical in which the article appears. If the periodical is abbreviated, the periodical index in the front of the book will have a list of periodical abbreviations and the full name of the journal for which those abbreviations stand. 6. Date of publication. 7. Volume and number of periodical. 8. Pages of the article. 9. This article has a bibliography with four references.

FIGURE 7–1. An entry from the *Cumulative Index to Nursing and Allied Health Literature.*

tion. The library receives monthly updates of information from all vendors. Summaries of important points in the texts of articles are presented and can be printed out for student use. CINAHL CD-ROM includes access to information from selected journals on AIDS, cancer, diseases, healthcare, nursing, occupational therapy, physical therapy, public health, and rehabilitation. For an additional fee from the institution, CINAHL is also available as an on-line service.

Because of computer technology, the process of "keeping up-to-date" has been simplified as far as finding information is concerned. All you need is time! CD-ROM databases are expensive sources of information. If your LRC has this technology available for student use, be sure to use it. The systems are user friendly. Combined with a helpful LRC staff, you cannot lose! Here are some hints when using these systems.

1. Read the directions that appear on the screen and are posted around the terminal.
2. When doing subject searches, be sure to narrow the topic. Provide the computer with key words so it can make a search that fills your needs.
3. Review suggestions for accessing the online catalog.
4. Avoid confusing the online catalog terminals (holdings of the library) with the CD-ROM database terminals (contains summaries and full text of articles, newspaper stories, and so on).

Helpful Miscellaneous CD-ROMs

CD-ROMs are also a source of textbook-type information for practical/vocational nursing students. Check your LRC to see whether any encyclopedias are available on CD-ROM. Some textbooks, including drug books, come with CD-ROMs. Some texts have a separate CD-ROM edition. Some of these resources provide audio pronunciation of terms and generally enhance learning. Some provide a testbank of questions to allow you to test your learning.

Merriam-Webster's Medical Dictionary, Deluxe Audio Edition

This CD-ROM includes more than 57,000 entries of medical terms. An audio component allows students to hear the pronunciation of medical terms.

Pronunciation Tutor on CD-ROM (Medsite Publishing)

This CD-ROM requires a computer with a sound card. Students can hear the pronunciation of more than 30,000 medical terms.

Encyclopedia of Nursing Skills CD-ROM: Set 1 (Concept Media)

This CD-ROM presents demonstrations of drug administration techniques and vital signs that can be used as a review by students as well as practicing nurses. The text of entire procedures or a specific step can be printed out.

 ### Learning Exercise: Locating Useful CD-ROMs

Locate specific CD-ROMs in your Learning Resource Center that would be (1) useful resources for keeping current in practical/vocational nursing and (2) would supplement textbooks and reference books.

 ### Learning Exercise: Using CD-ROM Databases

Identify one nursing problem or topic area to research on a CD-ROM database. Print out one article or newspaper story about this problem or topic.

Suggestions: Write an objective sentence describing the problem or topic. Then pick key words from the sentence and type these for the subject search.

Example: You have been assigned to do a report for Personal Vocational Issues class. You need information about health and illness beliefs of various ethnic groups, and you choose Korean-Americans (problem statement). Key words that apply to this statement would be ethnic groups, Korean-Americans, health beliefs, and illness beliefs.

Citing CINAHL

CD-ROM databases are costly. Some schools of practical/vocational nursing may share a computer system with other health care institutions. Student use of these databases may be restricted. Understanding how to use a periodical index is still a necessary skill. How well do you understand the information found in a periodical index entry? The beginning of each CINAHL book contains directions for using the source. Use the CINAHL entry below to test your understanding of CINAHL citing. Answer the questions found underneath the entry. Refer back to Figure 7–1 if you need help in reading the CINAHL citation.

 Learning Exercise: Using CINAHL

Freedom from the Chain of Septic Flow: handwashing in infection control (Kovach, TL) (CEU, exam questions, tables/charts) *The Journal of Practical Nursing* 1999 March; 49(1): 34–42 (11 ref)

Author_____

Title of article_____

Volume and number of periodical_____

Name of periodical_____

Date of article_____

Pages_____

Additional information found in article_____

Are there references in the article?_____

If so, how many?_____

Nursing Organizations

Nursing organizations frequently organize speakers, seminars, and workshops on up-to-the-minute nursing topics and related health care topics. These programs are frequently made available to students. Specific nursing organizations are discussed in Chapter 17.

Community Resources

The city library and museums sometimes sponsor programs and exhibits on topics of interest and use to practical/vocational nursing students. Health care facilities such as hospitals and clinics offer lecture series.

Guest Speakers

Nurses and other health professionals are frequently invited to visit nursing classes as **guest speakers.** These speakers donate their time to present current information on their areas of expertise and updates on specific nursing topics. Often they are released by their employers to visit nursing classes. Students need to treat these speakers with respect.

Summary

☐ The hints for using learning strategies and resources found in this chapter will help you obtain the information you need to get better grades on tests and achieve your goal of becoming a practical/vocational nurse. The PQRST method of reading a textbook is an effective technique for storing information in your long-term memory so that it is available for recall for tests and can be applied in the clinical area.

☐ Specific course learning strategies that most probably will be used by the practical/ vocational nursing student, in addition to textbooks, include minilectures, lecture-discussions, and cooperative learning. New ways of delivering instruction, such as distance learning, make learning more student-oriented. Additional learning resources include articles from periodicals, the syllabus, course outlines, audiovisual materials, the Internet, computer-aided instruction, computer simulations, and the Learning Resource Center.

☐ Staying current in practical/vocational nursing is made possible by using periodical indexes, CD-ROM databases and programs, the Internet, skills lab, nursing organizations, community resources, and guest speakers. After learning the information you need to be a practical/vocational nurse, you must demonstrate that learning has taken place by your performance in the clinical area and on tests.

Review Questions

1. If a student uses the PQRST textbook study method but skips the State step, what benefit is missed?
   A. The opportunity to identify weak areas to correct before examinations.
   B. Noting all main ideas in the reading material and storing information in long-term memory.
   C. Knowing what to look for when reading, instead of treating everything as "must-know."
   D. The opportunity to increase understanding by organizing the information and relating facts to each other.

2. Select the benefit of a minilecture during class time.
   A. A minilecture can clear up a difficult reading assignment.
   B. Minilectures keep students actively involved in the learning process.
   C. Much time is saved by having the instructor present all the information the student needs to know.
   D. Minilectures give the instructor the op-portunity to teach students what they need to know to be good practical/vocational nurses.

3. Select the strategy that would best help a student locate information in the Learning Resource Center.
   A. Make an appointment with the counselor.
   B. Arrange for a tour of the Learning Resource Center.
   C. Visit the lab and see what they have to offer.
   D. Make an appointment with the Head Librarian and discuss the problems you have finding pertinent information.

4. Select the best strategy to obtain an article quickly when the Learning Resource Center does not have the periodical.
   A. Demand the LRC subscribe to the nursing journal STAT.
   B. Order the periodical from Amazon.com on the Internet.
   C. Place an order for the article through interlibrary loan.

D. Try to find the article on one of the many CD-ROMs in the LRC.
5. When using the Internet to obtain information for a nursing class, it is most important for the practical/vocational nursing student to be aware of
   A. The time involved in obtaining the information.
   B. The search engine that will be used to obtain needed information.
   C. The type of computer that will be used to obtain access to the World Wide Web.
   D. The fact that the Internet is not regulated at this time and anyone can publish anything he or she wants.

References

Staton T. *How to Study,* 5th ed. Circle Pines, MN: Publisher's Building, American Guidance Service, 1959.

Bibliography

Chenevert M. *Mosby's Tour Guide to Nursing School.* St. Louis: Mosby–Year Book, 1995.

DeYoung S, Adams E. Study groups among nursing students. J Nurs Educ 34(4): 190–191, 1995.

Jensen E. *B's and A's in 30 days: Strategies for better grades in college.* New York: Barron's Magazine, 1997.

Levine J. *The Internet for Dummies.* Foster City, CA: IDG Worldwide Books Inc, 1998.

Meltzer M, Palau S. *Learning Strategies in Nursing: Reading, Studying, and Test-Taking.* Philadelphia: W. B. Saunders, 1997.

Pauk W. *How to Study in College,* 5th ed. Boston: Houghton-Mifflin, 1997.

Rose C. *Accelerated Learning for the 21st Century: The Six-Step Plan to Unlock Your Master-Mind.* New York: Dell Publishing Co., 1998.

Sternberger C. Moving past memorization. J Practical/Vocational Nurs 45(2): 12–15, 1995.

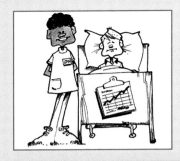

PART **THREE**
Knowing Others

Chapter 8

Straightforward Communication Skills

Outline

Key Terms

active listening
affective communication
belittling
chiding
closed-ended questions
commitment
communication blocks
empathy
false reassurance
feedback

focused questions
honesty
humor
knowledge
message
nonverbal communication
one-way communication
open-ended questions
patience
probing

purpose
receiver
respect
self-worth
sender
sensitivity
therapeutic communication
trust
two-way communication
verbal communication

Objectives

Upon completing this chapter you will be able to:

1. Explain the sender-receiver process in
   a. One-way communication
   b. Two-way communication
2. Discuss how nonverbal and affective communication can support or cancel the meaning of verbal communication.
3. Provide an example of how you use communication strategies in nursing.
4. Give an example of blocking therapeutic communication.
5. List two common differences in male/female communication that have biologic roots.
6. Give an example of a cultural communication difference in the area you live in.
7. List two common factors related to role change for a hospitalized client that can create distress.
8. Identify a communication difference for clients in two separate age groups.
9. Explain how common characteristics apply to straightforward communication with all persons.

Communication Process

Sara walked into the client's room without knocking on the door. "I'm going to measure your blood pressure. Give me your arm," she said. The client gave her a quizzical look, but he put out his arm. This was Sara's first contact with a client. When she finally got the cuff on, her face was flushed, and her own heart was beating so hard, she could not hear the client's heartbeat.

1. What kind of communication did Sara engage in with the client?
2. Who was Sara's focus?
3. What steps did Sara skip that resulted in showing disrespect for the client?

Sara engaged in **one-way communication,** in which the **sender** (Sara) controlled the situation by telling the **receiver** (client) what she was going to do (the **message**). Sara offered no opportunity for **feedback** (response) from the client. Feedback would have provided the client an opportunity to question, agree, or refuse the procedure. Sara was so focused on herself that she omitted common courtesies: a knock on the door, addressing the client by name, and introducing herself, her position, and reason for being there. His unspoken response may have increased Sara's discomfort.

One-Way vs. Two-Way Communication

One-way communication is used to give a command, as in the military service, or information with no expectation of feedback. Sometimes, one-way communication must be changed to **two-way communication** in which there is feedback or discussion. During an emergency, a doctor may give an order. Take the few seconds to change to two-way communication by repeating the order to the doctor so that it is verified for accuracy. Two-way communication is the usual form of conversation. Each one contributes equally, and feedback is both expected and respected.

Types of Communication

Three types of communication are identified: **verbal communication** (spoken or written word), **nonverbal communication** (body language), and **affective communication** (feeling tone). They may or may not all occur together. When they do occur together, all three must mirror each other (be congruent) for the communication to be honest. See Figure 8–1.

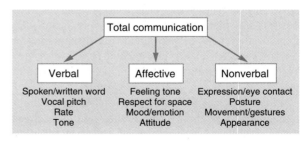

FIGURE 8–1 Communication.

Verbal Communication

The spoken word is powerful. A client may accept what you say as completely as though the team leader or doctor had spoken. Know in advance what you can or cannot discuss with a client. Sometimes your response will be, "I am not qualified to discuss that" or "I do not know, but I will find someone who does." Speak as clearly as possible, using proper grammar. Slang is usually not appropriate and may have a different meaning depending on age and culture. Medical jargon is rarely helpful. If you truly understand the terms, you can translate them into everyday language.

Some illnesses also affect a client's interpretation of verbalization. For example, clients diagnosed with schizophrenia interpret words concretely (literally). They experience difficulty with abstract (inferred) meanings. For example, after using a stationary bicycle, a client was asked by the nurse, "How do you feel now?" He grabbed his buttocks and responded, "My butt is numb. That's how." The nurse was trying to determine change in his stress level.

Nonverbal Communication

Commonly known as body language, nonverbal communication either supports or cancels out verbal communication. Expressions, posture, movements, and gestures, whether your own or the client's, give important clues to the truth of the verbalization. Careful observation of body language may clue you in to client discomfort, even though pain has been denied verbally. Gathering additional data will help clarify the real issue creating the discomfort.

It works both ways. Clients tend to observe you closely, also. They look for clues regarding the seriousness of their illness. For example, your distressed look may be interpreted as disapproval or serious concerns about their health. How are they to know that you brought your personal life worries to work?

Physical appearance is a part of nonverbal communication. The client's appearance upon admission provides signs of personal care plus important clues

about the illness. Clients also quickly evaluate you and, based on what you project, even before you speak, draw conclusions about your competence as a nurse. This is a major reason why most nursing schools continue to have a dress code. It is also the reason why your instructors model appropriate dress and behavior.

Affective Communication

Affect refers to mood or emotion. The feeling tone that you pick up on as you approach a person or step into a room is as significant as verbal and nonverbal communication. We are made up of energy; therefore, we emit energy. The tendency may be to ignore this level of communication because we cannot see, hear, or read it. Affective communication is as significant as verbal and nonverbal communication. Truly honest communication integrates verbal, nonverbal, and affective communications so that they all express the same message.

   ### Critical Thinking Exercise

Give an example of a time that you have stepped into a room or approached a person and, before anyone spoke, experienced a feeling of excitement, happiness, sadness, anger, or some other emotion.

Communication Strategies

Please do not interpret the term "strategies" to mean predetermined script, as in telemarketing. In real life, this would be awkward, even boring. You might even lose track of where you are in your conversation because of the focus on strategies. Work to understand the meaning of active listening, active listening behaviors, and types of questions discussed.

Active Listening

This is probably the most important part of any **therapeutic** (health-related) **communication.** Key factors in **active listening** include purpose, disciplined attention, and focus. *Purpose* refers to the health-related reason for gathering data or giving information. *Disciplined attention* means that you do not assume accuracy of information without checking it out. Clarify what you think you understand the client to say and ask further questions as needed. This applies both to gathering data and giving health-related information. *Focus* means that all your senses are alert to clues that the client may be communicating.

Active Listening Behaviors

The most commonly used *active listening behaviors* include restating, clarification, reflection, paraphrasing, minimal encouraging, silence, summarizing, and validation.

Restating refers to repeating what the client has said in a slightly different way. For example:

Client: "My chest hurts. I can't sleep at night."

Nurse: "You've been unable to sleep at night because of chest pain."

Clarification is asking a closed-ended question in response to a client's statement to be sure you understand. For example:

Client: "My chest hurts."

Nurse: "Exactly where does it hurt?"

Reflection is putting into words the information you are receiving from the client at an affective communication level. For example:

Client: "I'm sick of seeing doctors and not getting answers."

Nurse: "You seem upset with the lack of answers to your health problems."

Paraphrasing refers to expressing in your own words what you think the client means.

Client: "I don't think I'm being told the truth about my condition."

Nurse: "You think you may be more ill than what the doctor is telling you."

Minimal encouraging involves using sounds, words, or short phrases to encourage the client to continue. For example:

Client: "It just happened so fast —."

Nurse: "Yes — go on — and then what — hmmm — uh huh —."

Silence involves pauses used with skill. The tendency is to fill silence with chatter or your speculation. This may cause the client to "turn off" or shift the story. Maintaining disciplined attention and focus during silence lets the clients tell the story in their own way.

Summarizing means briefly stating the main data you have gathered. *Validation* provides the client with an opportunity to correct information, if necessary, at the time of summary.

Types of Questions

Three types of questions are commonly used in therapeutic communication. They are open-ended, closed-ended, and focused questions. **Open-ended questions** permit the client to respond in a way most meaningful to him or her. The questions often begin with what, where, when, how, or why? For example: "What happened to your leg?" **Closed-ended questions** require a specific answer. For example: "When did you first notice the pain?" **Focused questions** provide even more definitive information. For example: "On a scale of 1 to 10, with 10 as the worst possible pain, how do you rate your pain right now?"

Nurse/Client Communication Evaluation

Communication is far more complex than just talking. Some of the many contributing characteristics are listed below with a brief description. Self-evaluate according to those characteristics that are working for you and those you need to work on.

Self-Evaluation of Personal Characteristics

Characteristic	Desirable	Self-evaluation
Eye contact	Usually 3–5 seconds. Cultural variations	
Respect for personal space	About 1.5 feet except for personal care. Cultural variations	
Appropriate touch	Gentle, but firm. Cultural variations	
Attitude	Nonjudgmental. Practices unconditional love	
Voice/tone	Moderate or according to growth and development needs. Example: Newborns	
Rate	Paced according to client's ability to comprehend	
Appearance	Models positive nursing image. Looks healthy	
Posture	Open, without folded arms or hands on hips. Stand or sit tall	
Gestures	Moderate to enhance conversation	
Language	Speaks effectively and at client's level of understanding. Correct grammar	
Expression	Congruent with topic. Nonjudgmental	

Blocks to Communication

It is sometimes easy to slip into communication styles that block communication. Perhaps the client reminds you of someone you know or you have history with the client. Sometimes you don't like the client or are just plain tired. Whatever the reason, it is worth thinking about the possibility in advance. As a nurse, you want to continue to give every client the best care possible regardless of your personal response. Common **communication blocks** involve false reassuring, probing, chiding, belittling, giving advice, and providing pat answers.

Avoiding Blocks

False reassurance involves telling the client "Everything will be OK," "You'll be just fine,"

"Don't worry about anything," "We'll see to it that you get well," "This experience will make you stronger," "You'll see the good in this some day," and so on. There is no way you can guarantee what you have just finished saying to the client. **Probing** means pushing for information beyond what is medically necessary to know. Curiosity takes over and the client's privacy is no longer respected. Ask yourself about the value of the information and how you will use the information once you have it. Think twice before continuing with statements like "Let's get to the bottom of this once and for all." **Chiding** (scolding) for behavior such as smoking is of limited value for the client with severe emphysema or lung cancer. Your information is hardly an "alert." You can be sure that she or he has heard the message over and over again. Without supporting the behavior, you can continue to be therapeutic to the client.

Belittling involves mimicking or making fun of the client in some way. It may include down-playing the importance of the symptoms. For example: "You could be having heart surgery! This is just wart removal." As a physician pointed out, "If *you* have a tonsillectomy, it's minor surgery; if *I* have a tonsillectomy, it's major surgery." It's all a matter of perspective. *Giving advice,* when you know what someone else should do, is so tempting. Unsolicited advice is rarely beneficial and closes the door to having the client problem-solve. A more beneficial response, even when the client asks what you would (or he or she should) do, is to say, "What ideas do you have? I'm sure you've thought of ways you might solve this problem." Listen carefully, summarize what the client has said, and then ask, "Which one of your ideas do you want to begin with?" After the client's response, you could say, "When do you think you'll start?" *Pat answers,* like "Everyone feels this way," come so easily. Clients feel dismissed and misunderstood. They do not really care that everyone else feels this way. As far as they are concerned, these feelings are theirs, are different, and need comforting words or touch. If you can, offer something you know you can deliver, like "I'll be with you the entire time" or "I'll be in the room when you return."

Male/Female Differences

Being equal does not mean being the same. Men and women communicate differently for biologic reasons. While there are examples of similarities in both sexes, most males and females follow certain patterns. According to Sieh and Brentin (1997; pp. 10–12), four areas that relate to nursing communication are conversation patterns, smiling, head movements, and posture.

Conversation

Men tend to approach conversation with an eye to maintaining status and independence, to report or to get information, and to solve problems. They express their ideas more assertively; women do so with less certainty. Therefore, male opinions are often valued more highly without validation. Women seek to establish intimacy and develop rapport, share feelings, and establish relationships. Men ask fewer questions but readily interrupt during conversations without apology. Women use questions to encourage conversation. They wait for a pause to seek clarification and apologize for the interruption. Men apologize for a wrong; women say "I'm sorry" to indicate regret, sympathy, or concern. Men rarely say "I don't know"; women often phrase ideas as questions, such as "Have you thought of—?" Men make decisions; women are looking for agreement. Men make demands more often, whereas women express preferences with reasons. Men's sentences are shorter and fewer; women create longer, more complex sentences linking more ideas together. Men make declarations, whereas women often end a statement with a question like "Don't you think so?" (Tannen, 1990).

Head Movements

Men nod if they are in agreement. Women nod to show they are listening. A man may be surprised to discover that a woman does not agree at all with what he said. Men hold their heads erect while speaking; women frequently assume a lower status position by tilting their head to the side or placing their chin down with eyes gazing upward (Sieh and Brentin, 1997, p. 10).

Smiling

Smiling by a woman may or may not denote happiness. A smile is also used to mask unhappiness and other emotions. Reactions by others to her smiles may leave her feeling unheard. Men tend not to show an outward reaction when criticized, making them seem strong and in control.

Posture

A rounded posture with chest in, chin down, gives an appearance of being threatened. Standing tall, with shoulders back and head held high, speaks of confidence and control.

Looking at differences in the way men and women communicate has important implications in working with clients, staff, and instructors. Smiling and nodding by a woman does not have to mean she understands the instructions. A lack of questions from a male client may not mean he knows what the surgery entails. Gather all three types of communication data. Ask the client to tell you what he or she understands—summarize—validate. Make use of the skills you are learning.

Cultural Differences

Members of subcultures within our cultures embrace and value their beliefs and practices. In order to be respectful and respond therapeutically, we have to know what the differences are. We briefly review communication differences for Native Americans, African-Americans, Mexicans, Filipinos, Chinese, and Japanese. Be sure to read Chapter 9 for a more complete understanding of cultural diversity. Mark the chapter and use it as a reference when questions arise.

Native American

Periods of silence during conversation show respect. Native Americans may not ask questions but expect the health provider to know and direct them in health issues. Eye contact may be minimal, and insisting on it may be considered disrespectful.

African-American

Touch is common within the family and extended family. Use of black dialect may cause misunderstanding between the nurse and client. Speaking in loud voices is common among friends and family.

Mexican

Touch is common, especially among members of the same sex. Touching the arm or shoulder when making a point shows trust or rapport. Shaking hands is a common greeting when saying hello or good-bye. Sustained eye contact is considered rude or immodest. Personal space is closer than usual. Pain is sometimes suppressed, sometimes not. Grief may be overtly expressed.

Filipino

Touch is important. Pain medication needs to be offered more than once; Filipinos tend to accept pain. There may be some fear of eye contact. However, if it is initiated, return and maintain it.

Chinese

Touch by strangers may cause concern. A slight nod or bow acknowledges an introduction. Avoidance of direct eye contact while listening is considered respectful and polite. Direct eye contact is accepted by the elderly. Personal space is preferably greater than an arm's length. Expressing negative feelings and emotions is considered weakness. Offer pain medication more than once since it is not considered proper to accept something the first time it is offered.

Japanese

Handshakes are all right, but a pat on the head is not considered proper. Japanese people may bow as a greeting. Personal space is preferably more than an arm's length. Direct eye contact is considered disrespectful. They tend to withstand pain without complaint, so look for physical signs. Public expression of grief is unacceptable. They avoid confrontation and saying "no" directly. Laughter may be used to mask embarrassment, bereavement, and rage. Happiness may hide behind a straight face.

Learning Exercise: Cultural Differences

List two cultural differences of someone in the area in which you live.

1. _____

_____

2. _____

_____

The characteristics described here are brief and cover a small number of the cultures within the country. Wherever you work, it is important to learn as much as possible about the cultures of your clients. Remember also, that just because you can identify someone's ethnic background, their families may have been in this country for generations. Differences may be nonexistent.

Role Changes for the Client

What happens to clients who find themselves in a dependent position after having been in charge of their lives? The concerns they have go beyond the physical realities into areas we consider next.

Critical Thinking Exercises

Imagine yourself being hospitalized. List four immediate concerns.

1. _____

_____

2. _____

_____

3. _____

_____

4. _____

_____

It Begins with "Hello, My Name Is _____"

Whatever you communicate verbally, nonverbally, and affectively sets the tone for rapport with the client. You have some preliminary information (a name), even if the client is just being admitted. Knock on the door or side of the doorway, pause briefly to collect data *before* walking in. You begin to pick up nonverbal and affective communication clues. Address the client as Mr., Mrs., Miss, or Ms, or by professional title if it applies. Extend your hand (unless culturally improper). Give your name, identify yourself as a student practical/vocational nurse, plus the name of the school and what your purpose is for being in the room.

It may sound like this: "Mrs. Hill, my name is Mr. Fry. I am a practical nursing student from the Middle American Technical College. I am here to measure your blood pressure, pulse, and respiration. It is a part of the admission procedure." The client may request that you address her by her first name, but do not assume this without permission. Some hospitals and other health agencies limit staff use of name to first name only. This will dictate how you introduce yourself.

Nursing Jargon

Remember how time-consuming it was to learn all those medical terms and abbreviations? Using the terms may sound impressive to you now and involve a feeling of having arrived. However, use of unknown terminology can serve to increase client fears and cause misunderstanding. "What does it mean that I will have an I.V. started, have a WBC stat, and you'll be doing vitals q2h for now?" When you really know something you can explain words and symbols in terms understood by a lay person. Now *that's* really impressive!

Fear of the Unknown

Clients frequently have numerous unspoken fears about tests, procedures, and possible outcomes. These include, but are not limited to, pain, sleep, needle sticks, thirst, hunger, and being treated respectfully. A pat answer of "Everything will be OK" shows lack of understanding of the depth of the fears. Clients may not ask questions because of fear of embarrassment—"Silly question," "Everyone is so busy." An open-ended question from you like, "What question do you have? If I don't know the answer, I'll try to find out for you," can open the way for expression of fears. When you make a promise to a client, follow through.

Personal Factors

A client's illness rarely affects the client alone. Thoughts and concerns may extend to family, work, finances, and so on. For example, the mother of a newly hospitalized child was irritable and inattentive when the nurse was explaining the unit rules. Finally, the nurse stopped in mid-sentence and said

to the mother, "Tell me what is troubling you," and paused. The mother looked at her, then blurted out that she had a sick child at home, her husband worked nights and slept days, she had been up most of the last three nights. "Where should I be? Both kids need me, and my neighbor can only come in for two hours a day. I'm at my wit's end!" The mother could not begin to focus on the unit rules until there were solutions to the home problems. You may not have a solution, but you can be a catalyst to make needs known to the instructor or team leader. They are aware of additional resources.

Environmental Factors

A health care setting, whether a clinic, hospital, rehabilitation center, or nursing home, is so different from home. There is no true opportunity for privacy. A variety of staff show up at different times, 24 hours a day; lights are on day and night; the staff makes more noise than they realize; machinery is humming, buzzing, or beeping; staff check out different parts of your body, they pick and poke: you get the picture. The client may have put the light on because of a need to go to the bathroom *now*. By the time someone arrives, it may be too late, much to the client's embarrassment.

Advance communication and planning does not take as long as it sounds. You may find out that the client always has a snack of toast and tea at 9:00 PM, always gets up to go to the bathroom at 11:00 PM, always has bran cereal and banana at 6:00 AM, and so on. Notes of this nature in the client's care plan assist in continuity of communication and care.

Communicating with Instructors and Staff

Communication characteristics involve **trust, honesty, empathy, respect, sensitivity, humor, knowledge, patience, commitment,** and **self-worth.** These characteristics are equally important in communicating with clients, instructors, and staff.

Trust

This characteristic begins with confidence in your ability to make decisions. You communicate this to instructors and staff by consistently doing the required preliminary preparation for assignments.

Honesty

This implies that you will not deliberately deceive in order to present yourself in a more favorable light. Asking the instructor to repeat a procedure for more practice is an example of this characteristic in communication.

Empathy

The ability to understand and appreciate what someone else is feeling without experiencing the emotion itself separates empathy from sympathy. This permits you to maintain control and think clearly. You may offer to help a staff member do client care (something practical), instead of getting pulled into an "Isn't it awful" conversation.

Sensitivity

Tuning in on nonverbal and affective communication helps you verify verbalization or lack thereof. Picking up at these levels permits you to check it out with the staff or instructor. "Is there something else I need to know?"

Humor

Healthy humor at the client's level of appreciation can help "lighten up" a situation. Offensive humor, poking fun at the client or at other cultures or races, is unacceptable. Staff sometimes privately get involved in "gallows humor," which is laughing at something very serious or medically gross. Look for examples in movies and television programs with medical themes.

Knowledge

The cornerstone of gathering data and other health-related communication is knowledge. Instructors and staff quickly determine your level of knowledge. Instructors communicate the significance of this characteristic by making assignments early enough for you to research the information. You communicate back to the instructor (and staff) by following through.

Respect

This involves both self-respect and respect for others. You communicate self-respect by doing your best each day. When you treat yourself with respect, it becomes easy to extend this to your instructors, staff, and clients. Clients quickly pick up on this during conversation and physical care (verbal and nonverbal communication).

Patience

In this modern world, we are often accustomed to instant results and/or gratification. It is sometimes difficult to provide the time needed to learn, receive explanations from instructors, or follow staff orders. This extends to our work with clients, in whom illness and growth and development levels dictate the need to slow down or repeat directions. The client (or you) may be tempted to say "I know," when such is not the case. The characteristic of patience takes time to perfect. You may initially feel like you are moving backward in your communication attempts with clients.

Commitment

Commitment means incorporating all the previous characteristics as a part of your nursing communication. Decide that you are in nursing because you really want to be here. Then do the work that needs to be done. It shows and it pays off. Take time to appreciate the uniqueness of each client.

Self-Worth

Self-worth is earned. No one can give it to you or take it away. It is that special sense that it is OK to receive, and that you have something very special to offer in nursing communication—that you are usually able to "connect" with clients and other health workers.

Life Span Communication

Growth and development levels, male/female differences, and medical conditions all affect communication with clients. Each age group, whether infant, preschooler, school-ager, teen-ager, adult, or elderly, each has somewhat different communication needs.

Infant

Infants' communication includes crying, cooing, and body language. They act out their feelings with total body language. As their recognition of words grows, certain words act to soothe or to trigger reaction. Up to that time, they are most influenced by the sound of the voice. As one dad pointed out, "I used to put my baby to sleep each night by rocking her and reading the *Wall Street Journal* aloud in a soothing voice." Newborns respond favorably to a high-pitched voice, but that changes by the end of the first month. After that, calm, low tones are more soothing.

Parents (caretakers) are the best source for learning the meaning of different cries. They learn quickly to differentiate between wet, hungry, and uncomfortable. Rely on them for specific information on communication style.

Preschooler

We are including toddlers in this category as early preschoolers. They are usually known for magnificent tantrums. Little wonder: they have learned some words but, when frustrated, may not be able to put them together effectively. Hence, the body acts out what the words cannot tell. Laughing at or reasoning with the preschooler is counterproductive. Removing the child from the immediate situation and audience helps. Once preschoolers are more composed, they can communicate by pointing or showing on themselves or in a picture what is upsetting. During procedures, explain briefly and simply what is going to happen. Tell them what they can do to help.

School-ager

The vocabulary of school-age children has increased considerably. They are ready to be a part of most (not all) discussions with the parents. Drawings or pictures can be used to explain an illness or procedure. Ask for feedback to avoid misconceptions. "Tell me in your own words what—." The child may not be privy to all information. In that case, go to a separate area so that the child will not overhear the conversation or parts of it. Whispering and misinterpretation can evoke new problems. Remember that most younger people think better in the afternoon.

Teen-ager

Teen-agers are the easiest or the most difficult to communicate with, depending on your perspective. When ill, they need to believe that someone knows more than they do and that someone is in charge. Deal with them with the same courtesy that you extend to adults. Have similar expectations of them. Encourage expression of feelings, fears, and concerns. Their sense that nothing will happen to them has been shaken. Answer questions within your role. Seek out answers as appropriate. Avoid hiding behind nursing jargon. Use of teen slang usually does not work out. Without real knowledge of its meaning, you may end up appearing foolish instead of "hip."

Adult

Many of the issues discussed in the chapter apply to adult communication. Collecting data at all three levels of communication is essential. Remember to limit your questions to areas that are medically related. Pushing and probing based on curiosity may open Pandora's box. It does not work to probe and leave the client to pick up the pieces.

Elderly

What picture do you hold of elderly people in your "mind's eye"? Unresolved parental issues, for example, can get in the way of quality care. If you can see aging as just another part of the life cycle, you may be able to work effectively with elderly clients. "Boys and men take in less sensory or proximal data than girls and women. They smell less, taste less, get less soothing and input from tactile information, hear less and see less" (Gurian, 1997, p. 16). Most elderly people think more clearly in the morning.

Lower frequency sounds are easier to hear for both men and women when hearing begins to diminish. As with younger men, check with the elderly man as to which ear hears the best. Remember that the left eye, even without loss of vision, has more acuity for a man. It works best for explanations and table games to be focused on the left side. Women see and hear equally well with both eyes and ears. Women also differentiate sounds easier from background noises. The elderly man may not hear you if you call when the TV is on. The male brain shuts on and off according to load. Part of it must remain functioning in order to continue vital functions. Men may continue to have reading problems. Read directions out loud for the male client without visual problems. You will continue to find that many female clients are orderly and satisfied with a smaller amount of space. The male client is generally the opposite, and you may have to seek additional space for games and puzzles in the day room.

Electronic Communication

Use of facsimile (FAX) machines, computer client charting, and electronic mail (e-mail) are all valu-

able modern methods of communication when used effectively and appropriately. FAX machines, for example, often shorten the time in which information can be sent between agencies and departments. Computer client charting ideally provides a location where the most recent client information is entered by all agency professionals involved in client care. Computer charting may be a part of your basic education for learning to enter medications and treatments. Each facility may have slightly different protocols. E-mail is a popular way of communication with administration and other departments. Before getting involved in sending e-mail, it is important to review the basics of e-mail etiquette. According to Lauchman (1999, p. 11), some people are sending in e-mail things they would never write in a memo or say directly to someone. Box 8–1 includes some e-mail essentials suggested by Lauchman.

Box 8–1 E-mail Etiquette

1. *Take it seriously.* Consider the content of the message and to whom you are sending it.
2. *To emphasize a point, let the sentence stand alone.* Special effects, such as boldface, may not show up on someone else's screen.
3. *Keep your sentences and paragraphs short.*
4. *Skip a line to separate topics.*
5. *Send your message to the right person.*
6. *Be especially careful filling in the "subject" line.* People read this first to decide whether the message is worth reading.
7. *Be specific.* Avoid useless information.
8. *Determine whether e-mail is the best way to send your message.*
9. *Be cautious with humor.* The person sees only the written word.
10. *Check your spelling and punctuation.* Proofread all messages before sending them.

Summary

☐ Communication can be one-sided or two-sided. Both involve a sender, a receiver, and a message. In one-sided communication, the receiver does not have the opportunity to provide feedback. During two-sided communication, feedback is an expectation.

☐ Communication involves verbal, nonverbal, and affective communication.

☐ The most important part of therapeutic communication is active listening. It involves purpose, focus, and disciplined attention.

☐ Common active listening behaviors involve restating, clarification, reflection, paraphrasing, minimal encouraging, silence, summarizing, and validating.

☐ Common blocks to communication involve false reassuring, probing, chiding, belittling, giving advice, and pat answers.

☐ Male/female differences do exist. Some differences are "hard wired" biologically. Characteristics can be modified if desired.

☐ Cultural differences in communication exist, especially with individuals who are new to the country and/or continue to have strong cultural ties.

☐ Role changes for the client during an illness experience can be distressing. Staff attitude, nursing jargon, fear of the unknown, plus personal and environmental factors are all involved.

☐ Communicating with the instructor and staff involves the same characteristics as communicating with a client. They include trust, honesty, empathy, respect, sensitivity, humor, knowledge, patience, and commitment. Self-worth is earned as your knowledge and skill in application grow.

☐ Life span communication differences are related to growth and other issues, male/female differences, and medical problems.

☐ E-mail etiquette is essential for effective and efficient electronic communication.

Review Questions

1. What is the sender–receiver–message–feedback process in one-way communication?
   A. It concludes when the message reaches the receiver.
   B. It utilizes verbal, nonverbal, and affective communication.
   C. Once feedback has been provided, the message is final.
   D. It is a short-hand communication, useful in close relationships.

2. What is the effect of smiling at someone when you share feelings of anger?
   A. Lightens up the message.
   B. Shows your depth of caring,

   C. Cancels the verbal message.
   D. Invites immediate feedback.

3. What accounts for basic male/female differences in communication?
   A. Socialization
   B. Environment
   C. Acculturation
   D. Biology

4. Which communication characteristic is earned?
   A. Commitment
   B. Sensitivity
   C. Self-worth
   D. Honesty

5. How is affective communication expressed?
   A. Through gentle, persistent probing.
   B. Through feeling tone.
   C. Through open-ended questions.
   D. Through a sympathetic response.

References

Gurian M. *The Wonder of Boys.* New York: Jeremy P. Tarcher/Putnam, 1997.

Lauchman R. Using e-mail for effective and efficient communication. Vitality, June, 1999, p. 11.

Sieh A, Brentin L. *The Nurse Communicates.* Philadelphia: W. B. Saunders, 1997.

Tannen D. *You Just Don't Understand.* New York: Ballantine Books, 1990.

Bibliography

Arnold E, Boggs KU. *Interpersonal Relationships; Professional Communication Skills for Nurses,* 3rd ed. Philadelphia: W. B. Saunders, 1999.

Balzer-Riley JW. *Communications in Nursing,* 4th ed. St. Louis: C. V. Mosby, 2000.

Battaglia C. The language of being. Reflections, First Quarter, 1999.

BonDurant P. Emma without words. Reflections, First Quarter, 1999.

Brown C. Nurses at the bedside. Am J Nurs 97(11), November, 1997.

Carson VB. The vehicle for healing: Communication as part of a therapeutic relationship. In *Mental Health Nursing, The Nurse-Patient Journey,* 2nd ed. Philadelphia: W. B. Saunders, 2000, Chapter 10.

Charles P. Meeting Ben. Am J Nurs 98(6), June, 1998.

Davidhizar R, Shearer R. Improving your bedside manner. Pract Nurs 48(3), March, 1998.

Giger JN, Davidhizar RE. *Transcultural Nursing,* 3rd ed. St. Louis: C. V. Mosby, 1999.

Hahn J. Cueing in to patient language. Reflections, First Quarter, 1999.

Nicoteri J. Critical thinking skills. Am J Nurs 98(10), October, 1998.

Ward-Collins D. "Noncompliant"—Isn't there a better way to say it? Am J Nurs 98(5), May, 1998.

Chapter 9

Cultural Uniqueness, Sensitivity, and Competence

Outline

What We Share in Common
Basic Daily Needs
    Personal Care and Hygiene
    Sleep and Rest
    Nutrition and Fluids
    Elimination
    Body Alignment and Activity
    Environment
    Emotional and Spiritual Support
    Diversion and Recreation
    Mental Hygiene
Definition of Culture
Characteristics of Culture

Danger: Ethnocentrism, Prejudice, and Discrimination
    Avoiding False Assumptions
Cultural Diversity
    Importance of Cultural Diversity
    Philosophy of Individual Worth and Celebration of Our Uniqueness
    Learning About Cultural Diversity
    Areas of Cultural Diversity
    Concept of Time
    Communication

    Educational Background
    Economic Level
    Wellness and Illness Beliefs and Practices
    Increasing Your Knowledge of Culturally Diverse Clients
Categories of Major Health Belief Systems
Developing Plans of Care for Culturally Diverse Clients
Developing Cultural Competence in Health Care Situations

Key Terms

acculturation
assimilation
biomedicine
cultural bias
cultural diversity
cultural pluralism
cultural uniqueness
cultural universality

culture
customs
discrimination
ethnic groups
ethnocentrism
melting pot
naturalistic system

nonjudgmental
personalistic system
prejudice
repatterning
stereotype
wellness and illness
world view

Objectives

Upon completing this chapter you will be able to:
1. Explain in your own words nine basic daily needs of all persons.
2. Define in your own words the following terms:
    a. Culture
    b. Cultural uniqueness
    c. Cultural diversity
    d. Ethnocentrism
    e. Cultural bias
    f. Cultural sensitivity
    g. Cultural competence

3. Explain the importance of the following in developing an ability to provide culturally competent care:
    a. Awareness of your own cultural self
    b. Attainment of knowledge about culturally diverse groups
    c. Negotiation of plans of care for culturally diverse clients
4. Explain in your own words the philosophy of individual worth as it applies to health care.

5. Describe your culture in the areas of
    a. Family
    b. Religion
    c. Communication
    d. Educational background
    e. Economic level
    f. Wellness and illness beliefs and practices
6. Describe specific differences between cultural groups in your geographic area that may have importance in client care situations.

In the nineteenth century, waves of immigrants from throughout the world entered the United States. The United States was referred to as a **melting pot.** This term indicated that the immigrants had given up their native cultures and adopted the culture of the people already in the United States. In the 1990 U.S. census, a write-in blank for racial ancestry was provided on the census form. Americans reported nearly 300 "races," 600 Indian tribes, 70 Hispanic groups, and 75 combinations of multiracial ancestry (Morganthau, 1995, p. 65). Obviously, the U.S population has not "melted."

You have chosen a career that will give you an opportunity to meet people who are different from you! Some of these people will be your clients. Some will be your coworkers. Some will be a different age than yours. Some will belong to a different social class. Some will have disabilities. Some will have different health care beliefs about what causes them to get sick. Some will have different values. In addition to all these differences, some of your clients and coworkers will have different cultural backgrounds owing to ethnic group status. Regardless of cultural background, some differences will be the result of a growing diversity in individual and family life styles. It may come as a surprise when you discover that people think, feel, believe, act, and see the world differently from you and your family and friends.

Review the code of ethics of the National Association of Practical Nurse Education and Service (NAPNES) and the National Federation of Licensed Practical Nurses (NFLPN) (see Chapter 18, Nursing Ethics and the Law). You will note that both organizations have embraced statements that describe the need of the practical/vocational nurse to provide health care to all clients regardless of race, creed, cultural background, disease, or life style. This is an ethical expectation. Review your state's nurse practice act. You might find that failing or refusing to render nursing services to a client because of the client's race, color, sex, age, beliefs, national origin, or handicap is listed as unprofessional conduct. The ethical expectation now becomes a legal mandate. Leininger (1994) reports

that some nurses face legal suits because of their ignorance of the culture of the client and resulting poor nursing judgment.

This chapter has three purposes. The first is to encourage you to identify how all persons, despite observed or assumed differences, are similar (**cultural universality**). The second is to encourage you to identify how all persons, despite similarities, are unique (**cultural uniqueness**). The third is to help you develop a sensitivity to **cultural diversity** among people. Not only do practical/vocational nurses need to provide care for all persons, they also need to provide culturally *competent* care. When differences are identified in a health care situation, the practical/vocational nurse should suggest adaptations to the plan of care so that the plan recognizes these differences. In doing so, the client will be encouraged to follow suggestions, avoid treatment failures, and return to health as quickly as possible. Practical/vocational nurses then will be able to say that they have truly met the clients' needs.

What We Share in Common

Because of our genes, each individual the world over is different from every other person. The only exception is identical twins. Before you start to think about the differences among people, it is a good idea to think about what people share in common.

When you are among a group of your peers (for example, in class, eating lunch in the cafeteria, walking to the parking lot), take a few minutes to play the "what we have in common" culture game. Excluding sex, age, marital status, and culture group, try to find five items you share in common with *each* member of the group. This activity is especially helpful when the group includes classmates you perceive as "different" from you. Discuss the items you have in common in a class situation. Were you surprised by any items you share in common with other members of the group?

Basic Daily Needs

All people share the same basic daily needs regardless of age, sex, economic status, life style, religion, country of origin, or culture. Chapter 13 discusses human needs as understood by the psychologist Abraham Maslow. Many years ago, Vivian Culver, a registered nurse, listed nine essential daily needs of all persons (1974, pp. 375–376). This list has stood the test of time. These essential needs are a good place to start in learning to understand that all people, regardless of background, share some things in common.

1. Personal care and hygiene
2. Sleep and rest
3. Nutrition and fluids
4. Elimination
5. Body alignment and activity
6. Environment
7. Emotional and spiritual support
8. Diversion and recreation
9. Mental hygiene

These nine basic daily needs can form the basis for planning client care. However, you need to understand the meaning of these basic needs for well persons, including yourself, before you can apply them to individuals in the clinical area. Once you gain understanding, the application of these needs to clients will be easier. As you read about the nine basic needs of all people, think about how you specifically meet each need in your own daily life. Could it be that some of your peers meet their daily basic needs in different ways than you meet your needs?

Personal Care and Hygiene

Clean hair, skin, nails, teeth, and clothing serve two general purposes: protection from illness and promotion of well-being. Skin constantly secretes sebum, the cold cream–like substance of the body, to keep the skin supple. Daily, epidermal skin cells (the outer layer of the skin) are shed as new cells push toward the outer layer. Skin eliminates fluid in the form of perspiration to help keep body tempera-ture stable. Sebum and perspiration are odorless substances. Ever-present bacteria on the skin are responsible for the body odor we associate with the body's oils and perspiration. We meet personal care and hygiene needs by bathing, shampooing, hand-washing, maintaining oral hygiene, and grooming. Do you prefer a shower or a bath or another method of cleansing your body? How often do you cleanse your body? During what part of the day do you cleanse your body? How often do you sham-poo? What grooming products do you use to style your hair? How often do you visit the dentist?

Sleep and Rest

Sleep is needed to refresh ourselves. The actual number of hours of sleep required varies with the individual. Rest and periodic relaxation are just as important because they also help the body restore itself. How many hours of sleep do you get each night or day? Where do you rest or relax? What do you do to rest or relax?

Nutrition and Fluids

Preparing meals from the basic pyramid food groups, as you studied in nutrition, is needed to stay healthy. We all need a variety of food daily from the food pyramid. A minimum of six to eight glasses of water each day is recommended to help our body complete its many chemical reactions, transport nutrients, regulate temperature, and lubri-cate body parts. These six to eight glasses are in addition to the food and other beverages we eat and drink. How many calories do you consume each day? How many glasses of fluid do you drink each day? What fluids do you prefer to drink?

Elimination

Elimination of wastes from the body is primarily accomplished by the kidneys (in the form of urine) and the large intestine (in the form of feces). The skin is not as good at elimination as these organs, but it does eliminate some body wastes through perspiration. What do you consider to be "normal" time intervals for urinary and intestinal elimination?

Body Alignment and Activity

Body alignment, or the relationship of the body parts to one another, is better known as posture. When posture is "good," the body can be used in a comfortable manner without danger of injury. Good posture also enhances the functioning of the respiratory, gastrointestinal, and circulatory systems. You will not get tired as quickly if good posture is maintained. The function of these body systems can also be enhanced by exercising the body daily. Exercise also helps maintain muscle tone. Have a peer evaluate your posture while you are sitting and walking. How much exercise do you get each day? How do you get your exercise?

Environment

Environment refers to the space that surrounds us. Our environment changes many times during a day. Regardless of our specific environment, the most essential component of our surroundings is oxygen. After that environmental need has been met, the next most important need is safety. When oxygen and safety needs have been met, the individual can focus on changing his or her environment to accommodate comfort and personal taste. Describe your home environment. Do you feel safe in your environment?

Emotional and Spiritual Support

Our emotions greatly influence our health because the body and the mind are linked. This linking enables the body to influence the mind and the mind to influence the body. All emotions, including excitement, fear, anger, worry, grief, joy, surprise, and love, can influence our bodies positively or negatively. Spiritual and emotional needs are closely related, yet different. People meet their spiritual needs in a variety of ways that are unique to their personal beliefs (see Chapter 10). Also, see Emotions and Feelings and Their Expression later in this chapter.

Diversion and Recreation

We all need to turn aside (diversion) from our usual activities and refresh our bodies and minds with activities other than work (recreation). What is work to one person can be play to another. How much time do you spend studying each week? How many hours do you work outside school? What type of recreation do you engage in each week? How many hours do you devote to recreation each week?

Mental Hygiene

Mental hygiene involves the care and hygiene of the brain. Just as there are good health habits for the body, there are also good daily health habits for the mind. You need to strive to understand and accept yourself, be happy, work well with others, accept criticism, know your abilities and limitations, trust and respect others, and accept responsibility for yourself. Who is responsible for your success in the practical nursing program? What is your attitude toward constructive evaluation? What kind of a team member are you in the clinical area?

Definition of Culture

Culture is a way of life. Culture is the total of the ever-changing ideas, thoughts, beliefs, values, communication, actions, attitudes, traditions, customs, and objects that a group of people possess and the ways they have of doing things. Culture also includes standards of behavior and sets of rules to live by. The generally accepted ways of doing things common to people who share the same culture are called **customs.**

Characteristics of Culture

An important point about culture is that it is *learned behavior.* The culture of a group is passed on from generation to generation. From the moment you were born you began to learn about the culture of the group into which you were born. The process of learning your culture (the way your group does things) is called **acculturation.** You are socialized (acculturated) to the ways of the group. Right now you are being socialized into the career of practical nursing. You are learning how to think and act like a nurse. The result of acculturation is a **world view** that is generally shared by persons with the same cultural background. The world view, or similar ways of thinking and seeing, becomes the reality of the group. This reality fills every aspect of life. It is a **cultural bias** (a mental leaning) that is never proved or questioned. The worth of everything, either within or outside of the group, depends on whether it fits the world view of the cultural group. One's world view can lead to ethnocentrism, prejudice, and discrimination.

Danger: Ethnocentrism, Prejudice, and Discrimination

People who belong to the same cultural group may develop the attitude, through their world view, that their way of doing things is superior to that of groups with different cultures (**ethnocentrism**). The group uses their culture as the norm against which to measure and evaluate the customs and ways of others. When intolerance of another cultural group occurs, **prejudice** results. When rights and privileges are withheld from those of another cultural group, **discrimination** is the result.

Avoiding False Assumptions

Nursing students sometimes think that somewhere there is a cookbook that will tell them how to care for people who are different from themselves. This type of approach can lead to stereotyping. A **stereotype** is an inaccurate generalization used to describe all members of a specific group without exception. Stereotypes ignore the ever-present individual variations that occur within every cultural group. When texts and articles present highly specific information about a cultural group, stereotypes may be perpetuated about that group because individual variations are ignored.

Did you discover any stereotypes present in your group of classmates when you played the "what we have in common" culture game?

Critical Thinking Exercise

During a seminar on business practices, the presenter, while talking about a specific business practice, singled out an engineer in the group who was of Japanese descent. He used the engineer as an example of someone who thinks differently from "Americans" because he is Asian. The engineer was a third-generation American and had no clue what the presenter was talking about. What is your reaction to this situation?

Cultural Diversity

The process of giving up your own culture and adopting the culture of the dominant group is called **assimilation.** Culturally different groups do adopt some of the culture of the dominant group. Although assimilation does occur, members of the generations that follow the original immigrants usually retain some elements of their original culture.

The concept of the melting pot has been replaced by the concept of cultural diversity. The many differences in the elements of culture (**cultural pluralism**) in groups of people in American and Canadian society are called *cultural diversity*. Traditionally, examples of groups that have been identified as culturally diverse are Asians, blacks, Hispanics, Native Americans, and whites. As a practical/vocational nurse, you need to define this concept more broadly. Defined more broadly, examples of culturally diverse groups include single parents, people who live in poverty, homosexuals, bisexuals, the wealthy, and people with disabilities.

The concept of race as a means of categorizing people by biologic traits has come under attack by scientists. These scientists suggest using ethnicity as a more accurate means of capturing the great diversity found in the 6 billion people in the world. Members of **ethnic groups** are a special type of cultural group composed of people who are members of the same race, religion, or nation, or speak the same language. They derive part of their identity through membership in the ethnic group. Examples of ethnic groups in the United States include Irish-Americans, African-Americans, Asian-Americans, German-Americans, Hispanics, Jews, Native Americans, Arab-Americans, Greek-Americans, and many more.

Importance of Cultural Diversity

As a practical/vocational nurse, you must be aware that cultural diversity is ever-present in the clinical situation. Failure to develop sensitivity to and competence in handling this diversity could lead to misunderstanding between the client and you. Stress can result. The plan of treatment for the client could fail. You could make false assumptions. You might label clients as difficult or uncooperative when their lack of cooperation with the plan of care could be related to a conflict with their personal health belief system. Less-than-adequate care could be experienced by clients when cultural diversity and the differences it represents are overlooked or misinterpreted.

Philosophy of Individual Worth and Celebration of Our Uniqueness

The philosophy of individual worth is the belief shared by all members of the health care team in the uniqueness and value of each human being who comes for care regardless of differences that may be observed or perceived in that individual. As a practical/vocational nurse, you need to realize that each individual has the right to live according to his or her personal beliefs and values *as long as they do not interfere with the rights of others.* Each individual deserves respect as a human being.

Many factors are responsible for differences in clients. They may think and behave differently because of social class, religion, ethnic background, or personal choice. Regardless of these differences, all clients have the right to receive high-quality nursing care. As a practical/vocational nurse you cannot decrease the quality of the care you give because of differences you observe or perceive.

Practical/vocational nurses need to guard against making judgments about people who are culturally different. This does not mean you must accept for yourself the differences you observe. It means being open-minded and **nonjudgmental.** It means taking the difference at face value, accepting people as they are, and giving high-quality care. Be aware of your own attitudes, beliefs, and values as they affect your ability to give care. If you do identify biases, see them for what they are. Become sensitive to cultural differences, and acknowledge that they exist. Gather knowledge about them so that you can work on trying to modify your biases and provide more culturally competent care.

Learning About Cultural Diversity

How to Begin

Unless you understand your own culture, it will be difficult to understand the culture of others. For starters, you need to look inside yourself to learn about your own cultural beliefs, values, and world view and how they influence how you think and act. Some elements of your culture are obvious— for example, your language, arts, celebrated holidays, and how and what you eat. However, much of your culture is hidden. Elements such as aspects of communication, beliefs, attitudes, values, sex roles, use of space, concept of time, and family ties and dynamics are more difficult to perceive and discuss.

How Many Hats Do You Wear? Or What Roles Do You Play?

Each of you fills many roles in your daily life. Sometimes you refer to this situation as wearing many hats. Some of these roles are played out individually, one at a time. Sometimes you play many roles at the same time. The exercises that follow will give you the opportunity to identify your personal cultural background.

Learning Exercise: Identifying the Roles You Play in Your Daily Life

The following categories describe the roles you play in several areas in your everyday life.

Category 1   Economic Status Role

Although standards are available to assign persons to each of the following economic classes, people generally place themselves in one of the following categories by how they perceive their economic status. Place a checkmark next to the economic class that best describes you. I am in the

_____ Lower economic class

_____ Middle economic class

_____ Upper economic class

Category 2   Political Role

Put a checkmark next to the word(s) that best describes the political role you play in society. I am

_____ Republican

_____ Democrat

_____ Independent

_____ Liberal

_____ Conservative

_____ Moderate

_____ Indifferent

_____ To the left of liberal

_____ To the right of conservative

Other _____

Category 3   Racial or Ethnic Role

Place a checkmark beside the racial or ethnic term that best describes you. Be sure to read the complete list before you choose. I am a(an)

_____ African-American

_____ American

_____ American-Indian

_____ Amerindian

_____ Anglo-Saxon

_____ Anglo

_____ Asian-American

_____ Asian

_____ Black

_____ Chicano

_____ Ethnic

_____ Gypsy

_____ Hispanic

_____ Indian

_____ Latin-American

_____ Latvian-American

_____ Native American

Learning Exercise: Identifying the Roles You Play in Your Daily Life *Continued*

_____ Spanish-speaking

_____ White

Other _____

Category 4   Social Role

Circle the social roles that best describe you.
I am (a)

female, male
married, single
separated, divorced
blended family
wife, husband
significant other
mother, father
daughter, son
sister, brother
stepmother, stepfather
stepdaughter, stepson
stepsister, stepbrother
half-sister, half-brother
godmother, godfather
godchild
grandmother, grandfather
granddaughter, grandson
aunt, uncle
niece, nephew
cousin
Other _____

Category 5   Work Role

Place a checkmark beside each work role you play
in your life.

_____ Blue-collar worker

_____ Business person

_____ Laborer

_____ Professional

_____ Service provider

_____ Skilled worker

_____ Student

_____ Technician

_____ Unemployed

_____ White-collar worker

Other _____

Summarize the hats you wear by listing the items
you have checked and circled in the categories below.

Category 1   Economic status role _____

Category 2   Political role _____

Category 3   Racial or ethnic role _____

Category 4   Social role _____

Category 5   Work role _____

Make up a sentence using all the words you listed
in the five categories. This sentence describes you
by the roles you play in your life. Each student
should write the sentence on a piece of paper and
put it in a paper bag. Someone can read each sentence, and the class can guess who the sentence
describes. (Adapted from Randall-David, 1992.)

What Makes Me Unique?

During class time, take a few minutes to play the What Makes Me Unique? culture game. The class divides into small but equal-sized groups. This activity is especially helpful when classmates you perceive to be "the same as" you are in the same group. Seek to find one item that makes you unique from other members of the group. This culture game was played by one of your authors with a group of people she had worked with for years and thought she knew inside out. What a surprise it was to find out that one person was a twin, another had worked with the lepers in Hawaii when she was very young, and another had a relative who was in a crowd scene in one of the Diehard movies. When discovering your uniqueness, it is not time to be humble. Let your uniqueness show. After your small-group work, share with the class the item that makes you unique.

Areas of Cultural Diversity

Areas of cultural diversity that might ordinarily be taken for granted in client situations as well as everyday life include family, food preferences, religion, communication, educational background, economic level, and wellness and illness beliefs and practices. After reading the following general information about each area, you will be given an opportunity to develop an awareness of your own cultural patterns in these areas by answering a group of statements or questions. Sharing this information with peers can be a good learning experience. Sharing will highlight the cultural diversity that exists in your nursing class, regardless of cultural background. See Table 9–1 for profiles of five culturally diverse groups.

Family Structure

No matter what culture is being discussed, the family is the basic unit of society. The role of the family is to have children, if desired or as they come, and to raise them to be contributing members of the group. Actual child-rearing practices vary from culture to culture. Families generally socialize the young to the culture of the group. They meet the physical and psychological needs of the young in culturally specific ways. Some cultures expect the nuclear family (mother, father, and children) to live in the same house. Others may expect the extended family (the nuclear family plus the grandparents and other kinsmen) to do so. Some Vietnamese families are examples of extended families, with three or more generations living in the same house. In many of these families, ties are strong. Behaviors that enhance the family name are encouraged, for example, obedience to parents and those in authority.

The traditional nuclear family is being challenged by the single-parent family. According to the 1990 statistics of the U.S. Bureau of the Census, approximately 25% of all households in the United States were single-parent families. A parent may become a single parent on the death of a spouse, by electing not to marry at the time of pregnancy, or by divorce. Health care workers who have not been in the same situation may be unaware of and insensitive to the special way of life of this type of family. Respond to the following statements. Your responses will help you discover your own cultural patterns in regard to the family.

1. Describe your family structure (nuclear, extended, or alternative life style).
2. Describe the role of children, if any, in your family.
3. Discuss who gives permission for hospitalization in your family.
4. List factors that influence the decision of your family members to visit or not to visit the hospital when a member is ill.
5. Describe the effect that your hospitalization today at 4 PM for surgery tomorrow would have on you and your family.

Food Preferences

All cultures use food to provide needed nutrients. However, what they eat, when they eat, and how they eat differ vastly by cultural group. Knowledge of nutrition as a science differs by culture. It is interesting that the soil of some cultures, for example, Mexico, encouraged the growth of two complementary proteins (corn and beans) that became staples of that culture's diet. Specific foods in different cultures have different meanings. All cultures use food during celebrations. Through generations of experience, different cultures have learned to use different foods to promote health and cure disease. To assist you in identifying your own cultural patterns in regard to food preferences, respond to the following statements or questions.

1. State your favorite food.
2. Identify one special occasion in which your cultural group participates. What foods, if any, are part of this celebration?
3. State your favorite "recipe" from your mother and from your grandmother. What special ingredients or techniques are used to make this food? Is there a written recipe?
4. List a food that is a comfort to you or makes you feel good. In what situation do you use this food?

Religious Beliefs

Religious beliefs are personal to the individual. Religion is an important aspect of culture. Religion can have different meanings in people's lives. For some, religion is a brief, momentary, and sporadic part of daily life. For others, it may influence every aspect of life and have a profound effect on personal outlook and on how one lives. Chapter 10 deals with religious differences. This aspect of life cannot be excluded from the present chapter. There is a close relationship between religious beliefs and the concept of wellness and illness in some groups. Practical/vocational nurses should be aware of their own religious beliefs, obligations, and attitudes. They should know whether these beliefs and attitudes influence the care that is given to clients. The questions that follow give you the opportunity to discover your own cultural patterns in regard to religion.

1. Do you have a religious affiliation? If so, state it.

2. What role does religion play in your life?
3. Is prayer helpful to you?
4. What is your source of strength and hope?
5. What rituals or religious practices are important to you?
6. What symbols or religious books are helpful to you?
7. What dietary inclusions or restrictions are part of your religious beliefs?
8. How does your religion view the source and meaning of pain and suffering?

Concept of Time

Some persons follow clock time. An hour has a beginning and an end (after 60 minutes). People who follow clock time eat, sleep, work, and engage in recreational activities at definite times each day. Some persons live on linear time. Time for them is a straight line with no beginning and no end. People who follow linear time eat when they are hungry and sleep when they are tired. The questions that follow give you an opportunity to discover your own cultural patterns in regard to time.

1. What determines when it is time for you to eat or sleep?
2. Do you wear a watch if you are not in the clinical area?
3. Are you on time for appointments?

Communication

Chapter 8 introduced you to some types of communication and some barriers to the communication process. A major barrier to communication in health care is a different language spoken by the client or nurse. A person's language gives a view of reality that may differ from yours. For example, in English the clock runs, but in Spanish it walks. This illustrates the different concept of time between the two cultures. For a person with English as a first language, time could move quickly, and there may be a rush to get things done. For those with Spanish as a first language, time may move more slowly. The following is a list of areas of communication that may vary for people who are culturally different.

TABLE 9–1: Cultural Diversity Profiles

These profiles reflect only one person's perspective of the culture discussed and are intended to be a general sketch of the culture.

	African Americans	Hmong	Latinos	Native Americans	Northeastern Wisconsinites
History/ Traditions	Origin: Africa. Elders pass on history and tradition and are held in high esteem	Refugees from Vietnam	Women carry on the family and religious traditions	Traditions passed on through ceremonies	Predominantly of German and Belgian origin. Home of the Oneida and Menominee Indians. Also home to Hmong, Hispanic, African-Americans, and Arab-Americans
Family Structure	Strong kinship bonds with extended family	Immediate family plus father, mother, brothers, sisters, uncles, aunts, nieces, nephews considered one family	Family not always defined by blood or marriage. Godparents are important part of family structure	Biologic extended family. Also includes those who are not blood relatives	Emphasis on extended family and large families. Newcomers may have problems being accepted. Emphasis on privacy
Religion	Catholic, Episcopalian, Baptist, African Methodist Episcopal Church, Muslim, and Pentecostal	Animism: worship of deceased ancestors. This worship helps bless the living family	Catholicism most common religion	Spiritual rituals important. Religion and spirituality are different. In addition to practicing Indian spirituality, many belong to traditional Christian religions	Traditionally Catholic and Lutheran but ecumenical in spirit. Live by motto "Help thy neighbor." Green Bay Packers are a regional religion

Food	Chicken, pork, fish. Prefer natural foods such as vegetables, fruits, nuts, beans, peppers, onions, greens, yams, cornbread	Rice the main food—served at breakfast, lunch, and dinner	Red meat, rice, vermicelli, rice, pinto beans, tortillas, potatoes, tomatoes, chilies, onions, garlic, limes, oranges, bananas, mangoes. May not trim or drain off fat when cooking meat	Each Indian ceremony is associated with a specific food that conveys a meaning. Bread, meat, fish, natural fruit, and potatoes are served. Soups are important. Sweets not a part of the traditional diet	Chicken booyah, Belgian pie, bratwurst, beer, brandy, cherry bounce, kneecaps. Live in a state with one of the highest intakes of snacks in the United States (excess salt and fat intake)
Health Beliefs	Illness results from bad spirits, eating poisoned foods, angering the creator, or putting off the creator's warnings. May treat illnesses with home remedies. May wait until illness becomes too serious before seeking medical care. May visit a spiritualist	Natural plants and roots used to cure a sick person. Shaman can be called on to sham a client	Illness a consequence of behavior or the will of God. Therefore, a person is tempting fate by going to the doctor when there is nothing wrong. Sobadores work with complaints of stress, mood swings, or depression. The "bad spirit" in the body must be exorcised or massaged to bring body, mind, and spirit back in sync. May use herbs, roots, and ointments for body ailments. Curanderos have knowledge of homeopathic remedies	Illness is seen as being out of balance or harmony. Spiritual well-being affects physical well-being	Illness due to accident, germs, or may be a punishment from God. Folk remedies. Use traditional medicine

Adapted from Reinhardt E. *Through the Eyes of Others—Intercultural Resource Directory for Health Care Professionals.* Minneapolis: University of Minnesota School of Public Health, 1995, pp. 5–6, 8–14.

139

FORMS OF GREETINGS AND GOODBYES. You may greet your client and want to get right down to business, but the client might expect some light conversation before getting down to the matter at hand. In some cultural groups people take an hour to say good-bye, whereas, in others, people may get up and leave without saying anything.

APPROPRIATENESS OF THE SITUATION. Some groups prefer people to sit, not stand, while they converse. In some groups the sharing of food is a good way to relate to others and get them to verbalize.

CONFIDENTIALITY. All information the client gives the nurse is considered confidential. Some clients do not want their spouse questioned or informed about their problems of the reproductive organs because they fear the spouse may think they are less desirable sexually.

EMOTIONS AND FEELINGS AND THEIR EXPRESSION. Emotions are universal, but the cues to those emotions vary considerably. A lack of awareness of this fact can cause unnecessary stress between the client and the nurse. In some cultural groups people cannot display affection in public, show disapproval or frustration, or vent anger. Some cannot take criticism. You may show dissatisfaction with other members of the health care team by approaching them directly, whereas some team members may show dissatisfaction with you by being polite to your face but then complaining about you to the rest of the staff.

PAIN EXPRESSION. Pain has two parts, sensation and response. All individuals experience the same sensation of pain. However, one's culture influences the definition of pain and the response to the sensation. Pain is whatever the person says it is. It exists whenever the person says it does. One's culture provides guidelines for approved ways of expressing one's response to the pain sensation and ways to relieve the pain. Some cultures teach individuals that it is acceptable to cry, moan, and ex-

hibit other behavior that calls attention to the pain. These behaviors may also be a cure for pain. Other cultures encourage uncomplaining acceptance of pain and passive behavior when pain is experienced (stoic behavior). Discuss some nursing situations in which these two different reactions to pain could have negative consequences if a practical/vocational nurse lacked knowledge of cultural differences in pain expression (for example, a woman in labor or a client having a heart attack).

TEMPO OF CONVERSATION. You may tend to speak quickly and expect a quick response. The client may be accustomed to pausing and reflecting before giving a response.

THE MEANING OF SILENCE. Silence can mean anything from disapproval to warmth, but generally it does not indicate tension or lack of rapport. Silence can be difficult for some persons to tolerate. Resist the temptation to jump in at a pause in the conversation by forcing yourself to meditate or even by biting your tongue (not literally, we hope).

Now develop an awareness of your own cultural patterns in communication by answering the following questions:

1. What facial or body habits are you aware of in yourself while you are talking?
2. How do you greet people and how do you say good-bye?
3. How do you express
   a. love?
   b. hate?
   c. fear?
   d. excitement?
   e. disappointment?
   f. dissatisfaction?
   g. humor?
   h. anger?
   i. sadness?
   j. happiness?
4. Do you make eye contact when you talk to people?
5. Do you touch people while talking?
   a. If so, how do they react?

b. How do you react when people touch you while they are talking to you?

See Box 9–1 on Hints for Using Interpreters.

Box 9–1. Hints for Using Interpreters

Interpreters provide an invaluable service when clients do not speak English or do not have sufficient experience with the English language to understand complex medical information. To decrease the possibility of difficulties in an interpreter situation, follow these suggestions.

1. The ideal interpreter should be trained in the health care field, proficient in the language of the client and the nurse, and understand and respect the culture of the client.
2. If the ideal interpreter is not available, make sure that the individual chosen has training in medical terminology, understands the health matter that needs to be translated, and also understands the requirements for confidentiality, neutrality, and accuracy.
3. Use family members as interpreters cautiously. Clients of specific cultures may be embarrassed to discuss intimate matters with family members who are younger or older or of the opposite sex. Family members may censor information to protect the client or the family.
4. Make sure the interpreter is acceptable to the client.
5. Look and speak directly to the client.
6. Speak clearly and slowly in a normal voice. Use short units of speech.
7. Avoid slang and professional jargon.
8. Observe the nonverbal communication of the client.
9. Be patient. Remember that interpretation is difficult work.

Adapted from Reinhardt E. *Through the Eyes of Others—Intercultural Resource Directory for Health Care Professionals.* Minneapolis: University of Minnesota School of Public Health, 1995.

Educational Background

Approximately 27 million persons in the United States have literacy skills below the fourth-grade level. These persons are called functionally illiterate. The functionally illiterate have trouble reading and understanding simple directions. Some adults have literacy skills below the eighth-grade level. Differences in educational background need to be taken into consideration when one is teaching clients. It has been estimated that one of every three Americans has some difficulty with reading or writing. Adapt your explanations to the client's level of understanding. Responding to the following statements will help you identify your own beliefs and practices in regard to education.

1. Calculate the number of years of education you have had.
2. State your ultimate educational goal.
3. Discuss the role education plays in your life.
4. Describe your feelings toward a person who has less education than you have.
5. Describe your feelings toward a person who has more education than you have.
6. Describe your feelings if you were referred to your school's skills center.
7. Discuss the impact of your cultural background on your values and practices with regard to education.
8. Who in your family has graduated from high school, technical school, junior college, or college or university?

Economic Level

Economic level is frequently related to educational background. Sociologists use these two factors to determine the social class of individuals. You will meet clients who are very wealthy and clients who are at or near the poverty level. Others have mid-level incomes. A client's annual income determines the type of house he or she lives in, the neighborhood where he or she lives, the availability of food, and the ability to participate in certain types of preventive health care. Practical/vocational nurses have to take economic level into consideration when they make suggestions during client teaching and should adapt the suggestions accordingly.

Identify your personal patterns in regard to economic level by responding to the following statements or questions.

1. Describe how your economic background affects your daily life in the following areas:
   a. Availability of food
   b. Availability of shelter
   c. Availability of clothing
   d. Amount and type of recreation
2. Discuss your feelings toward a person who has less money than you have.
3. Discuss your feelings toward a person who has more money than you have.
4. Describe how these feelings fit with those of your cultural group.
5. Discuss your ability to afford to go to a physician when you get sick.
6. If you work, do you have health insurance benefits?

Wellness and Illness Beliefs and Practices

Wellness and illness can have different meanings for persons who are culturally different. Wellness and illness are relative terms. What is good health to one person can be sickness to another. Wellness may not be a high-priority matter to some clients. Some clients believe that illness can be prevented; they practice elaborate rituals and engage special persons to carry out those rituals in an attempt to prevent disease. Some rituals may be used to cure disease. Other clients look at prevention as an attempt to control the future. They may consider this an impossible feat in the way they view their lives. Some people may think prevention is tempting fate or the gods; to follow through with prevention would be risky. Others wonder about the necessity of making a trip to a health care provider for preventive care, for example, immunizations.

When disease does strike, some people blame pathogens (germs), others spirits, and others an imbalance in the body. Generally, death and dying bring out strong emotions in most people. Be aware that some cultures have special taboos and prohibitions when death occurs. Roles that family and friends carry out at the time of death may vary.

Some cultural groups attach a stigma to mental illness and psychiatrists. They may not attach the same stigma to impairments of physical health. Some groups may feel that the mental symptoms manifested are a healthy reaction to an emotional crisis. Some cultural groups believe that the mind and body are united and are not separate entities. These cultures may have traditional healers who are expert at healing both the mind and the body. Some people may seek out traditional healers to heal the mind while at the same time consulting Western medicine to heal the body.

In the area of nutrition, some groups believe that special foods or food combinations can prevent or cure illnesses. Others see no relationship between the diet and health. Individuals in some cultures are embarrassed when they have to discuss bodily functions or allow certain body parts to be examined. Others are not bothered by this. Hygiene practices vary according to beliefs, living conditions, personal resources, and physical characteristics. To assist you in identifying your own cultural patterns in regard to wellness beliefs and practices, respond to the following statements and questions.

1. Describe what it means to you to have good health.
2. What are some of your own practices or beliefs about staying well?
3. Describe what it means to you to be sick.
4. List some foods in your diet that you think help prevent illness.
   a. How does eating these foods prevent illness?
   b. What are some foods you must avoid to prevent illness?
5. List some foods in your diet that help you recover when you are sick.
   a. What foods are they?

b. What illnesses do they cure?

c. How do they cure illness?

6. How do you care for your skin and hair?

7. Describe the customs you follow when there is a death in your family.

a. Who makes the burial arrangements?

b. Who should be present when the death occurs?

c. Describe what you believe happens to a person after death.

d. Do you have a get-together after the burial? If so, for whom?

e. How does your family remember the dead?

8. Describe your attitude toward mental illness.

9. Describe what you think causes mental illness.

10. Who do you think should treat mental illness?

■ It is hoped that some of these exercises have started you thinking about the many ways you and your peers differ, regardless of which cultural group you belong to. And along with that awareness a tolerance may be developing for ways of doing things that may be different from yours. No particular way or world view is correct. *It merely is.* ■

Increasing Your Knowledge of Culturally Diverse Clients

Before discussing how to increase your knowledge of specific cultures, it must be said that no one can be an expert on every culture in the world. Even "experts" of one culture are cautious about being labeled an expert. These people are aware of the ever-changing nature of cultures and of the important individual variations that occur within any cultural group. Experts are always cautious about stereotyping persons in any particular cultural group.

There are strategies that can help you increase your knowledge of different cultures. First, avoid applying the information you gain automatically to all individuals in that group. This may be called the cookbook method of learning about different cul-

tures. To apply information in this way makes you guilty of stereotyping individuals—assuming that everyone in that cultural group is the same. You have already learned that classifying people as being the same just because they share the same religion, life style, or ethnic background is stereotyping. Leave room for personal variations within each cultural group about which you gather information.

Suggestions for Learning More About Culturally Diverse Groups

1. Identify the different cultural groups in your community.

2. Read about the different cultures to which you are personally exposed. The list of suggested readings on pages 150 and 151 can help you get started. Use the suggestions given in Chapter 7 to find additional information about specific cultural groups through your learning resource center.

3. A helpful class activity is to hear reports from peers about various cultural groups. Remember to think beyond the more traditional cultural groups based on ethnicity. Include the disabled, aged, single parents, different sexual life styles, and so on. And remember to allow for individual variations and the fact that cultures are always changing.

Categories of Major Health Belief Systems

Anthropologists are scientists who study the physical and cultural characteristics of human groups. A helpful framework for generally discovering and understanding health belief systems has been developed by these scientists. They divide systems of health beliefs into three major systems: biomedicine, personalistic, and naturalistic.

Biomedicine is the primary belief system of the United States and is also called Western medicine. There is a movement in nursing education at all levels to transform curriculums so that they reflect multicultural concepts in nursing. However, it is possible that the curriculum of your school of practical/vocational nursing is set up to reflect biomedicine.

The **personalistic system** is found among groups native to the Americas as well as those south of the Sahara and among the tribal peoples of Asia (Jackson, 1993, pp. 30, 32). The **naturalistic system** of beliefs developed from the traditional medical practices of the ancient civilizations of China, India, and Greece. Variants of this belief system are found today in the Philippines and among low-income blacks and poor white southerners (Jackson, 1993, p. 37). Rarely does a group ascribe to all the beliefs in one system. You might see elements of each of the three systems at work in one individual. With this in mind, Table 9–2 compares these three health belief systems according to: (1) location of the belief system, (2) cause of disease, (3) how disease is diagnosed and treated,

TABLE 9–2: Categories of Major Health Beliefs

	Biomedicine	Personalistic	Naturalistic
Location of belief system	United States, Western countries	Native Americans, Africa south of the Sahara	Japan, China, Vietnam, Korea, Taiwan
Cause of disease	Abnormalities in structure and function of body organs by pathogens (germs), biochemical alterations, environmental factors	Sick person punished by a deity, ghost, god, evil spirit, witch, or angry ancestor; punishment may include poisoning, stealing of soul, witchcraft	Imbalance of body elements caused by excessive heat (yang) and cold (ying)
How disease is diagnosed	Physical exam, x-ray, identification of pathogens by lab studies	Agent is identified by magical powers, trances, and so on	Cause is identified as excess heat or cold
How disease is treated	Drugs, surgery, diet	Curing rituals, relief of symptoms by herbs	Restore body balance: "hot" illness treated by cold, "cold" illness treated by hot; also, acupuncture, coining, cupping
Who cures the disease?	Physician	Diviner, herbalist	Physician or herbalist
How disease is prevented	Avoidance of pathogens, preventive life styles including diet, exercise, moderation, safety, immunizations	Faithful obedience to rituals (e.g., wearing amulets), protective spells	Maintain balance of hot and cold in body, mind, and environment

Adapted with permission from Jackson L. Understanding, eliciting and negotiating clients' multicultural health beliefs. Nurse Practitioner, 1993; 18(4): 30–32, 37–38, 42. © Springhouse Corporation.

(4) who is responsible for curing disease, and (5) how disease is prevented.

Developing Plans of Care for Culturally Diverse Clients

Jackson (1993) offers suggestions for discovering the health beliefs of clients, along with guidelines to develop plans of care that incorporate those beliefs through a process of negotiation with the client. Jackson points out that discovering specific health beliefs is easier if the nurse is familiar with a specific culture, but this is not absolutely necessary. She suggests ways of negotiating a treatment plan when dealing with culturally diverse clients. The practical/vocational nurse can collaborate with the professional nurse to incorporate these beliefs into the client's plan of care:

1. Discover the health beliefs of the individual. Be respectful and open-minded when you question the client about the cause of the problem, when it started, its severity, its course, the problems it has caused in the client's life, and the treatment the client thinks will cure the disease. Avoid assuming anything. When you are unsure of anything, ASK! In situations of cultural diversity, our clients are the teachers and we are the students.

2. Negotiate treatment plans with the client. Avoid trying to change clients' beliefs. This is an impossible feat. Cultural health practices are deeply ingrained. Tradition means more than your word does, even though you are a person representing a health profession. Instead, involve the client in making decisions about his or her own care. Do so in a way that does not threaten the client's beliefs and practices or conflict with them. Explain from the biomedical point of view the cause of the disease, how the body is altered by the disease, the role of treatment, and the expected outcome. Then compare the client's belief system with that of biomedicine. All clients need to have this information to help ensure their cooperation with the plan of care. See Box 9–2 for an example of negotiating treatment plans with the client.

Box 9–2. Negotiating Treatment Plans with the Client

Situation

Nancy Thai, a Cambodian refugee, resides in Chicago with her husband and three children. She delivered an 8-pound boy early this morning at St. Mary's Hospital. The practical/vocational nurse who was assigned to Mrs. Thai on the day shift reported to the evening staff that the client was "uncooperative." Specifically, Mrs. Thai refused to eat and take her pills. In frustration, the nurse stated, "I just don't know what to do with her."

Cultural Health Beliefs in This Situation

Mrs. Thai's health beliefs include the belief that pregnancy and birth weaken the body. Also, blood loss during delivery is considered a ying (cold) condition. Mrs. Thai believes that for one month after delivery a mother must have a yang (hot) diet to restore strength, keep the stomach warm, counteract heat loss, prevent incontinence, and prevent itching at the site of the episiotomy. Among preferred foods are rice, pork, and chicken. Cold foods (for example, beef, salad, sour foods), as well as cold water, are bad for the stomach and the teeth.

Negotiating Treatment Plans

The nurse assigned to Mrs. Thai on the evening shift informed Mrs. Thai that the doctor had ordered pills to help prevent bleeding after delivery. After discussing this, Mrs. Thai agreed to take her pills with warm water. In a respectful manner, the evening nurse asked if Mrs. Thai did not like the hospital food. Mrs. Thai smiled and explained her need for a yang diet. The evening nurse said that she could arrange to have the dietary department send rice, chicken, or any other food Mrs. Thai would find helpful after childbirth. Mrs. Thai said her husband would bring rice and chicken from home. The nurse canceled Mrs. Thai's food order but requested a pot of hot water, silverware, and napkins for her use.

3. Preserve the beliefs and practices that are helpful to the client. Starting in 1993, the Office of Alternative Medicine of the National Institutes of Health began to identify, study, and bring together the best healing practices of other cultures with those of Western medicine. Many of the beliefs and practices of non-Western systems of health beliefs have proved beneficial. Examples are acupuncture and acupressure. More are about to be approved. Other practices of your client may not yet have been researched or found effective. Collaborate with your professional nurse about these practices. If they seem to help the client and do no harm, in-clude them in the plan of care, regardless of your ability to see the benefit of the practice. These prac-tices have special significance and meaning to some individuals despite the fact that you may be unable to see how or whether they help. See Box 9–3 for an example of preserving the beliefs and practices that are helpful to the client.

4. Repattern harmful practices. Harmful practices prevalent in Western society include lack of exer-cise, smoking, and diets high in fat and refined sugar. In Burma, when a woman is pregnant, ex-treme dietary restrictions are imposed. In Cambodia, mud is placed on the umbilicus of newborns. Both

---

Box 9–3. Preserving the Beliefs and Practices That Are Helpful to the Client

Situation

Ted Washington, a 72-year-old African American, lives in a rural area of South Carolina. He was admitted to Brent Hospital with pneumonia and advanced osteoarthritis. An LPN, John, is his nurse. John cannot understand how anyone can get to such a state of ill health without seeing a doctor. John is especially upset because Mr. Washington could have prevented much of his disability from arthritis if he had followed a preventive program when he first developed symptoms of this disease.

Cultural Health Beliefs in This Situation

Mr. Washington has been poor during his entire life. As with any person experiencing poverty, his main concern in life has been the present and getting through his problems on a day-to-day basis. Mr. Washington's time orientation is the present, not the future, so preventive regimens have not been central to his way of thinking. Persons with similar backgrounds and situations delay care until the disease interferes with their ability to work or results in a disability.

It cannot be said that Mr. Washington ignored his condition. He participated in self-treatment by using cultural health practices in the form of topical application of oils and ointments to his aching joints. These self-treatments helped Mr. Washington deal physically and psychologically with his condi-tion. Mr. Washington looks at his disability as a punishment from God who let something get into his joints. His belief stems from the wellness and illness beliefs brought to this country by slaves from Africa. These beliefs center on wellness as a state experienced when one is in harmony with nature and illness as a state experienced when disharmony with nature occurs.

Preserving the Beliefs and Practices That Are Helpful to the Client

John supported Mr. Washington's application of oils and ointments. He applied backrub lotion to Mr. Washington's joints at bedtime. John made arrangements for a friend of Mr. Washington's to bring his ointment from home. After clarifying self-treatment with the client, John realized that such applications could give psychological comfort to the client as well as relieve pain. In the future, John will make it a point to ask all newly admitted clients about self-treatment for their diseases.

Box 9–4. Repatterning Harmful Practices

Situation

Over a two-month period of time during the summer, a Chinese infant was seen in a New York clinic for diarrhea that did not respond to treatment. Stool cultures showed no unusual organisms. A change in formula did nothing to stop the diarrhea. During a home visit, the visiting nurse found a hot apartment with several bottles of home-prepared formula on the windowsill. Several other full bottles were in the refrigerator.

Cultural Health Beliefs in This Situation

The child's mother explained that she had recently given birth. Because of this she had to avoid cold. To avoid her exposure to the cold of the refrigerator, her husband would remove the bottles from the refrigerator that she needed during the day before he left for work, and line them up on the windowsill.

Repatterning the Client's Harmful Practices

The visiting nurse explained that by being exposed to the heat of the day, the formula would grow germs that could cause diarrhea. She asked if there was a way that the bottles could be kept cold till needed. After some thought, the mother said she could put on a hat, coat, and gloves before removing bottles from the refrigerator. The nurse agreed with this plan. The baby had no further episodes of diarrhea.

Reproduced with permission from Jackson L. Understanding, eliciting and negotiating clients' multicultural health beliefs. *Nurse Practitioner* 18(4):30–32, 37–38, 42, 1993. © Springhouse Corporation.

these practices are dangerous. If followed, these practices could lead to high blood pressure, heart disease, obesity, poor fetal development and maternal toxemia, and tetanus in the newborn. Explain your reason for opposing a harmful practice and offer alternatives. See Box 9–4 for an example of **repatterning** harmful practices.

Developing Cultural Competence in Health Care Situations

You have been given the opportunity to begin developing skills that will help you become a practical/vocational nurse who gives culturally competent care. You have been given the opportunity to identify your culture and its strengths and limitations. You can begin to see how your culture affects your thinking and behavior. Knowledge of the three major health belief systems increases your awareness of different world views about the cause, treatment, and prevention of disease. Awareness of ethnocentrism can help you gain respect for these health beliefs and practices even when they are different from yours. Your goal is to respond flexibly when your values and assumptions differ from those of your clients.

Follow Jackson's (1993) suggestions for negotiating client care with culturally diverse clients. Doing so will result in fewer dissatisfied clients and more compliance with the plan of care. Box 9–5 includes suggestions for the practical/vocational nurse working in a community with culturally diverse clients.

Box 9–5. Modifying the Environment to Accommodate Culturally Diverse Clients

The health care environment can be made more "welcoming" to culturally diverse clients. Many of these changes require little cost or time to implement. But the results can promote better health among culturally diverse clients.

1. Identify the various cultural groups that use the health care facility.
2. Post welcome signs in the languages of the groups you serve.
3. Arrange for messages on answering machines to include the languages of the clients you serve.
4. Place magazines in the waiting room that reflect the diversity of the clients you serve.
5. Play background music that reflects the diversity of the clients you serve.
6. Provide handouts, appointment cards, and client education materials in the languages of the clients you serve.
7. Decorate the environment (pictures, posters, objects, etc.) to reflect the diversity of the clients you serve.
8. Stock adhesive bandages that do not match any specific skin tone—for example, Walt Disney characters and fluorescent colors.
9. In waiting areas, provide books, toys, and multicultural videos for children that promote acceptance of diversity. Barney and Sesame Street themes are especially effective.

Adapted from Reinhardt E. Through the Eyes of Others—Intercultural Resource Directory for Health Care Professionals. Minneapolis: University of Minnesota School of Public Health, 1995, pp. 19–20.

Summary

☐ A good place to start learning about how people are different is to remind yourself that all persons have similarities. The nine basic daily needs are shared by everyone. How individuals meet these needs varies with their culture, the learned ways they have of doing things.

☐ One guideline in health care is the philosophy of individual worth, the belief that all persons are unique and have value regardless of the way they view their world, and they deserve the best nursing care you can give.

☐ Awareness of cultural diversity is important for practical/vocational nurses so that they can avoid false assumptions and misunderstandings about the clients for whom they care. The first step in understanding other people's culture is to understand your own. It is important to be aware of your personal beliefs and practices in the areas of family, religion, communication, educational background, economic level, and wellness and illness beliefs and practices. Some ways to learn about cultural diversity include reading about different cultures, especially those found in your geographic area, and hearing reports from your peers who are culturally different. *Always allow for individual variations within specific groups.*

☐ Understanding your own culture, gaining knowledge about other peoples' culture, attaining sensitivity to cultural diversity, and adapting the plan of care to reflect the client's health and illness beliefs puts you well on the road to providing culturally competent nursing care.

Review Questions

1. Select the statement that best illustrates the philosophy of individual worth.
   A. All individuals are unique and have value regardless of their differences.
   B. People belonging to ethnic groups and minorities have different daily needs.
   C. People of different cultures need to be approached as if their culture is the best culture.
   D. People of color are sensitive about their differences and need to have these differences downplayed in client situations.
2. What is the most practical way for a practical/vocational nurse to begin developing cultural awareness of different groups?
   A. Major in sociology.
   B. Ask friends to tell you about their cultures.
   C. Live with the cultural group that most interests you.
   D. Read articles and books about cultures with whom you have contact in your daily practice.
3. If an Asian-American resident in a nursing home does not want to follow the nursing care plan regarding diet, the best course for the nursing staff would be to

A. Insist the resident follow orders.
B. Document the stubbornness of the resident.
C. Avoid making an issue of his noncompliance.
D. Consider the possibility of cultural differences.
4. Select the trait practical/vocational nurses need to avoid when studying different cultures.
   A. Assimilating
   B. Stereotyping
   C. Acculturating
   D. Diversifying
5. Select the priority cultural concern of the practical/vocational nurse for administering pain medication to a client whose culture values stoic behavior.
   A. That the drug be kept in a dark container.
   B. That the drug is always kept with the client.
   C. That nonverbal signs of pain not be overlooked in this situation.
   D. That the client be asked at the beginning of each shift whether she has pain.

References

Culver V. *Modern Bedside Care,* 8th ed. Philadelphia: W. B. Saunders, 1974, pp. 374–384.

Jackson L. Understanding, eliciting and negotiating clients' multicultural health beliefs. Nurse Practitioner 18(4):30–32, 37–43, 1993.

Leininger M. Transcultural nursing education: A worldwide imperative. Nurs Health Care 15(5):254–257, 1994.

Morganthau T. What color is black? Newsweek 125(7):63–65, 67–70, 72, 1995.

Randall-David E. *Strategies for Working with Culturally Diverse Clients.* Bethesda, MD: Association for the Care of Children's Health, 1992.

Reinhardt E. *Through the Eyes of Others—Intercultural Resource Directory for Health Care Professionals.* Minneapolis: Hennepin County Medical Society, United Way Intercultural Awareness Task Force, Junior League of Minneapolis, and University of Minnesota School of Public Health, 1995.

Bibliography

Bartol, G. Using literature to create cultural competence. Image: Journal of Nursing Scholarship 30(1):75–79, 1998.

Bushy A. Ethnocultural sensitivity and measurement of consumer satisfaction. J Nurs Care Quality 9(2):16–25, 1995.

DeWit S. *Essentials of Medical-Surgical Nursing,* 4th ed. Philadelphia: W. B. Saunders, 1998.

Foster G. *Medical Anthropology.* New York: John Wiley and Sons, 1978 (now out of print).

Geissler, E. *Pocket Guide to Cultural Assessment.* St. Louis: C. V. Mosby, 1998.

Giger J, Davidhizar R. *Transcultural Nursing: Assessment and Intervention.* St. Louis: Mosby-Year Book, 1995.

Giger J., Davidhizar R. *Canadian Transcultural Nursing: Assessment and Intervention.* St. Louis: C.V. Mosby, 1998.

Hall E. *The Silent Language.* Westport, CT: Greenwood Press, 1990.

Hall E. *The Hidden Dimension.* New York: Peter Smith, 1992.

Informed consent, cultural sensitivity, and respect for persons. JAMA 274(10):844–845, 1995.

LaMarca K. Culturally competent cancer care? Cancer Pain Update: Wisconsin Pain Initiative, issue 37, 1995. Published in Madison, WI, by the Wisconsin Cancer Pain Initiative.

Leininger M. *Transcultural Nursing: Concepts, Theory, Research, and Practice.* Columbus, OH: McGraw-Hill and Greyden Press, 1996.

Lipson, J, et al. *Culture and Nursing Care: A Pocket Guide.* San Francisco: UCSF Nursing Press, 1996.

Ludwig-Beymer P. The cultural aspects of pain. HT: The Magazine for Healthcare Travel Professionals 2(4):34–37, 1995.

Rodriguez B. Understanding and integrating cultural awareness and related issues into specialized health curricula. Seminar at Northeast Wisconsin Technical College, Green Bay, WI, May 18, 1995.

Rosenbaum J. Teaching cultural sensitivity. J Nurs Educ 34(4):188–189, 1995.

Suggested Readings

African-Americans

Morganthau T. What color is black? Newsweek 125(7):63–65, 67–70, 72, 1995.

Asian-Americans

Fadiman A. *The Spirit Catches You and You Fall Down.* New York: Farrar, Strauss, and Giroux, 1997.

Kim M. Cultural influences on depression in Korean Americans. J Psychosoc Nurs 33(2):13–18, 1995.

Wong F. The integration of traditional Chinese health practices in nursing. Reflections 24(2):20–21, 1998.

Native Americans

Bell R. Prominence of women in Navajo healing beliefs and values. Nurs Health Care 15(5):232–240, 1994.

Erickson A. Back to basics: Practicing on a reservation. HT: The Magazine for Healthcare Travel Professionals 5(1):6–7, 9, 40–41, 1997.

The Family

Antai-Otong D. *Psychiatric Nursing: Biological and Behavioral Concepts.* Philadelphia: W. B. Saunders, 1995.

Betz C, et al. *Family-Centered Nursing Care of Children.* Philadelphia: W. B. Saunders, 1994.

Ignatavicius D, et al. *Medical-Surgical Nursing Across the Health Care Continuum.* Philadelphia: W. B. Saunders, 1999.

Smith C, Maurer F. *Community Health Nursing: Theory and Practice,* 2nd ed. Philadelphia: W. B. Saunders, 2000.

Varcarolis E. Blended families. In *Foundations of Psychiatric Mental Health Nursing,* 3rd ed. Philadelphia: W. B. Saunders, 1998.

Wong D, Whaley L. *Whaley and Wong's Essentials of Pediatric Nursing,* 5th ed. St. Louis: Mosby-Year Book, 1997.

Single Parents

Betz C, et al. *Family-Centered Nursing Care of Children.* Philadelphia: W. B. Saunders, 1994.

Ignatavicius D, et al. *Medical-Surgical Nursing Across the Health Care Continuum.* Philadelphia: W. B. Saunders, 1999.

Wong D, Whaley L. *Whaley and Wong's Essentials of Pediatric Nursing,* 5th ed. St. Louis: Mosby–Year Book, 1997.

Sexual Orientation

Betz C, et al. *Family-Centered Nursing Care of Children.* Philadelphia: W. B. Saunders, 1994.

Ignatavicius D, et al. *Medical-Surgical Nursing Across the Health Care Continuum.* Philadelphia: W. B. Saunders, 1999.

Misener T, et al. Sexual orientation: A cultural diversity issue for nursing. Nursing Outlook 45(4):178–181, 1997.

Stevens P. Structural and interpersonal impact of heterosexual assumptions on lesbian health care clients. Nurs Res 44(1):25–30, 1995.

Varcarolis E. *Foundations of Psychiatric–Mental Health Nursing,* 3rd ed. Philadelphia: W. B. Saunders, 1998.

Chapter 10

Spiritual Caring, Spiritual Needs, and Religious Differences

Outline

Spirituality and Religion
Spiritual Versus Emotional Dimension
  of the Individual
Who Needs Spiritual Care?
What Is Spiritual Care?
How Do I Meet the Spiritual Needs of
  My Clients?

The Pastoral Care Team
How the Client Meets Spiritual Needs
Religious Needs
Major Western and Eastern Religions
  in the United States and Canada

Major Christian Religions in the
  United States and Canada
Eastern Religions/Philosophies in
  the United States and Canada

Key Terms

agnostics
Allah
atheists
Buddha
Christ
emotional needs

pastoral care team
religion
religious denomination
religious needs
rituals
spirit

spirituality
spiritual caring
spiritual dimension
spiritual distress
spiritual needs
symbols

Objectives

Upon completing this chapter you will
be able to:
1. Differentiate between spirituality
   and religion.
2. Identify the difference between the
   spiritual and emotional dimensions
   of individuals.
3. Discuss the practical/vocational
   nurse's role in providing spiritual
   care to the client and the family.

4. Discuss nursing interventions that
   can be used to meet the spiritual
   needs of clients.
5. List members of the health care
   team who can help provide spiritual care for clients.
6. Discuss your personal religious
   beliefs or the absence of them,
   and how these will influence nursing practice.

7. Discuss the general beliefs that
   account for the differences. among
   various western and eastern religions.
8. Describe specific nursing actions
   that can be used to meet the religious needs of clients.

■ Jan L.P.N., the evening nurse, found Thomas
Berns, age 32, sitting up in bed crying and moaning
with what she interpreted as pain after a testicular
biopsy that was positive for cancer. After assessment, she volunteered to get Thomas some pain
medication but he refused. Tom shouts, "Why did I
have to get cancer? Why me?" Jan then volunteered
to call Thomas's minister. Tom replied, "I'll be fine.

Just let me meditate and pray and I will get rid of
the pain myself." Jan quickly and quietly leaves the
room so Thomas can be alone. ■

The Joint Commission on Accreditation of
Health Care Organizations (JCAHO) requires that
spiritual care be provided to all clients. The North
American Nursing Diagnosis Association (NANDA)

includes the following two nursing diagnoses in its listing:

1. Spiritual distress
2. Potential for enhanced spiritual well-being

In the foregoing client situation, Thomas was in spiritual distress. Thomas's minister might have been able to address Thomas's problem. But at the time, Thomas needed immediate spiritual care. It would have been helpful to Thomas if his nurse would have offered to spend time with him and encouraged him to talk about what he was thinking and feeling at that time. Nursing has always embraced a holistic approach to client care—care of the body, mind, and spirit. Despite the JCAHO mandates and NANDA diagnoses, some nurses are uncomfortable with matters of the spirit. Some have not had adequate education in how to deal with clients in this aspect of care. This chapter will (1) help you differentiate spiritual matters from religious matters, (2) provide interventions for the patient in spiritual distress, and (3) meet the client's religious needs.

Spirituality and Religion

Spirituality is an essential part of being human. The word comes from the Latin word **spiritus,** which means breath or air. The **spirit** is the very essence of a person, the innermost part of a person that provides animation. The spirit is a life force that penetrates a person's entire being. It includes the beliefs and value system that provide strength and hope to persons and give meaning to their lives. It is hoped that the spiritual self grows and matures throughout one's life. Oprah Winfrey provided a good look at the meaning of one's spirit with a segment of her daytime television show called "Remembering Your Spirit."

Spirituality and religion are related terms. But they are not words with the same meaning. **Religion** is a spiritual experience that contains specific beliefs and rituals. Religion includes spirituality. But spirituality, one's life force, does not necessarily include religion. Participation in a religion can include spirituality. But spirituality does not necessarily include participation in a religion.

Spiritual Versus Emotional Dimension of the Individual

The spiritual dimension of a client's life requires the same emphasis that other daily needs receive. When **spiritual needs** of clients exist and are met, practical/vocational nurses can say they have directed care to the total person. Meeting the spiritual needs of clients through spiritual caring differs from providing emotional support. The **spiritual dimension** of a person gives insight into the meaning of life, suffering, and death. This dimension refers to the relationship of an individual to a higher being. **Emotional needs** include how people respond and deal with feelings of joy, anger, sadness, guilt, remorse, sorrow, and love, among others.

Who Needs Spiritual Care?

An individual's spiritual dimension is a very private and personal area. Although all persons have a spiritual dimension, needs that arise in this area depend on a variety of situations and the individual's ability to cope with them. The goal of parish nurses is to keep their groups happy and healthy by treating the whole person—body, mind, and spirit. Parish nurses recognize the relationship between spirituality and health and encourage spiritual growth in their clients.

Crisis situations occur in all health care situations and frequently surface in acute health care situations. An individual's beliefs and values can profoundly affect his or her response to these crises, the attitude toward treatment, and the rate of recovery. Hospitalization, illness, pain, injury, and the prospect of death can intensify a person's spiritual needs. Be especially alert to the need for spiritual care in clients who are in pain, have a chronic or incurable disease, are dying, or have experienced the death of a loved one. Clients who are facing an undesirable outcome of illness (such as an amputation) or have lost control of themselves also may have spiritual needs. "When the body and mind are battered by time and use, the spirit, the very essence of the client remains" (Schoenbeck, 1994, p. 19).

What Is Spiritual Care?

Florence Nightingale encouraged nurses to be instruments of **spiritual caring.** Avoid waiting for crisis situations to occur to be concerned about spiritual care. As a practical/vocational nurse, you have the responsibility to provide spiritual care to all clients. In addition, practical/vocational nurses need to enhance the continued growth and maturity of the client's spiritual self in all client situations.

Perhaps the best place to start in providing spiritual care is to strive to be personally comfortable with spiritual matters. Be aware of your own spirituality and the spirit that is the essence of you. Take a spiritual journey and get to know yourself. The following questions can help you increase awareness of your personal spirituality as well as that of clients.

1. How do you cope?
2. Who is your source of support?
3. With whom do you laugh?
4. Do you feel loved?
5. Do you have someone to cry with?
6. What gives your life meaning?
7. What brings joy to your life?
8. Do you believe in the power of prayer?
9. Do you have a relationship to a higher power?
10. What is your philosophy of death?

Critical Thinking Exercise

Have you ever said or heard others say "my spirit is broken"? What does this remark mean?

How Do I Meet the Spiritual Needs of My Clients?

Once you know your spiritual self, you will be better able to help others meet their spiritual needs. *When you acknowledge that your beliefs are effective for you but not necessarily for others,* you will be able to set your beliefs aside when helping clients meet their spiritual needs. Respect for the client's belief system can give strength, hope, and meaning to his or her life. Ask questions to help clients verbalize beliefs, fears, and concerns, such as, "What do you think is going to happen to you?" "Who is your source of support?" Show interest through supportive statements. Listen with an understanding attitude. Respond as naturally to spiritual concerns as you do to physical needs. It is always a delicate matter to help clients face the reality of a terminal illness without abandoning hope. Encouraging the client's active involvement in self-care can help uphold hope. When a client faces death, you can help to make the remaining days meaningful by attending to needs and approaching the client in a supportive and empathetic manner. Feeling loved helps bring peace to the dying. Box 10–1 lists interventions that can be used by practical/vocational nurses when providing spiritual care.

The Pastoral Care Team

The **pastoral care team** is made up of ministers, priests, rabbis, sisters, and lay persons. All are educated to meet spiritual needs in addition to religious needs in a health care setting. The members of this team are allies with nurses in providing spiritual care. If a health care facility does not have a pastoral care team or a chaplain on the staff, a listing of religious representatives of area churches will be available. You can notify this team with a request for someone to see a client. Whenever members of the pastoral care team come to your unit, inform them of the client's background and condition. Describe the interventions you have incorporated into the client's care to provide spiritual care. Remember

---

Box 10–1. Spiritual Care Interventions

1. Ask open-ended questions.
2. Actively listen to the client. Sit beside the client. Make eye contact.
3. Be nonjudgmental of the client and her or his responses.
4. Avoid giving advice or a lecture to the client.
5. Be aware of nonverbal messages from the client.
6. Experience the feelings of the client but avoid adopting those feelings for yourself (empathy).
7. Expect to learn from clients.
8. Stay with the client after the person has received an unfavorable diagnosis.
9. When appropriate, offer to pray with clients.
10. After assessing the situation and when appropriate, offer to read scripture or other special readings to clients.
11. Assist the client to participate in religious rituals.
12. Protect the client's religious articles.

---

that the pastoral care team does not relieve you of your responsibility to provide spiritual care.

How the Client Meets Spiritual Needs

All clients have a spiritual self. Some clients help meet their spiritual needs by belonging to a specific religious denomination. A **religious denomination** is an organized group of persons who share a philosophy that supports their particular concept of God or a higher being. The different rituals and practices of a religion are stabilizing forces for the client. **Rituals** can bring the security of the past into a crisis situation. Concrete **symbols,** such as pictures, icons, herb packets, rosaries, statues, jew-

elry, and other objects can affirm the client's connection with God.

Prayer is a spiritual practice of some individuals whether or not they are members of an organized religion. Prayer can put a client in touch with a personal God and sometimes can decrease anxiety as effectively as a drug. Illness sometimes interferes with the client's ability to pray. Honor requests to pray with a client. In other situations, carefully assess whether there is an unexpressed need for prayer.

The value of rituals and religious practices is determined by the faith of the client and not by scientific proof of their benefit. Studies have found that people who have faith can recover more quickly from illness, surgery, and addiction and are less likely to die prematurely from any cause. When clients express an interest in praying, ask what prayer they would like to say. Try to accommodate the request. When clients are not allowed to practice their religious rituals, practices, and responsibilities, they may feel guilty and uneasy.

As a practical/vocational nurse, you need to develop an awareness of the general religious philosophy of the client's particular denomination. If membership is claimed in a specific denomination, be aware of the rituals and exercises that the client believes in and practices. **Spiritual distress** can be observed in clients who are unable to practice their religious rituals or who experience a conflict between their religious and spiritual beliefs and the prescribed health regimen.

Agnostics hold the belief that the existence of God can be neither proved nor disproved. **Atheists** do not believe that the supernatural exists, so they do not believe in God. Christians may find comfort and solace in their refuge in God, including passing into another life after death, but the atheist does not have this belief. It may be difficult for the nurse who believes in the supernatural to relate to a person with atheistic beliefs. The nurse may feel unsuccessful in meeting the total needs of the client who is an atheist because atheists do not believe in the supernatural. The nurse encourages this client to express personal feelings about life, death, separation, and loss and does not impose his or her own personal beliefs and values on the client.

Religious Needs

Spiritual needs are not the same as **religious needs.** The religious self refers to the specific beliefs held by an individual in regard to a higher being.

Major religions in the United States and Canada are Judaism, Catholicism, and Protestantism. The Jewish religion is approximately 3000 years old. The three major divisions of Judaism are (1) Orthodox Judaism, which is rigorous about observing rituals, including diet; (2) Conservative Judaism, which adapts traditions to the modern world; and (3) Reform Judaism, which stresses the ethical teachings of the prophets and autonomy of the individual, and regards Judaism as evolving and subject to change. Christianity is approximately 2000 years old. The two major divisions of Christianity are Catholicism and Protestantism. Catholics believe that their religion is the true religion and their dogma is infallible (incapable of error). Authority is traced from Christ through an unbroken line to the Pope, the representative of Christ on earth. Protestantism began in the sixteenth century, when Martin Luther separated from the Catholic church. The term *protestant* means a person who makes a solemn declaration to profess a conviction. Protestants contend that their convictions are closer to New Testament Christianity. During the second half of the nineteenth century, opposition to innovations in protestantism resulted in a conservative type of Protestantism called fundamentalism.

The remainder of this chapter will present the beliefs and practices of some of the numerous religions or groups found in the United States and Canada that evolved from the Judeo-Christian tradition as well as Eastern religions. The emphasis on nursing implications will serve as a reference to be used in meeting the religious needs of specific clients during your time as a student practical/vocational nurse and in your nursing career after you graduate. Although each religion has specific beliefs and practices, sometimes an individual will adapt them to fit his or her own circumstances. Do not assume that all Protestants, Catholics, Jews, for example, actually believe in all the aspects of their formal religion. Do not judge a client if there are variations in his or her beliefs. Clarify with the client which beliefs offer comfort and are preferred. Develop awareness of health issues and decisions that may involve religious beliefs. The references at the end of the chapter can be used to learn more about a specific religion when such information is needed.

Major Christian Religions in the United States and Canada

The Bible

Many Christian clients will find comfort in reading or having someone read to them selected passages from the Bible. Treat the client's Bible with respect. In addition to believing it contains the inspired word of God, some persons have received their Bibles as gifts commemorating special occasions, such as a wedding, graduation, confirmation, anniversary, or jubilee. Some Bibles list passages that can be used in specific client situations, such as pain, sorrow, sleeplessness, and so on.

Baptism

When a client who belongs to a religious group that believes that baptism is essential to salvation requests the sacrament, and death is imminent, the practical/vocational nurse may baptize him or her if the minister or priest has not yet arrived. When the dying client is an infant, baptism may be given if the religious beliefs of the parents include infant baptism. The procedure for baptism is as follows:

1. If the client is Protestant, have a witness present for the baptism if possible. This is not necessary for a Catholic client.
2. Allow water to flow over and contact the client's skin while saying the words: "[name, if known], I baptize you in the name of the Father, and of the Son, and of the Holy Spirit."
3. If the client is Catholic and it is uncertain whether baptism was received in the past,

TABLE 10–1: Baptism Beliefs and Practices

Denomination/Group	Age of Administration	Method	Comments
Assembly of God	Age of accountability	Immersion	The person needs to understand the meaning of baptism
Baha'i	—	—	No baptism
Baptist	Adult	Immersion	Not a means of salvation. Opposed to infant baptism. The person needs to understand the meaning of baptism
Christian Scientist	—	—	No baptism
Eastern Orthodox Churches	Infant	Immersion	Age of infant differs by group
Episcopalian	Infant	Sprinkle	Necessary for salvation
Jehovah's Witnesses	Adult	—	No infant baptism. Necessary for salvation
Lutheran	Infant or adult	Sprinkle or immersion	Infant baptism at 6 to 8 weeks
Methodist	Infant and adult	Sprinkle or immersion	An outward and visible sign of an inward and spiritual grace
Mormon	8 years or older	Immersion	Baptism causes remission of sins. Allows person to receive the gifts of the Holy Spirit. Required for salvation
Presbyterian	Infant	Usually sprinkling	—
Quakers	—	—	No baptism. At birth, infant's name recorded in official book
Roman Catholic	Infant or adult	Usually sprinkling, or immersion	Means of salvation and initiation into the community. Removes all sin. Person receives Holy Spirit
Seventh Day Adventist	Adult	Immersion	Opposed to infant baptism. Makes one a church member
United Church of Christ	Infant	Immersion	When baptized, people become church members

precede the above words with "If capable . . . ." These words indicate the client's desire for the sacrament if it has not been received before.

4. Report the baptism to the chaplain or pastoral care team and the family.
5. Record the baptism in the nurses' notes.

Table 10–1 summarizes the status of baptism in various Christian religious denominations and groups in the United States and Canada.

Communion

Various groups differ in their interpretation of the meaning of communion. Table 10–2 discusses the status of communion beliefs and practices for various Christian denominations and groups in the United States and Canada.

Nursing Implications for Major Christian Denominations and Groups

Table 10–3 lists specific features that have importance in client contact for the major Christian denominations and groups found in the United States and Canada. When meeting a client of a specific affiliation, use the nursing implications as a guide to increase awareness of differences. Avoid stereotyping the client. Question the client and family regarding specific practices. Table 10–4 provides nursing implications for clients who ascribe to Judaism and Islam. Remember not to stereotype a client claiming a specific affiliation. Question the client and/or family to clarify specific beliefs and practices.

Eastern Religions and Philosophies in the United States and Canada

The Western and the Eastern worlds contain different value systems, and the two represent completely different ways of thinking that have molded the culture, including the world view, of two different

TABLE 10–2: Communion Beliefs and Practices		
Denomination/ Group	Do They Have This Practice?	Comments
Assembly of God	Yes	—
Baptist	Yes	A remembrance of Christ's death
Christian Scientist	No	—
Eastern Orthodox Churches	Yes	Belief same as Catholic
Episcopalian	Yes	—
Lutheran	Yes	Believe the presence of Christ is real
Methodist	Yes	Open to everyone
Presbyterian	Yes	Believe Christ is present in spirit
Quaker	No	—
Roman Catholic	Yes	Believe the bread and wine are the body and blood of Christ
Seventh Day Adventist	Yes	Practice washing of the feet in preparation
United Church of Christ	Yes	—

TABLE 10–3: Christian Denominations and Groups

Denomination/Group	Special Features	Nursing Implications
Protestants	General practices to be clarified	Would client like to be visited by personal minister? Does client want Communion, anointing with oil, or time for Bible reading? If client is an infant and condition is serious, do parents desire baptism if child is not baptized? If client is dying, what are family's beliefs about death and dying?
Roman Catholics	General beliefs	If desired and condition allows, make arrangements for client to attend Mass. Ill Catholics are excused from this obligation on Sundays and holy days. If desired, arrange for the sacrament of Reconciliation and provide privacy when the priest hears the client's confession. If desired, arrange for the anointing of the sick, which offers hope, consolation, and peace and assists in physical, mental, and spiritual healing
	The dying Catholic client	Catholic clients facing death may want to receive the Last Rites, which includes the sacraments of penance, the anointing of the sick, and Viaticum (the last Eucharist before "passing over"). Make arrangements for the priest to administer the sacrament of Reconciliation, the anointing of the sick, and Holy Communion
	Observation of dietary rules	When sick, a Catholic is excused from fasting (giving up food for a specified period of time) and abstaining (giving up meat at certain times)
	Desire for religious objects	Catholic clients may request that religious pictures and objects be kept at the bedside or on their persons. These are reminders of God's presence in their lives and are sources of consolation
Jehovah's Witnesses	General beliefs	Jehovah's Witnesses will refuse to receive blood products, including plasma. To receive such products is viewed as a violation of the law of God

continued

TABLE 10–3 continued		
Denomination/Group	**Special Features**	**Nursing Implications**
Seventh Day Adventists	Observation of dietary rules	Adventists generally do not smoke or drink. Some Adventist clients may avoid beverages with caffeine. Many Adventists are vegetarians and use soybean products as a protein source. These dietary practices are not mandatory
	Observation of the Sabbath	Adventists observe the Sabbath from sunset on Friday to sunset on Saturday and do not pursue their jobs or worldly pleasures during this time
Mormons	General beliefs	Mormon clients may avoid tobacco, alcohol, coffee, and tea
Christian Scientists	General beliefs	Clients may believe that sickness can be eliminated through prayer and spiritual understanding. Healing is considered an awakening to this belief. Clients may want to have a Christian Scientist practitioner contacted to give treatment through prayer
Amish	General beliefs and practices	The Amish do not believe in health insurance and social security and rely on mutual aid in time of need. Clients may believe that sudden fright or blood loss may cause loss of the soul. Female clients may not approve of cutting their hair.

parts of the world. In the twentieth century, cultures and religious practices of other countries became more known to us due to travel, the mass media, and immigration of people from all over the world to the United States and Canada. The East (for example, India, China, Japan, and Korea) emphasizes self-discipline and control, the inner nature of self, moderation, nonattachment to worldly things, awareness that selfish desire is the cause of much suffering, tolerance to other religions and points of view, respect for family, elders and authority, and the principle of doing no harm to any living creature. The West (for example, Europe, Canada, and the United States) traditionally emphasizes the value of individual worth, religion as a personal commitment to one God, freedom and democracy, the scientific method, technology, emphasis on the need to satisfy desires, and a wide range of social services. Because of immigration and acculturation of Eastern peoples and interest in and adoption of Eastern philosophies by Western society, both traditions can be seen reflected in the other; for example, the large number of Christians among Eastern peoples and the adoption of meditation, yoga, complementary therapies (including use of herbs), and the focus on inner development in Western peoples.

TABLE 10–4: Major Non-Christian Religions		
Religion	**Special Features**	**Nursing Implications**
Judaism	Observation of Sabbath	If desired, provide time for rest, prayer, and/or study from sunset on Friday till after sunset on Saturday If desired, provide yarmulke (skullcap) or prayer shawl. Inform family of need for these items
	Observation of dietary rules (Kosher)	Clarify if client follows these dietary rules Make arrangements for separate utensils for preparing and serving meat and milk dishes, if desired. If separate dishes are not available, these foods can be served in the original containers or on paper plates. Meat may be consumed a few minutes after drinking milk, but 6 hours must pass after eating meat before drinking milk. Do not serve pork, ham, Canadian bacon, eel, oysters, crab, lobster, shrimp, or eggs with blood spots
	The dying Jewish client	Family and friends may want to be with the client at all times. Some Jews do not believe in autopsies, embalming, or cremation Some Jews may not want the nurse to touch the body of a deceased Jew and may request that the nurse notify the Burial Society for preparation of the body for burial
Islam	General beliefs	Some Muslims, members of the Islam religion, may desire to pray to Allah five times a day (after dawn, at noon, in midafternoon, after sunset, and at night). If client requests to face Mecca, the holy city of Islam, a bed or chair may be positioned in a southeast direction If a Muslim brings the Koran, the holy book of Islam, to the health care institution, do not touch it or place anything on top of it. If a Muslim wears writings from the Koran on a black string around the neck, arm, or waist, these writings need to be kept dry and need to remain on the client Rules of cleanliness may include eating with the right hand and cleansing self with the left hand after urinating and defecating
	Observation of dietary rules	Some Muslims might not eat pork and pork products, eel, oysters, crab, lobster, shrimp, and meats from animals that have not been bled to death by a Muslim. Some Muslims might not drink alcoholic beverages
	Observation of female modesty	Some Muslim females prefer to be clothed from head to ankle. During a physical examination, they may prefer to undress one body part at a time

Because of the variation in beliefs and history of Eastern groups, time interval since immigration and degree of acculturation, it is difficult to provide black on white examples of what a Japanese American or East Indian Hindu American believes and practices. Buddhism, from which much of Eastern beliefs has evolved, is an example of this difficulty.

Buddhism can be considered a religion, a philosophy, and a way of life. Well before Christianity, Buddhism originated in India, as did Hinduism, and shares much with Hindu philosophy but also radically departs from it (see Table 10–5). Buddhism spread to China, Japan, Korea, Tibet, Burma, Sri Lanka, Laos, Cambodia, and Vietnam. As Bud-

---

TABLE 10–5: Comparison of General Religious Beliefs/Practices of Buddhist and Hindu Clients

Belief/Practice	Nursing Implications
Not having a central authority or dictated doctrine, the approximately 550,000 **Buddhists** and 1.3 million **Hindus** in North America exhibit a variety of traditions, beliefs, and practices.	Clarify with the client his or her preference of practices to be observed.
Buddhists believe pain and suffering is due to actions in a past life.	Accept the client's right to this belief: neither agree or disagree.
Buddhist and **Hindu** clients accept traditional medical treatment. However, in order to maintain a clear state of mind, **Buddhists** may refuse drugs that alter the state of the mind.	Inform physician of client's concern. Explain to client/family the action of all medications before administering them. Report to physician and chart any medications refused and reason for refusal.
Generally, **Buddhists** do not believe in healing through faith. Healing for **Buddhist** clients may be promoted by awakening to the laws of Buddha, the Enlightened One. Buddhism was founded in the sixth century B.C. in India by Gautama. After many years of searching, Gautama finally found the truth of existence and became the Buddha—the Enlightened One. Many persons since then have become Buddhas by becoming enlightened.	Avoid references to "God" (for example, "God will help you get through this").
Most **Buddhists** and **Hindus** are vegetarians. **Hindu** clients may prefer a light diet in the morning and evening and a heavy meal at noon. Some **Hindu** clients may fast on a specific day of the week or month.	Allow client/family to select diet for each meal. Encourage client/family to write in preferences when not listed. Arrange for visit by dietician.
Hindus may practice the traditional Indian science of health, Ayurveda, which utilizes herbs to treat disease. Some **Hindus** also practice folk medicine.	As with clients of all cultures and in all settings: Question use of herbs in daily life so possible drug interactions can be avoided. Question use of folk medicine. If practice is not harmful, include practice in plan of care. If practice is harmful, repattern practice. (See Boxes 9–3 and 9–4.)

TABLE 10–5 continued	
Belief/Practice	**Nursing Implications**
Buddhist clients may use incense, images of Buddha, and/or prayer beads in worship.	Respect these objects if used by client. Provide these personal objects if client asks for them.
Hindu clients may have a thread on their torso or around their wrist to signify a blessing.	Avoid removing the thread.
Buddhist clients may have a visit from a Buddhist priest, monk, or nun to conduct a religious ceremony. **Hindu** priests generally are not involved with illness care.	Provide privacy for visit of priest, monk, or nun.
Buddhist families may perform traditions with client. Significant others of **Hindu** clients may do the same.	Arrange the environment to accommodate the family. Provide quiet and privacy.
Buddhist clients may chant or meditate to help calm and clear their minds.	Avoid interrupting the client during meditation.
Puja, the worship of **Hindu** deities, is preceded by outer purification. **Hindu** clients may request a daily bath.	Provide necessary equipment for bathing for ambulatory clients. If client requires assistance, give bath before meal. If bathing required in bed, add hot water to cold water. (Lipson, 1996, App. B-12).

dhism spread, the core beliefs were adapted to the culture of the host country. They were shaped and influenced by rituals and the belief system of each country. Two core beliefs of Buddhism remained constant. They are the Four Noble Truths and the Noble Eightfold Path leading to Nirvana. The **Four Noble Truths** are:

1. Life is suffering.
2. Suffering is caused by desire.
3. Suffering can be eliminated by eliminating desire.
4. To eliminate desire, follow the **Noble Eightfold Path***

---

* The exact order and description of the Noble Eightfold Path was taken from *How to be a Perfect Stranger: A Guide to Etiquette in Other People's Religion.* Arthur Magida. (Editor). Woodstock, Vermont: Jewish Lights Publishing, 1996.

a. Right understanding of the nature of reality.
b. Right thought—free from cruelty, ill will, and sensuous desire.
c. Right speech—avoid lies, harsh words, and useless chatter.
d. Right action—avoid killing, stealing, intoxicants, gambling, and wrong conduct in matters of bodily pleasure.
e. Right livelihood—avoid trickery or fraud in the service of one's trade. Carry out right speech and right action.
f. Right effort—encourages purifying the mind. Avoid generating new, unwholesome actions.
g. Right mindfulness—meditative practices that encourage greater alertness and awareness of self.
h. Right concentration—striving for "one-pointedness."

TABLE 10-6: Death Beliefs and Practices of Buddhist and Hindu Clients

Buddhists believe in many reincarnations until they achieve Enlightenment and are freed from worldly illusion, passions, and suffering. Until this is achieved, death provides the opportunity to improve in the next life. Understanding of the Four Noble Truths and the Noble Eightfold Path will allow one to achieve Enlightenment and enter Nirvana (a state, the absence of self, extinguishing of desire and suffering), at which time the cycle of re-births and re-deaths ends. Resources within the person to achieve Enlightenment are stressed rather than reliance on ancient gods.

Hindus believe in the wheel of birth, life, and death (reincarnations) until they break through the illusions of the world and participate in the manifestation of the true self (Atman, the deathless self, the soul). Meditation and grace will help the Hindu believer to realize the Supreme self, which is hidden in the heart. When this occurs, eternal peace or Brahman (the universal soul and source, the Absolute Truth) is the reward.

Belief/Practice	Nursing Implications
Buddhists and **Hindus** believe in re-birth and re-death *(reincarnation)*. They do not believe in the concept of an immortal soul.	Accept the client's right to this belief: avoid agreeing or disagreeing.
Buddhists and **Hindus** believe in *karma,* the law of cause and effect, by which thoughts, words, and deeds of each person create his or her own destiny. One reaps what one sows. Karma is carried over to the next life and determines the form of each new existence. **Buddhists** believe it is the state of one's consciousness at the time of death that usually determines one's rebirth.	For dying clients, make provision for rites and ceremonies by the family and/or spiritual leaders. Avoid disturbing praying, singing, and chanting. *Buddhist clients* Provide an environment for the dying client that will allow a clear, calm state of mind and a peaceful death. *Hindu clients* Allow the family/spiritual leader to place water in the mouth of Hindu clients.
Buddhist and **Hindus** treat the body with respect. Cremation is common for **Buddhists** and **Hindus.** The **Hindu** client's ashes are saved to be disposed of in a holy river, e.g., the Ganges. Family may want to wash the body in preparation for cremation.	Inform funeral director of client's religion. *Hindu client* When requested, provide family with equipment to wash the body.
Organ donations **Buddhists** may allow organ donation if it will help someone pursue enlightenment. **Hindus** allow organ donation.	Present possibility of organ donation to family in a private environment. Allow family to make decision. Follow agency policy for obtaining permission for autopsy.
Autopsies **Buddhists** and **Hindus** permit autopsies.	Follow agency policy for obtaining permission for autopsy.

Nursing Implications for Eastern Religions/ Philosophies

In client care, the licensed practical/vocational nurse can come in contact with a Japanese Buddhist, Korean Buddhist, and Tibetan Buddhist, among others, plus American/Canadian clients who have blended Buddhism with their chosen religion. Apply principles from Chapter 9, Cultural Differences. Develop awareness that not everyone sees the world as you do. Avoid stereotyping individuals and considering them all the same, because they are Buddhist, Shinto, Hindu, and so forth. Table 10–5 presents a comparison of general religious beliefs and practices that may be commonly found in Buddhist and Hindu clients and appropriate nursing implications.

Table 10–6 presents general death beliefs and practices of Buddhist and Hindu clients and appropriate nursing implications.

 Learning Exercise: Learning About Other Religions

Using Chapter 7, "Hints for Using Learning Resources," as a guide, gather information about a religion or group that interests you but of which you are not a member. Examples include, but are not limited to, Shintoism, Taoism, Confucianism, Wicca, and such others.

Summary

- ☐ The practical/vocational nurse has a responsibility to care for the total person, including physical, emotional, and spiritual needs. The spiritual self grows and matures throughout life. Practical/vocational nurses need to support this growth in clients. Spiritual needs of clients arise from their desire to find meaning in life, suffering, and death.
- ☐ Spiritual care is a part of all clients' care, not only in times of crisis. To meet the spiritual needs of clients, you need to be aware of the client's personal spiritual beliefs or the absence of them. Members of the health care team who assist the practical/vocational nurse in providing spiritual care to clients are the minister, priest, rabbi, chaplain, and pastoral care team.
- ☐ Many clients help meet their personal spiritual needs by their participation in an organized religion. Although spirituality can be part of religion, religion is not necessarily part of spirituality.
- ☐ Spiritual distress can occur when clients cannot fulfill the rituals and practices of their religion or when they experience conflict between their spiritual beliefs and their health regimen. For these reasons, you need to develop an awareness of religious differences and an understanding of the basic beliefs, rituals, and practices of the many religious denominations and sects that exist today.
- ☐ Although the majority of clients in the United States are Protestant, Catholic, and Jewish, you will encounter other denominations and groups such as Muslims and members of Eastern religions/philosophies, as well as persons who have no religious beliefs. By learning more about these groups, you will be able to accommodate their beliefs and practices and will be able to say you have met the needs of the total person.

Review Questions

1. Select the statement that best describes the role of the pastoral care team.
   A. The pastoral care team is the social services department.
   B. The pastoral care team works with the nursing staff to help meet the spiritual and religious needs of clients.
   C. Religious care is offered to seriously ill clients by pastoral care.
   D. Because of pastoral care, the nursing staff does not have to worry about meeting the spiritual needs of clients.
2. The God a Muslim client prays to is
   A. Christ
   B. Jesus
   C. Allah
   D. The divine redeemer
3. If a Catholic client requests "Last Rites" before surgery, the practical/vocational nurse responds by
   A. Reassuring the client that he is not going to die during surgery.
   B. Notifying the client's family that his condition has changed.
   C. Calling the client's physician to report his mental state.
   D. Contacting the pastoral care team and passing on the client's request for the Last Rites.

4. Select the statement that best reflects the role of faith and prayer in health care in the twenty-first century.
   A. Faith and prayer are important in the healing process of clients who believe in these interventions.
   B. Faith and prayer are not scientifically based interventions in health care.
   C. There is little time in health care to include considerations of faith or to pray with clients.
   D. Only mandates of accrediting agencies must be addressed in health care organizations.
5. If a client with a bleeding peptic ulcer is a Jehovah's Witness and refuses to receive an ordered blood transfusion, the licensed practical/vocational nurse needs to
   A. Notify the supervisor STAT.
   B. Encourage the client to accept the blood transfusion.
   C. Explain to the client that the transfusion is needed because of the blood she is losing from her condition.
   D. Alert surgery that the client may have to be restrained or medicated if she sees blood running into her veins.

References

Magida A (ed). *How to Be a Perfect Stranger: A Guide to Etiquette in Other People's Religious Ceremonies.* Woodstock, Vermont: Jewish Lights Publishing, 1996.

Schoenbeck S. Called to care: Addressing the spiritual needs of clients. J Pract Nurs 44:19–23, 1994.

Bibliography

Biddex V, Brown H. Establishing a parish nursing program. Nursing and Health Care Perspectives 20(2):72–75, 1999.

Bowker J. (ed). *The Oxford Dictionary of World Religions.* Oxford: Oxford University Press, 1997.

Brussat F. *Spiritual Literacy: Reading the Sacred in Everyday Life.* New York: Simon and Schuster, 1996.

Buddhist Churches of America, 1710 Octavia Street, San Francisco, CA 94109.

Carson V. *Spiritual Dimensions of Nursing Practice.* Philadelphia: W. B. Saunders, 1989.

Catechism of the Catholic Church. Liguori, MO: Liguori Publications, 1994.

Chilton B. Recognizing spirituality. Image: Journal of Nursing Scholarship 30(4):400, 1998.

Chopra D. *The Seven Spiritual Laws of Success.* San Rafael, CA: Amber-Allen Publishing and New World Library, 1994.

Dossey B. Holistic modalities and healing moments. Am J Nurs 98(6):44–47, 1998.

Dossey B. Attending to holistic care. Am J Nurs 98(8):35–38, 1998.

Giger J, Davidhizar R. *Transcultural Nursing: Assessment and Intervention.* St. Louis: Mosby, 1999.

Lipson J, Dibble S, Minarek P. *Culture and Nursing Care: A Pocket Guide.* San Francisco: The Regents of the University of California, 1996.

O'Brien M. *Spirituality in Nursing: Standing on Holy Ground.* Boston: Jones and Bartlett, 1998.

O'Neil B, Kenney E. Spirituality and chronic illness. Image: Journal of Nursing Scholarship 30(3):275–280, 1998.

Rupp J. *The Cup of Our Life: A Guide for Spiritual Growth.* Notre Dame, IN: Ave Maria Press, 1997.

Sumner C. Recognizing and responding to spiritual distress. Am J Nurs 98(1):26–30, 1998.

Titus H, Smith M, Nolan R. *Living Issues in Philosophy.* Belmont, CA: Wadsworth Publishing, 1995.

When clients refuse blood. Emerg Med 16(18):65, 69, 1984.

Wright K. Professional, ethical, and legal implications for spiritual care in nursing. Image: Journal of Nuring Scholarship 30(1):81, 1998.

Zimmerman P. Rest in peace, Rabbi Shapiro. Am J Nurs 98(4): 64–65, 1998.

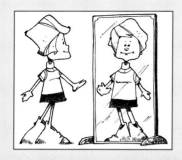

PART **FOUR**

Leading and Managing Others

Chapter 11

Assertiveness as a Nursing Responsibility

Outline

Key Terms

aggressive
assaults
assertiveness
automatic responses
burnout
choice

codependency
compensation
cultural differences
denial
empathy
harassment

impaired nurse
manipulation
nonassertive (passive)
problem-solving
projection
rationalization

Objectives

Upon completing this chapter you will be able to:
1. Explain why assertiveness is a nursing responsibility.
2. Differentiate between assertive, aggressive, and nonassertive (passive) behavior.
3. Describe three negative interactions in which nurses can get involved.

4. Maintain a daily journal that reflects your personal interactions and responses.
5. Develop a personal plan for change toward assertive behavior.
6. Discuss positive manipulation as a cultural choice.
7. Discuss a way to prevent burnout in nurses.

8. Describe abuse of alcohol or other drugs as a path to the label of Impaired Nurse.
9. Discuss codependent behavior as an attempt to control fears.
10. Discuss an assertive nursing response to violence in the workplace.

Assertiveness is an expectation in nursing—a responsibility for you as a client advocate. Once again you are requested to do a brief exercise before going on with your reading.

Critical Thinking Exercise

Directions: Imagine for the next few minutes that the nurse-client roles are reversed and that you are the client.

Question: What are your expectations of the nurse assigned to you? List the rationale for each expectation that you identify.

Expectation	Rationale
_____	_____
_____	_____
_____	_____
_____	_____
_____	_____
_____	_____

Completing this exercise has already begun to give you an insight into the need for assertiveness in the nurse. At the end of this chapter you are encouraged to do this exercise again. Evaluate any changes in expectations.

Three types of communication styles translate into three major behavior patterns. Because communication is verbal, nonverbal, and affective, you will *hear, see,* and *feel* the message acted out.

The most effective communication style is open and honest. It promotes positive relationships and a healthy sense of self. Ineffective communication or behavior is hurtful. It blames, attacks, or denies and is harmful to self as well.

An *assertive* style separates the person from the issue. Most important, you speak out of **choice.** With either an *aggressive* or a *nonassertive (passive)* style, you are caught by an emotional hook. Both types of responses are **automatic responses.** You no longer respond from choice.

Now let's take a look at the three major behavior styles: nonassertive (passive), aggressive, and assertive. We will also look at negative interactions specific to nursing and at how you can move toward truly assertive behavior.

Nonassertive (Passive) Behavior

Nonassertive (passive), fear-based behavior is an emotionally dishonest, self-defeating type of behavior. Nonassertive nurses attempt to look the other way, to avoid conflict, and to take what seems to be the easiest way out; they are never full participants on the nursing team. *Nonassertive individuals do not express feelings, needs, and ideas when their rights are infringed on, deliberately or accidentally.* The overall message is *"I do not count. You count."* This personal pattern of behavior is reflected in their nursing as well. Consequently, they are unable to recognize and meet the client's needs. A number of examples of nonassertive behavior observed in one nurse follow. With each, the type of behavior is given in parentheses.

- Tells another nurse how "stupid" the doctor is for ordering a certain type of treatment (indirect nonassertive behavior).
- Limits contact with a client she is uncomfortable with to required care only (indirect nonassertive behavior).
- Routinely tells clients who question her about an explanation for the illness, test, medications, or treatment to "ask the doctor" or "ask the RN." Although this answer is advisable some of the time, it certainly is a form of brushoff. Part of the nursing responsibility is to seek answers for the client (takes the easy way out).

- Experiences inability to continue with a necessary, uncomfortable treatment ordered for the client (interprets client's expression of discomfort personally ["He will not like me if I make him do this"]).
- May assume, without checking, that the client wants to skip the daily personal care when a visitor drops in (avoids conflict).
- Experiences a feeling of being "devastated" when a client, doctor, nurse, or other staff person criticizes his or her work (interprets criticism of work as criticism of self).
- Responds to client's questions about own personal life and that of other staff (afraid of not being liked).
- Client asks her to pick up some personal items on the way home. She frowns but agrees to do so (communicates the real message nonverbally).
- Becomes angry with the team leader and drops hints to others about own feelings (communicates real message indirectly).
- When asked by another nurse to take on the care of his clients, she responds by saying, "Well, uh, I guess I could," although she is already too busy (hesitance, repressing her own wishes).
- Needs help with his assignment but says nothing (refrains from expressing his own needs).
- After making an error, overexplains and over-apologizes (unaware of the right to make a mistake; should take responsibility for it, learn from the error, and go on).
- Plans on finding a new job because she is afraid of approaching the supervisor to tell her side of what has happened (avoids conflict).
- When "chewed out" by the doctor in front of the client, the nurse is angry but says nothing (refrains from expressing her opinion—internalizes anger).

By not taking risks and not being honest, nonassertive nurses typically feel hurt, misunderstood, anxious, and disappointed and often feel angry and resentful later. Because they do not allow their needs to be known, they are the loser.

Critical Thinking Exercise

What are some other examples of nonassertive behavior?

Aggressive Behavior

Outspoken people are often automatically considered assertive when in reality their lack of consideration for others may be a sign of **aggressive** behavior. Aggressive (anger-based) behavior violates the rights of others. It is an attack on the person rather than on the person's behavior. The purpose of aggressive behavior is to dominate or put the other person down. This behavior, while expressive, is self-defeating because it quickly distances the aggressor from other staff and clients. The overall message is, *"You do not count. I count."*

The following examples are some of the ways by which aggressive behavior can be recognized. An explanation is included in parentheses.

- You have asked to go to a workshop, and the supervisor tells you, "Why should you go? Everyone else has worked here longer than you have" (attempt to make you feel guilty for making a request).
- Another nurse points out your error in front of other staff and adds, "Where did you say you graduated from?" (attempt to humiliate as a way of controlling).
- A peer approaches you with a problem. You don't want to listen and say, "If it isn't one thing, it's another for you. Why don't you get your act together?" (disregard for others' feelings).
- A new rule is instituted without requesting input from or informing those whom it will involve. You protest but are told, "That's tough; this is the way it's going to be from now on" (disregard for others' feelings and rights).
- The client has had his call light on frequently

throughout the morning. You walk in and say, "I have had it. You have had your light on continuously for nothing, all morning. Do not put your light on again unless you are dying or I will take it away" (hostile overreaction out of proportion to the issue at hand).

- You attempted to express your feelings to a peer about her behavior toward you. Today she greets you with an icy stare when you say hello (hostile overreaction).
- The client tells you, "I thought this was a pretty good hospital, but none of you seem to know what you are doing" (sarcastic, hostile).
- You push yourself in front of others in the cafeteria line (rudeness).
- Another employee greets you with "I hear you are a real whiz kid. Show us your stuff" (put-down).

Critical Thinking Exercise

What examples of aggressive behavior have you experienced?

Aggressive behavior certainly is a way of saying what you mean at the moment. It often does produce temporary relief from anxiety. However, the feeling does not last. Very often the aggressive person is left with residual angry feelings that simmer until the next stressful situation or person comes along. It is interesting that sometimes an aggressive person was once passive and made a decision that "no one will step on me again." However, instead of practicing assertiveness, such a person practiced and became involved in another form of destructive, self-defeating behavior. Aggressive nurses, like non-aggressive nurses, are unable to function as true advocates for the client because they are too busy taking care of what they perceive to be their personal needs.

Assertive Behavior

Assertiveness is a current name for honesty—that is, it is a way to live the truth from your innermost being and to express this truth in thought, word, and deed. The concept seems simple enough, but to practice actually being truthful all the time is difficult. Assertiveness, according to *Webster's Dictionary,* is characterized by taking a positive stand, being confident in your statement, or being positive in a persistent way. You, the nurse, work in a setting that requires speaking frankly and openly to others in such a way that their rights are not violated. Assertiveness is a tool, not a weapon. "First attempts to use assertiveness are usually clumsy and may do some damage. Remember that in the process of becoming skilled with any tool, you are bound to suffer some cuts and bruises and a lot of swollen thumbs" (Chenevert, 1994, p. 18). Although it is not the nurse's right to hurt others deliberately, it is unrealistic to be inhibited to the point of never hurting anyone. Some people are hurt because they are unreasonably sensitive, and some use their sensitivity to manipulate others.

The nurse has a right to express her own thoughts and feelings. To do otherwise would be insincere. It would also deny clients and other staff the opportunity to learn to deal with their feelings. Assertiveness, then, is a way of expressing oneself without insulting others. It communicates respect for the other person although not necessarily for the other person's behavior. The overall message is *"I count, you count."* Being assertive does not guarantee that you will get your way. What it does guarantee is that you will experience a sense of being in control of your emotions and your responses. Win or lose, you gave it your best shot. The real bonus is freedom from residual feelings of fear and anger.

The following examples, with the rationale in parentheses, are expressions of assertive behavior. As an assertive nurse, you claim responsibility for your own feelings, thoughts, and actions. Use of "I" in the statements shows acceptance of responsibility for your thinking, feeling, and doing.

- The doctor orders a medication or treatment that seems inappropriate. You request to talk with him privately. Ask about expected outcomes. Present any new information you have that may potentially affect the decision to continue with the order (direct statement of information).
- The client has been giving you a bad time. Pulling up a chair and sitting down, you say, "Mr. Smith, I would be interested in knowing what is going on with you. I have noticed that whatever I do, you are critical of my work." Then listen attentively and with understanding and respond nondefensively (direct statement of feelings, does not interpret client's criticism as a personal attack).
- When the client requests information you are unfamiliar with regarding his illness and treatment, you say, "I do not know but I will find out for you." Follow through by checking with appropriate staff. Determine who is to inform the client (respects the client's right to know).
- The doctor has ordered the client to be walked for 10 minutes out of each hour. She complains that it hurts and asks you not to make her walk. You respond by saying, "I know it is uncomfortable, but I will walk along beside you. We can stop briefly any time you like. I will also teach you how to do a brief relaxation technique that you can use while you are walking." If pain medication is available, you will also make sure that this is given prior to walking and in enough time for the medication to take effect (respects client's feelings but supports the need to carry out doctor's order).
- Unexpected visitors arrive when it is time for you to help the client with his personal care. Ask the client directly if he wishes to have his care done now or to postpone it briefly. State the time that you will be available to assist with care (respects the client's right to choose as long as it does not compromise his care).
- You have just been criticized for your work. You respond by saying, "Please clarify. I want to be sure I understand." If the error is yours, ask for suggestions to correct it or offer alternatives of your own (separates criticism of performance from criticism of self).
- The client asks for personal information about you (or another staff member). You respond by saying, "That information is personal, and I do not choose to discuss it" (stands up for rights without violating rights of others).
- Your client asks you to pick up some personal items for him. This would mean doing it on your own time, which is already very full. You respond, "I will not be able to do the errand for you" (direct statement without excuses)
- The team leader has been "on your case" constantly and, you think, unfairly. You approach him or her and say, "I want to speak with you privately today before 3 PM. What time is convenient for you?" (direct statement of wishes).
- You are being pressed by other staff members to help with their assignments, but you are too busy to do so. You say, "No, I do not have the time to help today, but try me again on some other day" (direct refusal without feeling guilty. Leaves the door open to help at a future date).
- Your day is overwhelming. You approach your team leader and say, "I know you want all of this done today. There is no way I can get it all done. What are your priorities?" (direct statement of information and request for clarification).
- The doctor has criticized your work in front of the client. You feel embarrassed and angry. You approach the doctor and tell her you want to speak to her privately. Using I-centered statements, you begin by saying, "I feel both embarrassed and angry because you criticized me in front of the client. Next time, ask to talk to me privately. I will listen to what you have to say" (stands up for your rights without violating the rights of others).
- You are ready to leave work when a peer approaches you about a personal problem. You respond by saying, "I have to leave now, but I'll be glad to listen to you during lunch-time tomorrow" (compromise).

■ Another staff person moves into the cafeteria line ahead of you with a nod and a smile. You are in a hurry too and feel put-upon. You say firmly, "I do not like it when you get in line ahead of me. Please go back to the end of the line" (stands up for your rights).

Critical Thinking Exercise

What examples of assertiveness can you identify in your own behavior or in the behavior of people around you?

Three rules are helpful overall in being assertive:

1. Own your feelings. Do not blame others for the way you feel.
2. Make your feelings known by being direct. Begin your statements with "I."
3. Be sure that your nonverbal communication matches your verbal message.

Negative Interactions

With the availability of so many types of preparation for nurses and the lack of differentiation in roles based on preparation, nurses sometimes experience insecurity in their role and the worth of the role as they understand it. This negative interaction involves use of the coping or mental mechanism of **projection,** in which an individual attributes his own weaknesses to others. The interaction can be characterized as "my education is better than yours" or "I'm more competent than you are," or "you're only a practical nurse," and so on. Unfortunately, this negative, aggressive interaction uses up energy that could be used to provide the client with the care that is being alluded to. Nurses who are confident and assertive enhance each other's knowledge base and legal responsibility. The client benefits.

Another negative interaction is based on a previous unresolved incident between the client and the nurse. The nurse uses the coping or mental mechanism of **rationalization,** in which she offers a logical but untrue reason as an excuse for his behavior. The nurse quickly informs others that this client is a "troublemaker" or a "manipulator" or is "uncooperative." This is a nonassertive, indirect type of behavior on the part of the nurse. Obviously, if other nurses incorporate this information into their transactions with the client, the client will never be seen as his or her true self. Anything that he or she does can be interpreted within the context of the label given by the nurses. A vicious circle can ensue. If the client's needs are not met because of this obstacle, this increases his or her frustration. This in turn is a threat to self, resulting in anxiety. Depending on the client's personal strength at this time, the situation can lead to problem solving, use of coping mental mechanisms, or symptom formation. See Figure 11–1.

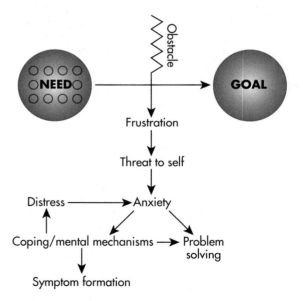

FIGURE 11–1. Bauer's model for goal achievement. (From Bauer B, Hill S. *Mental Health Nursing; An Introductory Text.* Philadelphia: W.B. Saunders, 2000.)

An honest, assertive response on the part of the original nurse involved would consist of dealing with the client directly in regard to the previous situation. It would not involve other nurses as allies in "getting this client." An example of an extreme situation resulting from just such a seemingly innocent rationalization occurred at a nursing home. A young man who was paralyzed from the waist down as a result of a car accident was being transferred from one nursing home to another. A transfer form arrived before he did. The information on the form created immediate anxiety for the nurses involved before they had even met the man. The form labeled the man as "manipulative." It explained that "he will be pleasant and polite at first, but watch out because it is a trick. When he has won you over, you will see his 'real colors.'" The nurses discussed the prospective admission. They expressed gratitude that they had been warned by their colleagues in the other nursing home. After all, that is what colleagues are for. And now they felt, "forewarned is forearmed."

When the client arrived and attempted to get acquainted, he was dealt with coldly and abruptly and made to wait. The nurses intended to show him that he could not manipulate them. As his frustration and his discomfort increased, he began to demand that his treatments be done on time. He shouted angry comments at the nurses when they finally arrived to assume his care. The nurses called him "demanding" and "hostile." The original title of manipulative was supported when the client asked his roommate to put on the call light to get help to take him to the bathroom. Each day seemed worse than the day before. The showdown finally came when a longtime nurse employee left, saying that she would not come back until the client was transferred to another facility. She would even volunteer to do the transfer note. Other nursing staff threatened to follow suit. Finally the administrator gave in. The client was transferred, and the nurses congratulated each other for having worked together!

Another negative transaction involves client rights. This transaction can be known by many titles, depending on the issue. It can be called

Critical Thinking Exercise

1. What factors contributed to the client's behavior? _____

2. What factors contributed to the nurses' response to the client? _____

3. How could this situation have been handled differently? _____

4. Was the behavior of the nurses passive, aggressive, or assertive? Explain your answer. _____ _____ _____

"I've got a secret," "it is not my responsibility," "she will be upset," or "she is too weak to know." The responsibility of informing the client about his or her condition or transfer plans is not carried out so that the present staff does not have to deal with the full impact of the client's reaction to the information. The coping or mental mechanism used by the nurses is **denial.** The nurse refuses to recognize the existence and significance of the client's personal concerns. The nurse further uses denial as a way of excusing her responsibility: "The doctor should tell him" or "It's the team leader's responsibility." Although the decision may not be entirely yours, it is clearly your responsibility to check out what portion of the information is yours

Critical Thinking Exercise

Is the nurse's refusal to take responsibility to seek out the information the client needs to know a passive, aggressive, or assertive transaction?

_____

to give. You also have the responsibility to check out who is going to present the information and when.

Although it has many possible negative interactions, certainly the passive or aggressive game of gossip—e.g., "Did I tell you?" or "I just found out"—is a destructive interaction that has the potential to ruin the reputations of both clients and personnel. The coping or mental mechanism is **compensation.** The nurse is covering for real or imagined inadequacies in his work by developing what he considers the desirable traits of observation, listening, and reporting. The energy is misguided because reputations are at stake, and time spent socializing while at work is time away from providing quality client care. A listener can squelch this game by saying assertively, "I will work on a relationship with you and me, but I do not wish to have you talk to me about others." Instead, if the listener, while calling the other nurse a gossip, listens with interest, she supports continuation of this behavior.

 Critical Thinking Exercise

1. What other negative interaction between staff or between clients and staff are you familiar with?
   _____

2. How is the continuation of this type of interaction supported by others? _____
   _____

Guidelines for Moving Toward Assertiveness

The following poem by an anonymous author captures the reason for working toward assertiveness—being able to feel good about yourself as you continue to grow as a person.

Myself

I have to live with myself and so,

I want to be fit for myself to know.

I don't want to stand with the setting sun

And hate myself for the things I've done.

I want to go out with head erect.

I want to deserve all men's respect.

But here in this struggle for fame and self,

I want to be able to like myself.

I don't want to look at myself and know

That I'm bluster and bluff and empty show.

I never can fool myself, and so

Whatever happens, I want to grow

More able to be more proud of me,

Self-respecting and conscience free.

Changing behavior is difficult. After all, the behaviors have been practiced and perfected for years. It is so much easier to tell others what *they* should do to change. The decision to change must come from inside yourself, so that it becomes yours alone.

Problem-Solving Process

It is easier to begin the **problem-solving** process before feelings and behaviors are deeply rooted. What you fear most is what you attract. The cycle of worry → fear → anger → rage can be resolved at any stage you choose. Make no mistake about it: problem solving is work!

The self tries to find relief of unresolved feelings through behavior such as codependency, self-medicating with alcohol and/or other drugs (or food), and projecting the anger toward clients (burnout). Prolonged, unresolved negative emotions such as worry, fear, and anger create changes in the body at a cellular level and can result in physical illness.

We first get clues in our thoughts of how we will become ill. Listen to your self-talk: "I'm sick of— I'm heartsick—I feel like I have the weight of the world on my shoulders—He's a pain in the neck (the butt)—Oh, my aching back—I'm so upset I can't speak—I can't stomach this much longer"— and so on. If your self-talk is negative, pay attention. These statements give clues to potential areas of involvement. We also read or hear news almost daily of mild-mannered, nice people who suddenly acted out of rage. No one wants to get there. Chenevert (1994, Preface) quotes the message on a button she saw as an incentive for becoming assertive: "I'm Damned If I Do. I'm Damned If I Don't. So Damn It, Just Do It!"

The problem-solving process is a conscious growth-producing method of dealing with this challenge in your life. It is important to note that problem solving is an active process and is more than simply developing an intellectual awareness of the challenge at hand.

Step 1: Define the Problem

Sometimes what is perceived as the problem is not the problem at all. Before making a commitment to change, it is important to look objectively at the gains and losses associated with the present behavior. Your present way of responding to others developed as a response to anxiety-producing situations in life. It usually has its roots in childhood.

Another consideration is that when you change the way you act toward others, you change the way they act toward you. What has been a predictable reaction will no longer be predictable. Initially, the "others" will test you. They will increase their old way of behaving as a way of getting you to give up the new behavior. If you persist with your new way of dealing with and responding to situations, their behavior toward you will also change. This is the only way to influence change in anyone's behavior. No amount of "telling" or "scolding" makes a difference as long as others can count on you to behave in a predictable way.

Defining the problem depends on collecting data for two or three days and writing your problem statement based on this information. Collecting data needs to be done in an objective manner, as though you were observing someone else. Keeping a daily confidential journal helps pinpoint specific situations. You can track what happened, when it happened, how you felt physically, the emotion you felt, what you would have liked to have done instead, and what kept you from doing it.

Reviewing the data you have collected will give you insight into the pros and cons of your present behavior. The problem statement you develop will have to be personal and specific.

Sample

I am afraid to say what I mean for fear that others will get angry with me.

This behavior is characterized by:

- Saying yes to requests to babysit when I need the time for homework.
- Not asking for help with household chores even though I am a full-time student plus homemaker.
- Saying yes to added requests not related to workload at school that I must complete on my own time.
- Feeling tired and resentful much of the time and eventually blowing up over something insignificant.

Step 2: Decide on a Goal

Review the problem statement, and form the question, "So . . . what?" In other words, what do you want to do differently? This can be stated as a single goal. Often it is more useful to break the goal down into a long-term goal and several short-term goals (sometimes called objectives), which are the steps needed to attain the desired long-term goal. All goals must be realistic, measurable, and time-referenced. At this time, write a goal for yourself: _____.

Sample

Long-Term Goal	Short-Term Goal
Within 6 months I will say what I mean without fear that others will be angry with me (give actual date—this is your best "guesstimate").	Within 2 weeks I will say "no" to babysitting requests when I need the time for homework (give actual date—this is your best "guesstimate").

As you read each of the goals you have written, ask yourself whether they are realistic. Are they reasonable to attain? Next, review each goal and ask whether it is measurable. Are they so specific that you can use the senses to detect the change? Note that each goal begins with the phrase "I will." This phrase signals a personal commitment to work on the goal. Note that the goals are to be attained within a designated period of time—that is, they are time-referenced. This is also the only way to give yourself a personal push to get started.

All the changes are not going to occur exactly by the projected date. You will have to revise the goal dates from time to time. But most important, they provide target dates to strive for. As you accomplish each short-term goal, cross it out and go on to the next one. Do not be alarmed if you find yourself working on more than one goal at a time. This is possible and even desirable when the opportunity presents itself. It is important to continue recording your progress in the confidential journal that was begun initially to obtain data. Its value now lies in keeping a record of the process you are going through and in seeing the changes taking place. Unless you do this, you may not fully appreciate your work and its progress. Many changes will be subtle and will not be accompanied by bells and claps of thunder.

Step 3: Choose Alternatives

Alternatives are the approaches that you will be using to attain each of the established goals. When you make a list of alternatives in your journal, let your imagination run wild. Consider all the possible solutions, from serious to humorous. This may even provide some comic relief to the serious challenge with which you are dealing. Remember to include "Do nothing" in the list of alternatives. Doing nothing is a *choice* and therefore an alternative. Look at each of the goals and think of specific things you can do or say to help support the goal.

Sample

Approach: Practice in front of a mirror. In an even tone of voice say, "No, I will not be able to babysit tonight, but try again another time." If the person persists, say, "No, I do not have the time tonight." Repeat as needed until heard. Compliment yourself for not giving in.

Do you see how the approach (alternative) corresponds specifically to the short-term goal?

Step 4: Try Out the Alternatives

The initial plan has been made. It is time to put the plan into action. For many of you the paperwork is far easier than taking the first step to make the "paper trip" become a reality. You may also have discovered that it is far easier to offer ideas to peers than to take the first step into action with your own plan.

Critical Thinking Exercise

What are you gaining from staying nonassertive? What are you losing from staying nonassertive?

The answer belongs in your confidential journal. Whether you are writing or tape recording a journal depends on your learning style. Regardless of the journal method used, it should by now have become an important part of the learning process.

It is a good idea to build in an incentive to continue using the new assertive approaches. Promise yourself something that is worthy of you (a worthy goal). As you go along, you will sometimes slip back into old familiar ways of behaving. Do not be dismayed. This is normal. Simply reinstitute the newly planned approaches immediately and continue. The more you practice the new approaches, the more they will become part of you. Ultimately, new assertive behaviors will replace old nonassertive or aggressive behaviors.

Step 5: Evaluate the Effectiveness of Your Approach

The evaluation mechanism is built into the overall plan for change by making the goals time limited. This tells you that each goal, along with the alternatives you have chosen, will be evaluated at the time indicated. Do not change a goal or approach too quickly. Give it at least two to three weeks. There are two reasons for this: (1) The negative behaviors of other individuals toward you will increase initially as they attempt to resist change created by the change in you. (2) It takes a minimum of two to three weeks for the new behavior to catch on. It takes approximately a year for a new behavior to become part of you. As a part of the evaluation process, review your entire confidential journal. This is an excellent source of information for what happened, how you dealt with it, and whether the present course is effective.

Step 6: Repeat the Process If the Solution Is Not Effective

Step 5 gives you information about whether or not to pursue the established course of action. If changes are needed, go back to step 3. Identify additional alternatives or perhaps choose alternatives that you originally identified but did not use. Then go through the rest of the steps as before.

As you pursue an assertive way of behaving, monitor your nonverbal messages. The nonverbal communication you provide is even more powerful than your words. It is possible to have the words just right but to sabotage them by hesitation, a sarcastic tone of voice, or emphasis on certain words. Practice in front of a mirror. Busy schedule? Try bath time. Listen to the way you sound. A tape is helpful, as is speaking into an empty corner and hearing your words bounce back. Try lowering your tone of voice. Be sure that the last word of a sentence is no higher than the one before. Listen for this in others. It makes a statement sound like a question.

Posture plays an important role. Sit up straight, walk with the shoulders back and a confident stride. Make eye contact when speaking. If this is new and difficult for you, look at the area between the eyes of the person you are addressing. This provides an illusion of eye contact. Periodically look away so that it does not look as though you are staring. Avoid annoying characteristics such as nail biting, finger or foot tapping or jiggling, playing with your hair, chewing on a pencil or glasses, and artificial laughter.

When someone asks you what you think of an issue or what you would like to do, answer the person instead of saying "I really do not know" or "Whatever you like. It does not matter." Life is an adventure. All of it, including your ideas, counts.

Cultural Differences

With feedback from valued teachers, students, and reviewers, we have learned that it is not safe to assume that all cultures are focused on moving toward assertive behavior. In some cultures, **manipulation** is an accepted norm. Although the term manipulation has a negative connotation in our society, manipulation in itself is not a maladaptive behavior. In some cultures it is taught and is accepted as a purposeful way of meeting one's needs. Skillful manipulation is especially applauded.

It is easy to jump to the conclusion that a manipulative person is trying to "trick" you because you do not share the same cultural background.

Make time to talk. The differences will be interesting and revealing for both of you.

Manipulation is considered maladaptive if (1) the feelings and needs of others are disregarded, or if (2) other people are treated as objects to fulfill the needs of the manipulator. The following examples of negative manipulative interactions show a lack of consideration for others' feelings and needs.

The *seducer* initiates a relationship with someone (for example, a nurse with a supervisor). They share what seem to be common goals and insights. Ultimately, the seducer asks for special favors or privileges. If denied, the seducer pushes the guilt button: "I thought you liked me," or "I thought we understood each other." The other person is left feeling guilty or angry or both.

The passive-aggressive manipulator focuses on the other person's weaknesses. He or she uses this knowledge to exploit or to create anxiety for the victim. For example, a physician might point out a nurse's errors or personal or professional problems in front of a client or other staff. The nurse is left feeling guilty, angry, embarrassed, or all of these.

The *divide-and-conquer* manipulator "confides" half-truths, rumors, gossip, and innuendo. A skilled manipulator can sever work relationships by sowing seeds of distrust. As the staff squabbles, there is less energy to unite and focus on common client issues. For example, a divide-and-conquer manipulator who is an established member of the community might "confide" to another department head that a newer employee cannot be trusted. By the time this information proves to be untrue, valuable time has been lost in client planning and care. Meanwhile, the divide-and-conquer manipulator has continued to tell the same story to other listeners. Because the feelings and needs of others are not considered, they are left with anger and seeds of distrust.

Dealing with a negative manipulator is difficult. An assertive approach is the best recourse. This will, however, be met with resistance and resentment. You may end up backing off if the problem cannot be worked out. Set limits on any inappropriate manipulative behavior toward you. Refuse to play the game any more.

Nonassertiveness (Passivity) and Personal Issues

As a nurse, you must learn to take care of yourself. In turn, you can be more effective in meeting clients' nursing needs. In taking care of yourself assertively, you serve as a positive role model for your coworkers, those you lead and manage, and your clients. How you view and deal with an event determines the outcome for you. Burnout, use of alcohol and other drugs, and codependency are possible outcomes that can be avoided and/or changed.

Burnout

Burnout is like looking at your career world through black glasses. The positive attitude you held about nursing, working with clients, and self-care begins to change. Attitude and behavioral changes may include:

1. Lack of respect for clients.
2. Blaming clients for their illness.
3. Taking a cynical view of clients, your place of employment, and management.
4. Personal feeling of emotional exhaustion.
5. Lack of self-care that may include an increase in the use of alcohol and other drugs.
6. A negative self-view.
7. More conflicts at home.

Differentiating between feelings of empathy and sympathy in regard to your client is a major consideration in preventing burnout. **Empathy** is a respectful, detached concern. As a nurse, you understand what your client is experiencing but do not experience the emotion with him. Clients entering a medical facility are out of their own element. The stress they experience can be picked up by you as a sympathetic response.

The client may be demanding a magical, dramatic change in his or her condition. Regression almost always is present in the client. Needs are often expressed indirectly, perhaps through irritable comments or requests. The client's emotional responses may elicit negative emotional responses in the sympathetic nurse.

Some clients do not respond to treatment no matter how hard they and you try. They may continue to go downhill to the point of death. Meanwhile, other clients may not cooperate, and your sympathetic response of anger and frustration will get in the way of a therapeutic relationship with them. Some clients are negative in their responses to staff or constantly ask questions in a challenging way. The families must be dealt with also, and at times they are equally challenging or more so than the clients. Maybe you are beginning to think in terms of who does and does not deserve care. Nonassertive and aggressive, verbal and nonverbal communication styles can have other devastating effects. The impaired nurse is another possible outcome as he or she attempts to self-medicate.

A sympathetic reaction leaves you vulnerable to identifying with and experiencing the emotion along with the client. This means that you are no longer in control of the situation, and your therapeutic value as a nurse will be limited. A long-term sympathetic response is very stressful. What starts out as a caring relationship can become detrimental to you and your client because of your overinvolvement.

Another significant step in preventing burnout is to develop a detached way of evaluating your daily personal performance. Waiting for a client, doctor, or nurse manager to notice your performance is rarely helpful or rewarding. Perhaps they notice only what is missing. However, a detached, daily evaluation of your performance leaves you free to credit yourself for what you have done well. Furthermore, it alerts you to areas in which you need more study, assistance, or practice. *You are your most effective boss!*

Time management is another important factor in dealing with both the personal and the professional areas of your life. Because of its significance, Chapter 4 is devoted to this topic.

Humor—do not forget humor. No matter how seriously you take yourself, you are never going to get out of this life alive. So lighten up. "1. Humor

Critical Thinking Exercise

What changes have you made using information from the chapter on time management? If you said none, read the chapter again. Repetition reinforces learning.

shows you care. 2. Nurses are accepted better when they have a sense of humor. 3. Humor shows you your client's personality with their defenses down. 4. Humor reduces tension and helps you get on with work. 5. Humor makes us equals, because we all laugh at the same things" (Balzer-Riley, 2000). Many things happen in a nursing situation that can be lightened up through humor. Case in point: The nursing instructor walked into the room to see how the student nurse was doing with her client. As he approached the client, he extended his hand and greeted the client by name. As the client opened his mouth to speak, he simultaneously expelled flatus— a thunderous clap! The client's eyes opened wide, there was a momentary silence, the student looked shocked, and then the instructor chuckled! "It happens," he said with a shrug. Soon all three were laughing; the embarrassment was gone. The real issue of the client's condition and nursing care was again the priority.

Maintaining nursing skills is essential. Even if you are in a situation that requires less hands-on care, make time to perform nursing procedures. Learn how to perform new procedures as they are introduced to your facility. This helps feed your self-worth and makes you a more valuable employee, an issue that is closely related to preventing burnout. Otherwise, you may develop a secret fear of being put on the spot and perhaps will lie your way out of requests to demonstrate or assist.

Some final tips for staying alive and well in nursing:

1. Set clear goals with realistic expectations.

2. Know your limits.
3. Work within your team structure.
4. Keep in mind that you cannot be all things to all people.
5. Maintain a clear understanding of what constitutes a professional relationship. Demonstrate professional—detached and somewhat limited—caring. A different kind will end in burnout because it becomes too burdensome.
6. Do not personalize the client's response to you. Keep the client in the client role. Maintain a professional outlook. See that the client responds out of the client's own needs. If you do this you will experience less guilt or anger.
7. Maintain a positive attitude, i.e., warm, caring, and hopeful, even if the client is dying. The client and the family will feel less hopeless.
8. Understand your own needs, both professionally and personally. You need to maintain a balance and a clear distinction between your work and your personal role.
9. Be alert to signs of burnout. Lack of caring is a real danger signal.
10. Maintain perspective about your work. Sometimes the whole world looks ill and grim! Remind yourself that you have a choice: Nursing can be a limited part of your life or the dominant goal in your life. You choose.

 Critical Thinking Exercise

1. Do you find yourself frequently focusing on home issues when at work?
2. Are you talking often about work when you are with your friends and family?
3. Name one change that you will begin to work on starting now.

Impaired Nurse

Impaired and **nurse** sound like contradictory terms. Some nurses, however, become chemically dependent on alcohol or other drugs. It often starts as a drink to unwind at the end of a work shift, then, two to three as more alcohol is needed for the effect.

Alcohol is a drug that acts like a depressant. Because of the loss of inhibition, the person who drinks may initially experience a sense of "loosening up." Unlike food, alcohol does not have to be digested. It is absorbed directly into the bloodstream from the stomach and small intestine. It reaches every tissue and organ of the body and slows the activity of the cells.

Alcohol is processed by the body at the rate of 1 to 1.5 ounces per hour. This is the amount of alcohol in one 12-ounce can of beer or one 5-ounce glass of wine. The liver processes most of the alcohol; a small amount remains unmetabolized and can be measured in breath and urine.

What is the difference between alcohol abuse and alcoholism? Abuse is drinking so much that you get drunk. Alcoholism is an addiction. The body craves alcohol, and physical effects result from its withdrawal. For you as a nurse, either way impairs your judgment and places your client in danger. Early intervention is essential. Not only are your health and life at stake, but so are the lives and health of your clients.

The most telling sign of any chemical dependency is a gradual decline in performance, which usually becomes noticeable in three to six months. Behaviors that need to be checked out include:

1. Complaints by staff and clients.
2. Accidents, errors in documentation, a greater number of injuries caused while moving clients or equipment, errors in practice.
3. Increased visits to the employee health department or emergency room.
4. Increased volunteering to take calls for others.
5. Arriving early or staying late to assist in the narcotic count.

6. Frequent absenteeism after days off and for personal emergencies, especially on a Monday.
7. Irritability and mood swings.
8. Performing only the minimum amount of work required.
9. Inability to perform psychomotor skills owing to intoxication or tremors.

Two emotional characteristics of chemical dependency make it difficult to begin treatment. The denial system is very strong, and the person who drinks is usually a skilled manipulator. A recovering alcoholic who is a commercial photographer explained, "I was always drinking with the finest professionals. My companions included a judge, a lawyer, the town's top surgeon, and the police chief. Obviously *they* weren't alcoholics. Anyway there was always someone in a more advanced stage than I was. As my alcoholism continued to progress I would point to someone in a more advanced stage and say, 'Look at him. I'm not doing that. I'm not an alcoholic.' And then one day I almost died after I fell down a flight of stairs. I finally heard when the doctor said, 'Either you quit drinking or you will die.'" Unlike in this case, it is not necessary to hit bottom to intervene.

Critical Thinking Exercise

1. Do I turn to alcohol and/or other chemicals for relief from pain or job stress on a regular basis? _____
2. If the answer to question one is yes, to whom will you go to seek intervention? _____
3. List the names of some facilities and persons in your area who assist with chemical dependency issues. _____
4. If you realize that a coworker or someone you supervise is drinking and is impaired while on duty, what is your responsibility to the client in this matter? _____

You can seek help from counselors, treatment centers, Alcoholics Anonymous, Moderation Management, Narcotics Anonymous, and other local resources. The yellow pages in your phone book list resource numbers under Alcohol Abuse Information and Treatment and Drug Abuse Information and Treatment. You can also look in the white pages under Business and Professional Listings for alcohol or drug abuse services and helpline and hotline numbers. It is worth the risk making a phone call to obtain information on your own or a friend's behalf.

Codependency

Before you read any further, answer the following questions:

1. What is your reason for making nursing your career choice?
2. Who supplies the most important critique of your day's work?
3. How do you feel if the client does not tell you that you did a good job?

Critical Thinking Exercise

"A codependent person is one who has let another person's behavior affect him or her, and who is obsessed with controlling that person's behavior" (Beattie, 1992, p. 36). What is your opinion about this statement and why?

Some writers have speculated that a significant number of nurses may be codependent. "For most codependents, helping others is a way to meet their needs. Although serving individuals and offering assistance are admirable endeavors, they become extreme in their efforts and in the level of involvement in others' lives" (Long, 1996, p. 20). Codependent nurses relate to their clients and their coworkers in unhealthy ways. For some, a painful childhood that included sexual abuse, violence, or chemical abuse may have paved the way to **codependency.**

Codependent people "fix" things and right wrongs. They react too quickly to feelings with a sense of intensity and urgency. Clients are viewed disrespectfully; i.e., they are thought to be incapable of participating in their own care. This viewpoint takes away clients' sense of personal control and may give them the message that they are more ill than initially perceived. Some characteristics of the codependent nurse are listed in Box 11–1.

Whenever a definition of a behavior provides a tinge of truth, it is followed by denial or harsh self-criticism. However, the intent is to inform—to allow you to evaluate yourself and modify codependent behaviors *if* they exist.

The following true incident illustrates codependency in a nurse. A man and his fiancée, both in their twenties, were involved in a car accident. The woman experienced serious injuries and was placed in traction. The man was admitted for observation. He was not placed on bed rest. The following morning a nursing student working as an aide during her summer break was assigned to him. Later in

---

Box 11–1

Codependent Nurse

1. Says "yes"—really means "no."

2. Feels the fate of nursing care rests on her shoulders.

3. Feels responsible for solving others' problems.

4. Competes for attention rather than supporting coworkers.

5. Often feels angry, unappreciated, and used.

6. Does not support client's need for autonomy and return to self-sufficiency.

7. Makes excuses and conceals negative practices rather than working for change.

8. Shows feelings of anger indirectly.

9. Perfectionistic: gossips and judges.

10. Avoids conflict.

Possible Behavior

Agrees to help another staff member and then complains to someone else about being taken advantage of.

Takes on non-nursing duties that belong to other departments.

Sympathetic, rather than empathetic, response to clients and other staff.

Engages in one-upmanship and intershift rivalries over client care.

Comes in early and works late. Works extra shifts to "help" coworkers.

Does for the client what the client needs to do in order to regain optimal health and self-confidence.

Feels powerless. Takes on extra duties because of chronic understaffing.

Pouts, procrastinates, forgets, gets sick, or is late.

Unrealistic expectations of others.

Too nice, loving, and forgiving. Smiles when having negative feelings.

the day, other aides were overheard talking about the male client's description of his morning care. "He told me that it was the best care he had ever received. She (the aide) insisted that he have a bedbath. She scrubbed him from top to bottom — and I do mean bottom! She even powdered his penis!" This aide interfered with the client's autonomy.

Using denial and manipulation to gain satisfaction in unhealthy ways has usually been practiced for many years. It takes special courage to really look at oneself to see whether any of these behaviors are present. Both self-help groups and books are available. How about codependency as a topic of discussion during class in relation to personal life or one's relationships with classmates? Replace the words "client," "coworkers," and "staff member" with "others" in the preceding characterization. Determine your codependency traits outside of nursing.

Beattie (1992, p. 83) compares codependent behavior to the sides of Karpman's drama triangle (victim, rescuer, persecutor). Since codependents are caretakers or rescuers, they rescue, then persecute, and ultimately end up feeling victimized.

Critical Thinking Exercise

1. Do your behaviors in regard to clients fit this pattern?
2. Are you looking for happiness through your relationship with the client?
3. Do you maintain focus on clients' needs, i.e., medical or nursing orders?

Beattie's self-help book *Codependent No More* (1992) has specific information on codependent characteristics and changing codependency behaviors. A 12-step program using only first names of members is available free. Inpatient therapy programs, including "Focus on the Family of Origin" and "Help for the Helpers: Co-dependency Treat-

ment for Professionals," are also available for a fee.

Aggressiveness and Work-Related Issues

Workplace violence has always been here. It is the increase in violence that is making nurses take notice. Homicide is the third highest work-related cause of death in the United States. The U.S. Department of Labor statistics reports homicide as the leading cause of death for women at work.

Violence is typed according to four categories:

1. Employee: Violence is directed toward supervisors or management.
2. Domestic: The issue is personal, but the violent act takes place in the workplace.
3. Property: Violence is directed against the employee's or employer's property.
4. Commercial: The employee engages in activities such as stealing from employers. Violence may ensue as a result of the activity.

Signs of Violence

Be alert to signs of violence. Early signs might include:

- Unusual behavioral change
- Lack of cooperation with nursing supervisors
- Cursing and other hostile forms of communications
- Short fuse and frequent arguments
- Spreading gossip or rumors to harm others deliberately
- Uninvited sexual remarks
- Hostile responses to other nurses, clients, or family members
- Sleep disturbances mentioned at work
- Increase in irritability and anxiety

The next stage might include:

- Conversation focused on "poor me, the victim"
- Notes with threats or violent or sexual content

- Verbalization that includes plans or a desire to harm someone
- Ignoring workplace policies
- Stealing workplace property
- Less interest in work and follow-through on assignments
- Increase in arguments
- Increase in physical accidents or injuries

As the anger intensifies and if conflicts remain unresolved, the result can be violence against self or others.

- Behaviors directed toward self might include depression or suicidal threats.
- Behaviors directed toward others might include physical fighting, property destruction, or use of a weapon to harm others.

Assault

Almost two-thirds of nonfatal workplace **assaults** occur in nursing homes and hospitals. According to the Department of Labor, the greatest number of hospital assaults is in the emergency department. Most of the assaults are done by clients, and almost three fourths of those assaulted are staff nurses. *At least part of the problem is related to nurses' accepting the possibility of violence as the norm.* As a nurse, you have the responsibility to act assertively together with other nurses to advocate for a safe workplace.

In March, 1996, the U.S. Department of Labor's Occupational and Safety and Health Administration (OSHA) released its first Act of Violence Prevention Guidelines geared toward protecting health care and social service workers on the job. The national guidelines are designed to protect employer and employees with a framework for deterring violence and increasing safety (Canavan, 1996, p. 3). The OSHA guidelines included recommendations for:

- Safer nurses' stations.
- Unit arrangement with staff safety in mind.
- No toleration of violence policy.
- At least two exits in rooms to prevent entrapment of staff.
- Adequate, qualified staff coverage at all times.

- Policies and procedures for protecting home care providers.
- Prompt medical evaluation and treatment regardless of severity of incident.
- Victims' right to prosecute perpetrators.
- Investigation of all incidents and installation of corrective action.

Not all agencies have complied. Therefore, some state nurses' associations have moved for legislative solutions. As of November 1998, Minnesota, New Hampshire, Ohio, and Washington are working toward increased penalties against people guilty of assaulting a health care worker or to establish task forces to study workplace violence (Slattery, 1998, p. 52).

 Learning Exercise: Workplace Violence

What is your state practical/vocational nurses' association doing to minimize risks of job violence in the workplace?

Contributing Factors

Although the research by Levine, Hewitt, and Misner (1998) focused on hospital-based emergency departments, many of their findings regarding contributing factors to violence apply to all of nursing.

PERSONAL FACTORS. These relate to verbal, nonverbal, and affective communication, including nurses' attitudes and behaviors. Attitude and body language were considered more significant than the sex and age of the nurse. The manner of approaching a client, such as with respect and confidence, emerged as important (p. 251).

WORKPLACE FACTORS. The quality, performance, and availability of security personnel emerged as important. The nurses believed they were safer when security officers wore police-type uniforms because then the officers better conveyed authority than when they wore a customer-friendly uniform of jacket and tie—a nonverbal form of communication. Incidents were also more common when nurses and security lacked aggression and management skills. Finally, not all administrators backed nurses on reporting incidents of physical and verbal abuse, including those involving supervisors and physicians.

ENVIRONMENTAL FACTORS. The type of client seen and the location of the care facility determine the type of clients admitted to a hospital. Many hospital workers cited substance use as a major factor in assaults. Substance-abusing clients (or families), psychiatric clients, and clients with dementia were those most likely to assault staff.

Counselling and Filing Charges

Levine et al. (1998) concluded that assault-related injuries are preventable. Only physical injuries are treated; all employees who have been verbally or physically assaulted should be referred for postincident debriefing. Hospital managers should implement violence prevention programs. If you are harmed or threatened by a client or his family member, you have the option to file charges. Some agencies will do this for you after a review board hearing, or they will support you filing charges yourself. Legal redress becomes an assertive stance for you and your fellow nurses (Carrol, 1997, p. 60.)

Harassment

Harassment is another form of aggressive communication. It is defined as any unwanted, deliberate, or repeated unsolicited comments, gestures, graphic materials, physical contacts, or solicitation of favors that is based upon one's group membership (Gregg, 1994, p. 1.) The person puts up with the harassment in order to remain employed. It affects the person's work or work environment. The key word is "unwanted." So your assertive response is to state this clearly to whoever is harassing you. Be sure that your response is firmly assertive. The message must

be congruent so that your verbalization, body language (nonverbal), and affective communication all say the same thing. Mere words do not justify a physical response on your part. Document for yourself what happened as well as what you said and did.

Wisconsin has a more detailed description of sexual harassment: unwelcome sexual advances, unwelcome requests for sexual favor, unwelcome physical contact of a sexual nature, or unwelcome verbal or physical conduct of a sexual nature (Gregg, 1994, p. 1.) The key word is "unwelcome." Employers have the responsibility to correct unwelcome behavior that they know about or should know about in the workplace. Once again, it is your responsibility to be assertive, to make known that the behavior is unwanted. Report to the employer with your documentation if the person does not stop the unwelcome behavior.

Prevention of Workplace Violence

Prevention begins when each nurse makes a personal commitment to practice prevention guidelines. There are policies in every workplace that cover forms of violence as well as harassment. Check them out. Be alert to warning signs. Think through what you can do. Take all threats seriously. Report them to management and advocate assertively for implementing. Some general safeguards include:

1. Doing your part to promote a supportive, congenial, yet professional work environment.
2. Whenever possible, resolve conflicts as they arise. Know that there are times when you have to back off. *However,* most of the time people want to have their point of view understood, to be listened to. A technique called *creative communication* encourages you to:
   a. Listen carefully to the other person's point of view.
   b. Ask questions to clarify what you do not understand. (Remember that this step is not a sneaky way to argue or to interject your own opinion!)

c. Tell the person what you think he or she said and what you think he or she is feeling. If your version is inaccurate, have the person repeat the explanation. When you can repeat back accurately what the person *thinks* and *feels,* it is your turn to present your view. Steps a, b, and c work for you as well.

3. Deal directly with unwanted or unwelcome behavior, including uninvited sexual advances. Review your own behavior to determine whether

   a. A clarification of the person's signals is in order, or

   b. Limits must be stated clearly and firmly on what you consider unacceptable behavior, or

   c. Supervisor or management intervention is needed.

4. Get to know your fellow workers and look out for each other.

5. Promote workplace integrity. Treat each other, your clients, and their families with respect, courtesy, and professionalism. Negative comments by clients and relatives usually are a response to their fear of the unknown. Rarely are the comments meant to be personal. Check out the fear. What are the questions? What can you do to help find answers?

6. Be alert to changes in behavior that may signal violence.

7. Avoid putting yourself in obvious danger. Make use of security guards for escort to parking lots and out-of-the-way areas. *Listen to your intuition.* This is making conscious use of effective communication.

 Critical Thinking Exercise

What are additional ways that you know of to defuse or prevent violence in the workplace?

Summary

☐ Communication translates into behavior. Assertiveness is honest and open behavior. It considers others' feelings and needs. It is based on *choice.* Both nonassertive (passive) and aggressive behaviors are based on *emotional hooks.* These styles are ultimately damaging to both parties involved. Be alert to unresolved feelings: worry → fear → anger → rage.

☐ Unresolved feelings from nonassertive behaviors can result in attempts to overplease (codependency), self-medication (alcohol and/or other drugs), burnout (negative response to clients), aggressive behavior, and/or physical illness.

☐ Undesirable behaviors and interactions can be changed through using the steps of the problem-solving process. Verbal, nonverbal, and affective interactions must be dealt with during this change.

☐ In some cultures, skillful positive manipulation is practiced successfully. Positive manipulation involves consideration of others' needs and feelings. Furthermore, other individuals are treated with respect rather than as objects to be used for personal gain.

☐ How you see your client gives you important clues about your needs. If you are able to separate your personal and professional lives, develop an empathetic approach to client care, and be your own best friend and boss, chances are that nursing will continue to excite you.

☐ Violence in the workplace has always been there, but it is on the increase in some areas. Most agencies have established policies and security measures for your benefit. Know what they are and follow them.

Review Questions

1. How is assertiveness different from aggressiveness?
   A. Focuses on the person, not the behavior.
   B. Indirect way of meeting needs.
   C. Is a tool, not a weapon.
   D. Recognizes others' needs as foremost.
2. How does nonassertiveness relate to burnout?
   A. Unresolved anger is projected onto the client.
   B. Being open and honest is difficult.
   C. Focus shifts to real needs of client.
   D. Burnout acts to equalize behavior.
3. What is an assertive response to a boss who is using divide-and-conquer manipulation?
   A. I agree. I noticed the same thing.
   B. Why don't we talk about this later?
   C. Let's just keep this between us.
   D. I'll talk with you about us, but *not* about Mary.
4. How does the impaired nurse use alcohol and/or other drugs?
   A. Self-medication, for fear and anger.
   B. To treat an inherited condition.
   C. To understand what client's experience has been.
   D. To separate from work responsibilities.
5. What are significant personal factors that may contribute to violence?
   A. Physical size and gait
   B. Attitude and body language
   C. Consumer-friendly environment
   D. Location of health facility

References

Balzer-Riley J. *Communications in Nursing—Communicating Assertively and Responsibly in Nursing: A Guidebook,* 4th ed. St. Louis: C. V. Mosby, 2000.

Beattie M. *Codependent No More,* 2nd ed. Center City, MN: Hazelton, 1992.

Canavan K. Nurses become political tour de force. Steps taken to protect health care workers from violence. American Nurse 28(3), April/May 1996.

Carrol V. Health and safety in workplace violence. Am J Nurs 99(3), March 1997.

Chenevert M. *Stat: Special Techniques in Assertiveness Training,* 4th ed. St. Louis: C. V. Mosby, 1994.

Gregg R. *Harassment Under Federal and Wisconsin Fair Employment Laws.* Madison, WI: Tom Linson, Gillman & Rikkers, 1994.

Levine P, Hewitt J, Misner S. Insights of nurses about assault in hospital-based emergency rooms. Image: Journal of Nursing Scholarship 30(3), 1998.

Long N. Co-dependency: Illusive and misunderstood. HT 3(5):18–45, 1996.

Peterson C. ANA calls workshop guidelines an excellent step. American Nurse 28(3), April/May 1996.

Slatterly M. The epidemic hazards of nursing. Am J Nurs 98(11), 1998.

Bibliography

Barker T. How to prevent violence in the workplace. Safety and Health, July 1994, pp. 32–38.

Bauer B, Hill S. *Mental Health Nursing, An Introductory Text.* Philadelphia: W. B. Saunders, 2000.

Bonneville G. Diagnosis violence. University of Minnesota Health Sciences. Spring 1995, pp. 2–7.

Branden N. *The Six Pillars of Self-Esteem.* New York: Bantam Books, 1995.

Cavello B. Codependency paints nursing's goals. RN 54: 132, 1991.

Grainger R. The genie in the bottle. Am J Nurs, March 1993, p. 18.

Hughes T, Smith L. Is your colleague chemically dependent? Am J Nurs 94:31–35, 1994.

Mallory G, Berkery A. Codependency: A feminist perspective. J Psychosoc Nurs 31(4):15–18, 1993.

Yates J, McDaniel J. Are you losing yourself in codependency? Am J Nurs 93:32–36, 1993.

Chapter 12

The Practical/Vocational Nurse's Role in the Nursing Process

Outline

Key Terms

ADPIE
APIE
current information
data collection (assessment)
evaluation

goals
historical information
interventions
NANDA
NIC

NOC
objective information
outcomes
strengths
subjective information

Objectives

Upon completing this chapter you will be able to:
1. Discuss how the nursing process has evolved from the 1950s to now.
2. Define your role in the nursing process according to the nurse practice act of your state.

3. Describe the four phases of the nursing process for the practical nurse:
   - Data Collection (Assessment)
   - Planning
   - Implementation
   - Evaluation

4. Describe nursing diagnosis as the exclusive domain of the RN.
5. Explain the purpose of NIC.
6. Discuss how NIC differs from NOC.

The nursing process is a problem-solving method. It is a way to plan client care. It helps clients reach the goals that have been set to care for their health problems.

Currently, unlicensed persons are doing all the tasks and skills that practical/vocational nurses do. It is the nursing process that separates practical/vocational nurses from the unlicensed persons. This makes practical/vocational nurses attractive to em-

ployers because they can solve problems and think critically.

As a student you will probably develop nursing care plans. Nursing care plans are learning tools. They are traditionally used in practical/vocational nursing programs to help students learn about client needs. Using your role in the nursing process to devise a care plan is a critical thinking exercise. The exact information fitting your client is not found anywhere. You compose it. This becomes easier plan by plan. And then—presto! You graduate. You are employed. You have internalized your role in the nursing process, and you are thinking critically as a nurse.

Nursing Process 1950s

Nursing process was originated in the 1950s to provide structure for thinking in nursing. "Nursing process was designed to organize thinking so that the problems encountered by patients could be anticipated and solved quickly" (Pesuit and Herman, 1998, p. 29). The four-step process included assessment (data collection), planning, intervention, and evaluation (**APIE**). The most important outcome of nursing process was for nurses to think before acting. The problem-solution (problem-solving) model became accepted. Nursing education programs and textbooks began to focus on the client's medical problem and nursing intervention. The interventions that were suggested varied in institutions and in nursing texts. Nursing did not yet see itself as having something unique to contribute to client care that was separate, and additional, to its dependent role to physicians.

Nursing Process 1970s– 1990s

When the American Nurses Association (ANA) published the standards of nursing practice in 1977, it established the five-step nursing process. Assessment (data collection), diagnosis (the new step), planning, intervention, and evaluation became **ADPIE.** The problem-solving format of the original nursing process was replaced with a reasoning model. Although nursing diagnosis was, and is, within the RN's legal role, the advances in nursing process challenge all nurses to think critically. Nursing process is a way for nurses to identify client problems they can respond to. It gives nurses a common language in which to communicate with each other and with other health providers.

What Does Your State Law Say About Your Role?

It is crucial at this time that, with the assistance of your instructor, you review the nurse practice act of your state. Your role in the nursing process is spelled out in this law. There are variations within the states and territories. Check it out. It is the basis of your nursing practice. Table 12–1, Nursing Process and Caregiver Roles, shows one model, developed jointly by the California Nurses Association and a union local (Local 250). The model roles are based on the California laws and educational requirements, which define the scopes of practice of RNs and LVNs and the tasks that can be assigned to nurses' assistants (NAs) and certified nurses' assistants (CNAs).

In developing the models, the organizations stated, "We recognize that skilled, experienced NAs, CNAs, LVNs, and RNs often contribute to patient care at a level beyond what their licensure or certification requires. We believe that nursing expertise must be encouraged and respected. But we must not permit employers to exploit the fear of losing a job or the need for recognition and job satisfaction in order to force speed-ups, impose greater responsibility for lower pay, and require nursing personnel to violate their legal scope of practice" (California Nurse, March 1995).

Phases of the Nursing Process for the Practical/ Vocational Nurse

As of April 1997, all steps of the nursing process are incorporated throughout the NCLEX-PN (National Council Licensure Examination for Practical Nurses) (National Council, 1998, p. 1).

The four steps that LP/VNs are responsible for are

1. *Data collection:* Participate in establishing a data base.

TABLE 12–1: The Nursing Process and Caregivers Roles

Assessment of Patient's Condition or Needs

RN Role	*LVN Role*	*NA/CNA Role*
■ Direct observation (see, auscultate, palpate, percuss)	■ Direct observation (see, auscultate, palpate, percuss)	■ Observation (seeing)
■ Data collection (measurements that require substantial scientific knowledge or technical skill)	■ Data collection (measurements, including those requiring LVN technical skill)	■ Data collection (basic measurements)
■ Information gathering shaped by theory, pattern recognition, or judgment	■ Recognition of abnormal values	■ Reporting
■ Verification/corroboration of data collected by other personnel	■ Collaboration with RN in nursing diagnosis	
■ Synthesis or interpretation of data		
■ Formulation of nursing diagnosis, including psychosocial and educational needs		

Planning or Coordinating Nursing Care

■ Application of theory to individual patient's findings	■ Collaboration with RN in planning care	
■ Three-way communication to enhance mutual respect or job satisfaction, or to promote coordination of care	■ Three-way communication to enhance mutual respect or job satisfaction, or to promote coordination of care	■ Three-way communication to enhance mutual respect or job satisfaction, or to promote coordination of care
■ Delegation, assignment, or clinical guidance for other caregivers		
■ Partnership with patient regarding plan of care		

Implementation, Not Fragmentation

■ Functions, including manual, requiring substantial scientific knowledge or technical skill	■ Technical or manual functions, including sterile technique or IVs with certification	■ Manual functions appropriate to education or skill level, or in accordance with RN and LVN regulatory rules
■ Functions requiring or closely related to patient's need for ongoing assessment	■ Ongoing data collection while implementing care	
■ Functions requiring RN assessment	■ Reporting or referral as needed	■ Reporting as needed

continued

TABLE 12–1 continued

Implementation, Not Fragmentation continued

RN Role	LVN Role	NA/CNA Role
■ Initiate/change treatment following standardized procedures		
■ Cooperation in implementation to promote peer support, unity, or patient or caregiver safety	■ Cooperation in implementation to promote peer support, unity, or patient or caregiver safety	■ Cooperation in implementation to promote peer support, unity, or patient or caregiver safety

Patient Education

■ Ongoing integration or application of new scientific knowledge to individual patient's signs or symptoms	■ Patient education based on licensed vocational nursing curriculum	■ Basic information regarding facility environment or facility procedures
■ Assessment of educational needs and delegation of implementation as appropriate to LVN	■ Appropriate implementation of patient education	■ Notify licensed personnel if patient needs additional education
■ Advice based on independent scope of RN and/or standardized procedures		

Evaluation

■ See assessment above	■ See assessment role above	■ Observation, data collection, or reporting as above

The RN is responsible for evaluation of patient's overall condition or response to treatment. This is achieved by the RN's direct observation or assessment, in addition to interpretation of the LVN's physical assessment, data collection, or recognition of abnormal values, or the NA/CNA's observations and measurements.

Patient Advocacy

■ Ethical or legal obligation or responsibility for active patient advocacy, which goes beyond observing patient's rights	■ Ethical obligation to use technical knowledge for patient's best interest	■ Ethical or legal obligation to respect patient's rights
	■ Ethical or legal obligation to respect patient's rights	

Developed jointly by the California Nurses Association and Union Local 250. Published in California Nurse, March 1995. Used with permission.

2. *Planning:* Plan to set goals for meeting clients' needs and design strategies to achieve these goals.
3. *Implementation:* Initiate and complete actions necessary to accomplish the defined goals.
4. *Evaluation:* Participate in determining the extent to which goals have been achieved and interventions have been successful.

What Differentiates Your Role from the RN Role?

The RN has the major responsibility for all five steps of the nursing process. As a practical/vocational nurse, you take an active part in four steps (phases) of the nursing process according to your skill level, as listed in the previous paragraph. You work from the established nursing diagnosis, one of the five steps of the nursing process, written by the RN. You turn *nursing diagnosis* to *nursing problems.* In this way you clearly understand the nature of the problems.

Nursing diagnosis, step two of the five-step nursing process, is a summary in nursing terms of actual problems or high-risk problems that nurses can respond to. It is considered the exclusive responsibility of the RN. When writing a nursing diagnosis, the nurse uses an established list of nursing diagnoses developed by the North American Nursing Diagnosis Association; called the **NANDA** list. Registered nurses are encouraged to use this approved diagnosis list to share a common language with other nurses. Nursing diagnoses are intended to create a communication bridge for all nurses, so that they can understand each other's terminology (see a medical-surgical nursing text for list).

RNs are taught assessment skills as part of their basic education; these skills include client interview and physical assessment of all body systems. Practical/vocational nurses may *choose* to learn more complex assessment skills as part of a postgraduate course. However, practical/vocational nurses learn to assess (collect data) the client and the environment during every encounter with a client. Data collection includes taking vital signs, checking therapeutic responses to medications and treatment, assessing for symptoms of health problems, and so on. The focus for data collection (assessment) is based in the current unit of study for the practical/vocational nurse.

The practical/vocational nurse acts in a more *dependent* role when participating in the planning and evaluation phases of the nursing process and acts in a more *independent* role when participating in the data collection and implementation phases of the nursing process.

Because of the depth of the RN's basic education, the RN functions independently in all steps of the nursing process. These actions do not need a physician's order. Both RNs and LP/VNs share an *interdependent* relationship with other health team members. For example, RNs and LP/VNs both carry out orders for treatments and medications written by a medical doctor, podiatrist, or dentist.

Data Collection (Assessment): Phase 1

Some states allow practical/vocational nurses to use the phrase "assist with assessment" in their job description. Other states permit use of the phrase "data collection." *Data collection* includes the following:

A. Gathering information relative to the client:

- Collect information from the client, significant others, and/or health care team members; and current and prior health records.
- Recognize significant findings.
- Determine the need for more information.

B. Communicating information gained in data collection:

- Document findings thoroughly and accurately.
- Report findings to relevant members of the health care team.

C. Contributing to the formation of a nursing diagnosis:
  ■ Assist in organizing relevant health care data.
  ■ Assist in determining a significant relationship between data and client needs and/or problems.

Your involvement in this step depends on the place of your employment and your skill level. The practical/vocational nurse usually has more responsibility in the nursing home where the client's condition is more stable. At the conclusion of your practical/vocational nursing program you have acquired strong, although incomplete, assessment (data collection) skills: "the tool box is not complete." An incomplete tool box is nothing to be ashamed of. For example, you take the temperature, pulse, respiration (TPR) and blood pressure properly. Be proud of your **data collection (assessment)** skills. They provide valuable data.

Most schools offer physical assessment as a course separate from the practical/vocational nursing program. Ask your instructor about the availability of such a course. It is an excellent way to learn interview, observation, and physical assessment skills. Whether you use part or all of these skills at work, the knowledge will improve the care you provide.

The *primary* source of information in data collection is the client. After all, clients know themselves and their bodies better than anyone else. All questions should be directed to the client unless he or she is unable to respond. *Secondary* information is available through family members, friends, and records that accompany the client. Clients need to be reassured that information will be considered confidential unless they give permission to share it with those not involved in direct care.

Data collection (assessment) begins on admission and continues with each client encounter. *The RN interviews the client to obtain his or her history and assess the body systems.* As *part of the one-year program, learning communication skills does not include learning the formal interview process.* Obtaining initial data such as vital signs is often

assigned to the practical/vocational nurse. It is important to separate the information gathered into *subjective, objective, historical,* and *current* data:

■ **Subjective information** is based on the client's opinion. It can include self-evaluation of pain, headache, nausea, feelings, and so on. Charting starts with the words, "Client states . . . ."
■ **Objective information** includes data that the nurse can observe and verify. Examples include vital signs, height, weight, appearance, personal hygiene, and so on. Use of the senses is required: seeing, hearing, smelling, touching, and, yes, sometimes even tasting. Objective information helps support or cast doubt on subjective information. Charting states what the nurse observes and measures, without judging or drawing conclusions.
■ **Historical information** includes the health history that relates to the current condition. Charting involves being as objective as possible.
■ **Current information** includes what is happening now. This is "where it's at" for the practical/vocational nurse who is *assisting with* data collection (assessment).

Words like check, observe, monitor, weigh, measure, smell, palpate, and auscultate are clues that this is an assessment (data collection) procedure. The practical/vocational nurse develops a list of data to be collected (assessed) to accompany the identified problems as a way to tell whether the client is meeting the goals.

Data collection (assessment) starts when you first see the client at the beginning of the shift. This is your baseline observation. It continues throughout your clinical shift. Florence Nightingale said that if you do not observe your client you should not be a nurse. With each contact the LP/VN must see, hear, smell, and touch the client when necessary and use all the senses to gather data about the client and the environment. Data collection is vital—the client changes throughout the day. This is why accuracy in taking vital signs; describing vomitus, bleeding, or a skin lesion; and determining level of consciousness, for example, is so important. "Has the client's skin lesion changed since the last time you checked the lesion? How? How much?" Sometimes LP/VNs do not understand that what they are assigned to do is a vital part of the total assessment (data collection). Data collection (assessment) starts during admission. It continues daily at the beginning of the shift for the baseline observation, then periodically during the shift, and right before leaving.

Data collection (assessment), whether partial or total, involves courtesy. Introduce yourself to the client and explain what you are going to do. Address the client as Mr., Mrs., Miss, or other title as appropriate. Avoid using a first name unless you have the client's permission. Remind yourself that this is a professional, not a personal, relationship you are building. The most common complaints put forth by clients are: "I don't know which one is the nurse," "I am treated with disrespect," "I am not their grandma," and so on. When in the client's presence, stand or sit where he or she can see you. Clients often experience fear on being hospitalized or transferred to a new facility. Confusion or lack of skills on the nurse's part serves to increase that fear. The focus of the nurse's job is to serve the client with the greatest skill possible.

Avoid asking questions that have been asked before. Be sure that you have looked at the record before entering the client's room. Explain why you are asking questions and reassure the client that he or she has the right not to answer questions that cause discomfort. Be a good listener. Encourage confidence. Request clarification rather than pretending that you understand: "I am not sure that I understand what you mean by that statement." Check out what you think you understand: "Am I correct in saying that you are worried about the kind of care you will receive here?" Avoid using reassuring promises that you cannot deliver: "Don't worry, everything will be just fine." Also avoid giving approval—for example, "That's right." This statement may make it difficult for a client to change his or her mind. Nursing responsibility does not involve judging the client's behavior, values, or decision. Finally, avoid showing or verbalizing dis-

approval or belittling the client: "You know you shouldn't do that." Chapter 8 elaborates on communication techniques that assist you in making the best use of the limited time you have to obtain needed data from the client.

In checking information for accuracy, it is necessary to validate it to differentiate between subjective and objective data. Subjective data is what the client feels. Sometimes it is demonstrated by objective signs. For example, the client may state that he or she feels very warm (subjective). The client has a temperature of 102°F (objective).

You must be alert to several possible barriers to data collection (assessment). These include insufficient time, poor skills in data collection (assessment), communication failure (such as a comatose client), the presence of distractions, or a client who is too sick to want to talk. If your personal values get in the way, what can happen is labeling the client before the interview is complete instead of basing decisions on facts. Respectful distancing is necessary if the nurse is to remain objective and use all senses clearly.

Physical assessment is an important part of data collection. RNs are taught how to perform physical assessment of clients as part of their basic education. They are taught assessment of all body systems. Practical/vocational nurses in basic programs learn assessment as part of each unit of study. Additional education in assessment, the acuteness or severity of the client's illness, and the area of employment all determine the extent of the practical/vocational nurse's involvement in physical assessment. The practical/vocational nurse is always assessing therapeutic responses to medications for side effects, symptoms of health problems, and so on (see Box 12–1).

When all the data are gathered, you will assist the RN in looking for gaps in information that will need further checking.

Charting data collection (assessment) information varies according to the guidelines of the specific facility where you work. Maintain a separation in your own mind about what constitutes subjective data, objective data, historical data, and current data. Remember that in a lawsuit, a nurse expert

---

Box 12–1. Examples of Data Collection

Examples of Practical/Vocational Nurse Data Collection

Examples used can apply to acute care or to the community

Observing results of a laxative or enema.

Observing for signs of congestive heart failure for a client taking furosemide (Lasix) and digoxin (Lanoxin).

Observing an ulcer on the lower leg of a diabetic: size (measure it), location, appearance, any drainage, and so on.

Observing the ulcer each time the leg is dressed.

Observing behavior for signs of disorientation or confusion.

Observing NPO client drinking water.

In acute care: observing position in bed; in community: observing gait, posture

Observing whether 76-year-old client is showing signs of ego integrity or despair. (Although the client should be at ego integrity, he is not capable of being there. Because of his cerebrovascular accident (CVA) he has to be washed, fed, and lifted everywhere. He is incontinent. His behavior reminds you of an infant. You will work at establishing trust in the client instead of ego integrity.)

Observing family interactions.

Observing the environment for need for safety factors—spills, bed rails, glasses on table, and so on.

Observing the urine for color, odor, amount, other characteristics.

---

reviewing a chart may interpret sloppy charting as sloppy nursing care. Refer to Chapter 18 for tips on charting.

Planning: Phase 2

Only the RN can develop the nursing plan. The practical/vocational nurse provides input into plan development. It is illegal for the practical/vocational nurse to write the plan and for the RN to initial it. The practical/vocational nurse's role in planning is to

A. Assist in the formation of goals of care:
   - Participate in the identification of nursing interventions required to achieve goals.
   - Communicate client needs that may require alteration of the goals of care.

B. Assist in the development of a plan of care:
   - Involve the client and health care team members in selection of nursing interventions.
   - Plan for the client's safety, comfort, and maintenance of optimal functioning.
   - Select nursing interventions for delivery of the client's care.

In the planning phase, practical/vocational nurses take the nursing diagnosis and state it as a nursing problem. Practical/vocational nursing students start here, state the problem, set goals, list interventions, and then list data collection (assessments). This process seems to reverse that of the RN, but remember that practical/vocational nurses do not have primary responsibility for assessment (phase 1) and rely on the RN for the nursing diagnosis. To demonstrate understanding of the nursing diagnosis, the practical/vocational nurse states it in objective specific terms as a nursing problem (see Table 12–2).

Whenever evidence of a new problem emerges, practical/vocational nurses collect data about the problem because of their good data collection skills. They collaborate with the RN, and the RN then formulates a new diagnosis.

For a nursing care plan to be a useful, realistic tool for the nursing staff, priorities must be established. A care plan will not include all the clients' problems. The most important problems, those that are potentially life-threatening, must be taken care of immediately. Maslow's hierarchy of needs (1943) is commonly used by nurses to assist in prioritizing client needs. The lowest level of needs according to Maslow (1943) is the physiologic (survival) needs. This means that in prioritizing client needs, attention is paid first to problems related to food, air, water, temperature, elimination, rest, and pain.

continued

TABLE 12–2: Student Assignment Sheet and Patient Care Plan

Student _____

Patient _____ Room _____ Doctor _____ Allergies _____

Age _____ Marital Status _____ Religion _____ Occupation _____

Admission Date _____ Date of Surgery _____ Diet _____

Medical Diagnosis _____ Surgical Procedure _____

Meaning in Own Words _____ Meaning in Own Words _____

Primary Nursing Problem _____

Categories of Human Function	Assessment	Nursing Problems	Goals	Nursing Intervention	Evaluation
Protective (e.g., personal care and hygiene, environment, surgery)	What you will: Check, observe, monitor, weigh, measure, palpate, auscultate. (1) Assess at beginning of shift for baseline, (2) periodically during shift, and (3) right before you leave	What is the problem in your own words? Be specific and objective. May use nursing diagnosis, but . . .	The patient will: (Reverse the problem and state positively what client will do—realistically, measurably, time-referenced)	The nurse will: (Be objective and specific. Care plans in texts rarely are. What the nurse will do to help client meet goals)	What progress is client making toward goals? Results of data collection and assessment in objective terms
Sensory-perceptual					
Comfort, rest, activity, and mobility (e.g., sleep and rest, body alignment)					
Nutrition					

197

TABLE 12–2 continued

Categories of Human Function	Assessment	Nursing Problems	Goals	Nursing Intervention	Evaluation
Growth and development (e.g., identify Erikson's developmental stage)					
Fluid-gas transport					
Psychosocial-cultural (e.g., emotional support, spiritual support, diversion and recreation)					
Elimination (e.g., urinary and gastrointestinal elimination)					
Need for community resources					

Critical Thinking Exercise

Write an example of a problem for each survival need.

1. Food _____

2. Air _____

3. Water _____

4. Temperature _____

5. Elimination _____

6. Rest _____

7. Pain _____

Possible answers: (1) not enough or too much food intake, (2) shortness of breath, (3) dehydration due to vomiting, (4) temperature seriously above or below normal, (5) diarrhea, (6) sleeping too little or too much, (7) pain that interferes with functioning.

It is not uncommon when working on several problems at the same time to find that a relationship exists between problems. Priorities may also change rapidly depending on the client's condition. The nurse has to remain flexible and to recognize the need to shift priorities according to client needs. The client will be far more cooperative with the care plan if he has been included in identifying the priorities of care. Remember that regression takes place during illness. The client advances on Maslow's hierarchy as he recovers. Cooperation is much more likely when the nurse understands this and respects it.

Think back to phase 1, data collection (assessment). What did the client say on admission about what she expects, wants, or needs during the time she is a client? (Check the chart: important information as you assist the RN in planning the care.) Did you also remember to collect data on client strengths (what she can do for herself)? **Strengths** are building blocks in developing a realistic plan.

Goal Setting

Specific **goals** provide direction for individualizing the care of the client. To be useful, goals must be client-centered and determined by the client and the nurse together. Goals must be (1) measurable, (2) realistic, and (3) time-referenced. The focus of the goal is the client, not the nurse. A goal is thought of as, "The client will do this or that." To get the best results, a goal must be set for each priority problem or need. To state a goal, *reverse the problem and state it in positive terms.* Terminology will vary to some degree. Some agencies use the terms goals, behavioral objectives, or expected **outcomes.**

The example in Table 12–3 shows how a client's care plan might look. A measurable, realistic, time-limited goal has been established for a *priority* problem. The goal statement specifically addresses the nursing problem. The stated time is an educated guess that becomes more accurate with experience. The examples show how the practical/vocational nurse *changes* the nursing diagnosis into a nursing problem.

Identifying the Interventions

The next step of the planning phase is to identify what nursing **interventions** (action, activity, treatment) will take place to achieve the goal. These are things the nurse will do to assist the client to reach the goals. Sometimes this means encouraging the client to do things for himself. This is also called nursing approach or nursing care. Interventions focus on the "related to (R/T)" portion of the nursing diagnosis. They tell all nursing personnel who, what, where, when, and how much. Anyone should be able to carry out your interventions. Check them out. Are they objective and specific? Interventions are based on courses you have taken, additional

TABLE 12–3: Nursing Problem, Goal and Interventions		
Nursing Diagnosis	**Nursing Problem**	**Goal**
Altered nutrition: less than body requirements. Related to (R/T) decreased calorie intake.	Eats only 5% of each meal. R/T loss of appetite and weakness.	The client will eat 1500 calories of ground foods and liquids during each 24-hour period. (The problem is reversed and stated positively.)

Interventions

1. Six small, ground meals at 8:00 AM, 10:00 AM, 12:00 noon, 2:00 PM, 4:00 PM, and 6:00 PM. Client seated in an easy chair with minimal assistance. Encourage self-feeding. Assist only if needed. Record time, amount, and type of food eaten.

2. Offer 240 ml of liquids at 6:00 AM, 9:00 AM, 11:00 AM, 1:00 PM, 3:00 PM, 5:00 PM, 7:00 PM, and 9:00 PM. Vary choices: likes Jell-O, ice cream, 7-Up, chocolate milk, and pineapple juice. Drinks herbal tea with meals. Record time, amount, and liquids taken.

reading, research, and so on. Interventions do not just come from the top of your head. See Chapter 7, Hints for Using Learning Resources.

Client and family strengths and weaknesses play an important part. The client and family are important partners with you in attaining the goal or goals. Building on client strengths provides a sense of contribution and some control. Maybe the client in the example given previously has the strength to feed himself but will not do so unless someone sits at the bedside. Rather than taking this strength away from the client and feeding him because it is "quicker and less messy," plan around it. The goal is to get him to take 1500 calories in 24 hours.

Different kinds of care plans are available. An individualized written care plan has been demonstrated. Some facilities use standardized care plans. These plans are based on research of the best possible options for a nursing diagnosis (nursing problem). To individualize a standard plan, cross out what does not apply and add appropriate interventions that apply to your client.

Computerized care plans are popular. Individualized plans can be entered into the computer. More commonly, standardized care plans are used and then individualized to deal with the nursing problem.

Multidisciplinary care plans work well in settings in which staff from varied professions and disciplines are frequently involved with the client. An example is a long-term care or psychiatric setting. These plans are developed by a multidisciplinary team and reflect specific interventions used by each discipline, e.g., physical therapist, nutritionist, nurse, and physician. Maintaining a separate plan for each profession is often considered repetitious. The focus of a multidisciplinary plan is client problems rather than nursing diagnoses. The language used must be common to all disciplines involved. All nursing interventions must be dated and signed.

Documenting (charting) the plan is essential. Legally, if it is not charted it is not done. Where the documentation takes place depends on the facility. It may be done on the computer or in longhand in the nurse's notes or on flowsheets. Some agencies have special care plan Kardexes or clipboards at the bedside. Eventually these become a part of the client's permanent record. Meanwhile, the plan is the recipe for meeting the client's nursing problems. Find it!

Implementation: Phase 3

The practical/vocational nurse's role in implementation is to

A. Assist with organizing and managing the client's care:

- Implement the established plan of care.
- Participate in a client care conference.

B. Provide care to achieve established goals of care:
- Use safe and appropriate techniques when administering client care.
- Use precautionary and preventive interventions in providing care to clients.
- Prepare client for procedures.
- Institute nursing interventions to compensate for adverse responses.
- Initiate life-saving interventions for emergency situations.
- Provide an environment conducive to attainment of goals of care.
- Provide care in accordance with client needs and/or preferences.
- Encourage client to follow a treatment regimen.
- Assist client to maintain present optimal functioning or to enhance it.
- Reinforce teaching of principles, procedures, and techniques for maintenance and promotion of health.
- Monitor client care provided by unlicensed nursing personnel.

C. Communicate nursing interventions:
- Document client's response to care, therapy, or teaching.
- Report client's response to care, therapy, or teaching to relevant members of the health care team.

The next stage is *initiating* the nursing interventions. What were those client strengths you identified? It is time to build on them as you begin to initiate the plan. Think back to the interventions listed on page 200.

1. Can the client move from the bed to the chair and back alone? With minimal support? With complete support?
2. Can he feed himself? Completely? With some assistance?
3. Does he eat best if someone is present? Alone? During conversation about family?
4. Are there any family members who can be instructed in how to act as partners in implementing the care plan?
5. Is the responsibility for the intervention within the licensed practical/vocational nurse role?

Once again, these are samples of the many questions that may be addressed at this time.

The implementation phase includes reporting and charting the shift activities. Reporting, to be useful, should be presented in an orderly fashion.

Your responsibility will vary according to the work area in which you are involved and whether you are functioning in a beginning or expanded role. In an acute care setting, your primary responsibility will be to use the care plan as a guideline for providing direct client care, continuing data collection, making verbal reports to the RN, and charting. In nursing homes and extended care facilities, you may be functioning in the role of a charge nurse and have responsibility for managing client care under the supervision of the RN.

The key for all your activity, regardless of your position and the agency involved, is to use the care plan as the basis for your nursing actions and reporting. For example, as a student you draw information from the care plan on how to provide individualized client care. While providing care you continue to make observations based on your knowledge of the client's strengths and disease conditions. You chart on flowsheets and nurses' notes following the priorities indicated by the nursing problem, plus any new observations you have made. You use the care plan as your guideline when reporting to the RN and offer information on any changes you have noted. Specifically, you focus on the nursing interventions outlined in the care plan: Do they continue to be appropriate? What changes or lack of changes have you observed? With this information the RN can update the plan of care and needs only to validate the data.

Evaluation: Phase 4

Evaluation is the fourth phase of the nursing process for the practical/vocational nurse. The practical/vocational nurse's responsibility in evaluation is to:

A. Compare actual outcomes with expected outcomes of client care:
- Assist in determining the client's response to nursing care.
- Assist in identifying factors that may interfere with the client's ability to implement the plan of care.
- Assist in determining the extent to which identified outcomes of the care plan are achieved.

B. Communicate findings:
- Document client's responses to care, therapy, or teaching to relevant members of the health care team.

Have you noticed how heavily dependent each step of the care plan is on the others, and how the steps are often going on simultaneously? Evaluation begins as soon as client contact occurs. The continual data collection (assessment) helps make daily evaluation part of the natural flow of good nursing care.

Evaluation is a way of measuring client progress toward meeting goals. You are not evaluating nursing behavior. Think of the client's goal. Look at daily data collection (assessment). If your data collection (assessment) list is complete, evaluation will be the results of your data collection. Compare this with goals. If progress is being made toward meeting goals, continue as is. If the client is not meeting goals, check the goals. Are they measurable, realistic, and time-referenced? If not, revise the portion that needs revision. Check the interventions or look for new interventions. If the goals meet the above

TABLE 12–4: Data Collection, Goal, and Evaluation		
Data Collection (Assessment) List	Goal	Evaluation
Check intake: ■ amount and type of liquid in milliliters ■ amount of food taken at each meal	The client will eat 1500 calories of chopped foods and liquids during each 24-hour period.	By day 2, client was able to consume 1500 calories, in ground meals and liquids, during a 24-hour period.

criteria, revise nursing interventions that are not working (see Leadership Hint #3 in Chapter 13).

When the goal is written in measurable terms and an appropriate data collection (assessment) list has been developed, the evaluation is built in. If you cannot evaluate the goal, it probably was not written accurately.

Nursing Process 1990s to Present

One of the exciting things about nursing is that it continues to grow as a profession. Nursing research and health industry focus and policy all drive the change from general to specific nursing interventions and measurement of outcomes. Two such well-researched projects are the Nursing Interventions Classification (NIC) and the Nursing Outcomes Classification (NOC). You may find yourself involved with one or both classifications sometime in your career.

Nursing Interventions Classification (NIC)

Have you looked in several nursing textbooks in preparation for a clinical assignment? Did you find yourself frustrated because the suggestions for interventions varied? What the *NIC* project is accomplishing is to develop a common, standardized language to describe interventions (treatments) performed by nurses. The lists are comprehensive and intended to assist all nurses. NIC is also a way to provide continuity of care between agencies. Some of the interventions listed need special training or special certification. Basic care is listed only if it is a required part of the intervention. Otherwise, you assume responsibilty to assist in basic care needs as taught.

NIC has been linked to the NANDA diagnoses (1996), but can be used independently. NIC's "concern with nursing interventions is *nurse behavior* or *nurse activity,* that is, those things that nurses do to assist patient status or patient behavior to move toward a desired outcome" (McCloskey and Bulechek, 1996, p. 4).

NIC clearly shows what nurses do and whether it is making a difference in the client's status. It also assists in defining what nurses need to learn to do the work of nursing. Students will have the opportunity to learn more decision-making as the currently medically oriented texts change to reflect nursing diagnosis and interventions.

Nursing Outcomes Classification (NOC)

NOC was developed to provide a common, standardized language for *measuring the degree of client response to nursing intervention.* It can be useful for interdisciplinary communication and with other care agencies. Currently, there are 16 measurement scales, of which 13 are most frequently used. Each is rated on a 1 to 5 continuum, with 5 as most positive (Johnson and Maas, 1997, p. 50).

For example, Scale 3 measures the degree of dependency for functional and self-care outcomes. These include (1) dependent, does not participate, (2) requires assistive person and device, (3) requires assistive person, (4) independent with assistive device, and (5) completely independent.

NOC differs from goals by identifying the degree of progress made or not made by the client. Many of the NANDA diagnoses have NOC linkages and are used to plan and evaluate nursing interventions for clients. Specific goals can be set for clients as needed to individualize cases. Bothe NIC and NOC are useful in teaching nursing students about decision-making and can influence the course of nursing education.

Summary

- ☐ Review the nurse practice act of your state or county to identify your role in nursing.
- ☐ Nursing process was originated in the 1950s to provide structure for thinking in nursing. The four-step process included assesment (data collection), planning, intervention, and evaluation (thinking model).
- ☐ The ANA standards of nursing practice, published in 1997, added nursing diagnosis to make a five-step nursing process (reasoning model).
- ☐ Nursing diagnosis is considered the exclusive responsibility of RNs because of their broad, science-based education.
- ☐ Nursing process, in the 1990s to now, continues to become more specific in identifying nursing interventions and measuring client behavioral and status outcomes. NIC (Nursing Intervention Classification) and NOC (Nursing Outcome Classification) are two current models.
- ☐ The RN, by virtue of a broad, science-based education, has the primary legal responsibility for the steps/phases of the nursing process. The nursing diagnosis is the RN's exclusive responsibility.

☐ The LP/VN, as a full partner in providing nursing interventions, must understand his or her role in the four phases of the nursing process. The practical/vocational nurse also participates in the nursing process according to assignment and skill level.

☐ Data collection (assessment), phase 1, includes participation in establishing a data base by (1) gathering information relative to the client, (2) communicating information gained in data collection, and (3) contributing to the formation of the nursing diagnosis. Data collection (assessment) occurs not only during admission but also during each nurse-client encounter. The client is the primary source of information.

☐ Planning, phase 2, includes participation in setting goals for meeting the client's needs and designing strategies to achieve these goals. This is accomplished by (1) assisting in the formulation of goals of care, and (2) assisting in the development of a care plan. Client problems are prioritized; realistic client-centered outcomes, and nursing interventions are established. The highest priority is always given to physiologic (survival) needs.

☐ Implementation, phase 3, involves initiating and completing the actions necessary to accomplish the defined goals. The practical/vocational nurse accomplishes this by (1) assisting with organizing and managing the client's care, (2) providing care to achieve established goals of care, and (3) reporting and recording nursing interventions.

☐ Evaluation, phase 4, includes participation in determining the extent to which goals have been achieved and interventions have been successful. This involves (1) comparing the actual outcomes with the expected outcomes of client care, and (2) communicating findings.

Review Questions

1. How did the origination of nursing process in the 1950s change the course of nursing care?
   A. Provided a reasoning model.
   B. Provided a specificity model.
   C. Provided a problem-solution model.
   D. Provided a critical thinking model.
2. Why is it important to understand how the state nurse practice act defines your nursing role?
   A. To prevent exploitation by employers.
   B. To learn under what circumstances you can assume an RN role.
   C. To review content of NCLEX-PN.
   D. To identify state variations in LP/VN role.
3. What makes nursing diagnosis the exclusive domain of the RN?
   A. RNs are taught client interview and assessment skills.
   B. LP/VNs can learn complex assessment through a postgraduate course.
   C. Practical/vocational nurses' data collection is undervalued.
   D. RNs and LP/VNs differentiate their roles in this way.
4. How does NOC differ from goals?
   A. Measures nursing treatments.
   B. Describes interventions performed by nurses.
   C. Describes standardized care.
   D. Measures degree of change.
5. How can nursing diagnosis, NIC, and NOC change nursing education?
   A. ANA standards of practice underlie all of nursing education.
   B. Texts will focus more on signs, symptoms, and medical treatment of illness.
   C. Texts will focus on nursing diagnosis and intervention.
   D. Education will become more problem-solution–oriented.

References

American Nurses' Association. *Nursing, A Social Policy Statement.* Kansas City, MO: American Nurses' Association, 1995.

American Nurses' Association. *Standards of Clinical Nursing Practice.* Washington, D.C.: American Nurses Association, 1977, 1991.

California Nurses Association and Union Local 250. Nursing Process and Caregivers Role. California Nurse 1995.

Iyer P, Taptich B, Bernocchi-Losey D. *Nursing Process and Nursing Diagnosis,* 3rd ed. Philadelphia: W. B. Saunders, 1995.

Johnson M, Maas M. *Nursing Outcomes Classification (NOC).* Iowa Outcomes Project. St. Louis: C. V. Mosby, 1997.

Maslow A. A theory of human motivation. Psych Rev 50: 370, 1943.

McCloskey JC, Bulechek GM. *Nursing Interventions Classification (NIC),* 2nd ed. Iowa Intervention Project. St. Louis: C. V. Mosby, 1996.

NCLEX-PN Test Plan for the National Council Licensure Examination. Chicago: National Council of State Boards of Nursing, 1998 (effective date, October 1999).

Bibliography

Ignatavicius D, Workman M, Mishler M. *Medical-Surgical Nursing: A Nursing Approach Process,* 3rd ed. Philadelphia: W. B. Saunders, 1999, Chap. 3.

Leahy JM, Kizicay PE. *Foundations of Nursing Practice: A Nursing Process Approach.* Philadelphia: W. B. Saunders, 1998. Chap. 2.

Linton A, Matteson M, Maebius N. *Introductory Nursing Care of Adults,* 2nd ed. Philadelphia: W. B. Saunders, 2000, Chap. 11.

McCloskey JC, Maas M. Interdisciplinary team: The nursing perspective is essential. Nursing Outlook, 46, July/August 1998.

National Council appoints new executive director. Issues 19(4), 1998. Chicago: National Council of State Boards of Nursing.

Pesuit DJ, Herman J. OPT: Transformation of nursing process for contemporary practice. Nursing Outlook 46, 1998.

Smith C, Maurer F. *Community Health Nursing: Theory and Practice,* 2nd ed. Philadelphia: W. B. Saunders, 2000, Chap. 10.

Varcarolis E. *Foundations of Psychiatric Mental Health Nursing,* 3rd ed. Philadelphia: W. B. Saunders, 1998, Chap. 6.

Chapter 13

Developing Leadership Skills

Outline

The Practical/Vocational Nurse as
First-Line Leader
The Organizational Chart
The Expanded Role of Practical/Voca-
tional Nursing
How You Are Already Preparing
for a Leadership and Man-
agement Role
The Difference Between Leadership
and Management
What Kind of Leader Are You?
Leadership Styles

Using the Leadership Continuum
as a Guide
Core Knowledge and Skills Needed
for Leadership
Understanding Motivation and
Human Needs
Applying Communication as an
LP/VN Leader
Applying Problem Solving as an
LP/VN Leader
Team Building

Stress Management
Additional Stress Control Skills
for the LP/VN Charge Nurse
Specific Knowledge and Skills Needed
for Leadership
Occupational Skills for First-Line
LP/VN Leaders
Organizational Skills for First-
Line LP/VN Leaders
Human Relationship Skills for
First-Line LP/VN Leaders

Key Terms

anger management
conflict resolution
continuous quality improvement (CQI)
continuum
empower
Health Care Financing Administration
(HCFA)
Howlett hierarchy

irrational thinking
Joint Commission on Accreditation of
Health Care Organizations (JCAHO)
leadership
management
mission statement
Omnibus Reconciliation Act of 1987
(OBRA)

patient outcome
performance evaluation
stress management
subjective versus objective
team building
time management

Objectives

Upon completing this chapter you will
be able to:
1. Describe the expanded role of
   the practical/vocational nurse as
   described in your state's nurse
   practice act.
2. Identify the location of the practi-
   cal/vocational charge nurse on
   the organizational chart of a
   long-term care facility.
3. Explain the difference between
   leadership and management.
4. Identify your personal leadership
   style.

5. Explain the following leadership
   styles in your own words:
   a. Autocratic
   b. Democratic
   c. Laissez-faire
6. Identify ways to attain competency in the five core areas in
   which knowledge and skills are
   needed to be an effective first-
   line leader:
   a. The ability to motivate team
      members to accomplish goals.
   b. The ability to communicate
      assertively

   c. The ability to problem solve
      effectively
   d. The ability to build a team of
      cooperative workers
   e. The ability to manage stress
      effectively
7. Identify ways to obtain competency in the three specific areas
   in which knowledge and skills
   are needed to be an effective
   first-line leader:
   a. Occupational skills
   b. Organizational skills
   c. Human relationship skills

8. Describe how the Howlett hierarchy of work motivators can help the practical/vocational nurse leader motivate nursing assistants.

9. Identify the importance of documenting objective, not subjective, charting entries in long-term care.

10. Use the problem-solving approach to set up a plan to solve a clinical problem.

11. Read the mission statement for your current area of clinical assignment.

12. Using suggestions in this chapter, write a plan that could be used to build a team to work on a unit in long-term care.

13. Develop a plan to decrease stress on the clinical area.

14. Using the A, B, C, D method of Ellis, identify an irrational thought you have had on the clinical area and convert it to a rational thought.

15. In your own words, explain specific skills required of the LP/VN charge nurse in long-term care because of OBRA requirements.

16. Prioritize tasks that need to be completed for your next clinical assignment.

17. Identify areas in which to improve efficiency in your current area of clinical assignment.

18. Explain techniques to discover the real issue when a conflict develops in the clinical area.

19. Develop a plan to control personal anger when working in the clinical area.

20. Practice giving positive and negative feedback in measurable terms to peers in a mock clinical situation.

21. Develop a plan for personal growth as an LP/VN charge nurse.

Polly Practical, LVN, charge nurse on the day shift, comes on duty in a frenzy. The staff shudders as she rearranges her uniform and papers. They murmur to each other, "Another day with Attila the Hun." Polly barks out the assignments after report. She reminds the staff (1) not to dawdle in their cares, (2) to have everything done by 10 AM, (3) to stay out of her way when she gives her meds, and (4) to give a thorough end-of-shift report because Polly has a headache and will be unable personally to check up on the residents that day.

Ann Assistant, NA, asks why everything has to be done by 10 AM. Polly takes off in a whirlwind of prose and assorted dramatics. Polly never answers Ann's question. This is unfortunate. The reason for getting cares done by 10 AM that particular day is because an entertainer from Branson, Missouri, and his entire orchestra will be visiting the nursing home. Had Ann and the other nursing assistants known the reason for the command, they would have worked twice as hard to complete their cares in time for one of the residents' favorite entertainers.

Because of the manner in which Polly conducts herself as a charge nurse, it could be said that Polly may be a manager, but she is not a leader.

The Practical/Vocational Nurse as First-Line Leader

Have you ever experienced an employment situation similar to the one just described with Polly Practical? Perhaps you received directions as a nursing assistant or in another job capacity and did not like the way you were approached by your supervisor.

Nurses at all levels need to manage client care. Some nurses will also be leaders. Licensed practical/vocational nurses have proved themselves effective as first-line leaders. First-line leaders are responsible for supervising nursing assistants who deliver care in long-term care situations. Such positions are referred to as charge nurse positions. If you are a manager of client care *and* a leader, you will be more effective in your expanded role in practical/vocational nursing

Practical/vocational nurses need to develop leadership and management skills so they can direct and supervise others in a manner that will effectively meet the goals of the employing agency. In your practical/vocational nursing program, you started to build a strong, solid base in these skills. The purpose of Chapters 13 and 14 is to help you continue

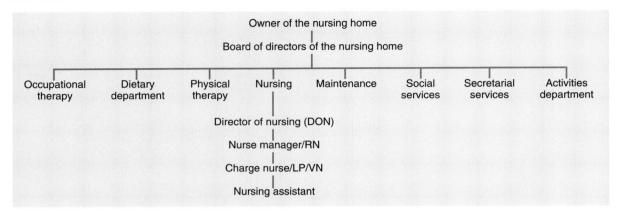

FIGURE 13–1. Sample traditional organizational chart for the role of the practical/vocational nurse in the nursing home/long-term care setting.

to develop skills to lead and manage. Chapter 13 will focus on the leadership role and provide 21 leadership hints and 6 leadership activities to get you started thinking in a leadership mode. Chapter 14 will focus on practical management tools to help you apply knowledge and skills needed to be a charge nurse. Chapter 14's interactive format will have you thinking as a new charge nurse and solving some of the problems new charge nurses face. Chapters 13 and 14 can be used as a reference tool of skills while becoming oriented to an LP/VN charge nurse position and in your future job when you function in your expanded role as an LP/VN charge nurse.

The Organizational Chart

The organizational chart is a picture of responsibility in an employment situation. In the *traditional* organizational chart, individuals lower on the organizational chart report to the person directly above them on the chart. See Figure 13–1 to visualize where the practical/vocational nurse fits into the organizational chart as a first-line leader in a traditional organizational chart. In Figure 13–1, the practical/vocational nurse reports to the nurse manager, who is a registered nurse. Nursing assistants report to the practical/vocational nurse. To whom does the nurse manager report?

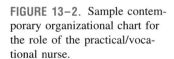

FIGURE 13–2. Sample contemporary organizational chart for the role of the practical/vocational nurse.

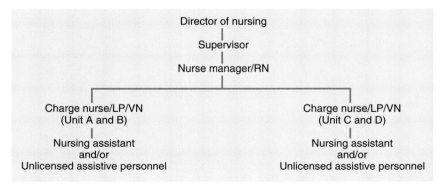

Because of changes in the structure of organizations, some organizational charts have become more horizontal than vertical in appearance. See Figure 13–2 for an example of a more *contemporary* organizational chart. This "flattening out" has eliminated some of the middle manager positions in organizations. As a result, remaining middle managers have taken on more responsibilities and are spread thin. Middle managers in this system have more persons reporting to them than in the past. Middle managers are depending on persons who report to them, such as the LP/VN charge nurse, to think critically and problem solve. Middle managers expect to be contacted when you have tried and are unable to solve your own problems. See Leadership Activity I.

Leadership Activity I: Examining Organizational Charts

Resources Needed:

Organizational charts from clinical sites used by students in your practical/vocational nursing program
Organizational charts may differ by regions of the United States. Obtain organizational charts of specific long-term care facilities in your area. Clarify specific levels of responsibility as they apply to the practical/vocational nurse. Identify whether these charts reflect a traditional or contemporary style of organization.

The Expanded Role of Practical/Vocational Nursing

It is important for you to review a current nurse practice act of your state. This law legally defines the exact role and boundaries for practical/vocational nurses. Also, review the following for more guidelines related to the expanded role of the practical/vocational nurse:

1. NAPNES Standards of Practice for Licensed Practical/Vocational Nurses, Appendix B.

2. NFLPN Specialized Nursing Practice Standards, Appendix C.
3. NLN Entry-Level Competencies of Graduates of Educational Programs in Practical Nursing, Appendix D. See Leadership Activity II.

Leadership Activity II: Determining Your State's Requirements to Assume the Position of Practical/Vocational Charge Nurse

Resource Needed:

Your state's nurse practice act

1. Obtain a current copy of your state's nurse practice act. Nurse practice acts can be purchased from your state's Board of Nursing for a nominal fee that covers printing costs. Identify the part of the act that addresses your state's position on the practical/vocational nurse assuming the charge nurse position in the following areas:
   • Requirements before assuming the LP/VN charge nurse position
   • Site of employment
   • Scope of practice
2. If your state's nurse practice act does not address the issue of charge nurse, how can this information be obtained?

An example of the expanded role of the practical/vocational nurse is the first-line manager position, also called charge nurse, in a nursing home/long-term care facility. In these situations, the practical/vocational nurse has the responsibility of supervising the care given by nursing assistants and other personnel. The practical/vocational nurse will direct, guide, and supervise these health care workers as they attempt to meet the goals of the resident's plan of care.

The most recent job analysis of entry-level practical/vocational nurses by the National Council of State Boards of Nursing Inc. occurred in 1997. This survey identified that 30% of all practical/vocational nurses who reported administrative responsibilities on the job named those responsibilities as their primary position. And a greater proportion of those practical/vocational nurses worked in nursing homes (National Council, 1997). To carry out the first-line manager/charge nurse role effectively, you will need the abilities found in a leader and a manager.

How You Are Already Preparing for a Leadership and Management Role

The topic of leadership and management for the practical/vocational nurse is a vast one. All practical/vocational nurses are managers in the sense that they consistently need to direct, handle, and organize care for assigned clients. It is worthwhile for you to review the ways in which your one-year program helps prepare you for a management position. The one-year practical/vocational nursing program encourages development of the following skills necessary for functioning successfully as a first-line manager:

1. Basic nursing skills, including the nursing process
2. Time management techniques for home and clinical time
3. How to learn new information, including use of resources for learning
4. The power of positive self-talk and thinking
5. Rules for assertiveness
6. Communication skills
7. Legal aspects of health care
8. Ethical aspects of health care
9. Problem solving and critical thinking
10. Stress management
11. Participation in clinical evaluation

Learning leadership and management is much more than taking one course or reading one chapter that turns you into a leader. Learning leadership is a process (continual development) that includes many skills and is something that evolves over time. This chapter will encourage you to think specifically of a leadership role, and it will provide leadership hints needed by practical/vocational nurses.

The Difference Between Leadership and Management

Management is the organization of all care required of clients in a health care setting for a specific period of time. The focus of management is planning and directing to meet client goals. Employers appoint managers to their position. Management is a formal role given to a person by the employer. The tools needed for management could be written in a step-by-step manner and given to you to follow. Following the directions for using the management skills would possibly get the job done in an efficient manner.

Leadership is the manner in which the leader gets along with coworkers and accomplishes the job. The focus of leadership is to produce changes in the workplace that will meet the goals of the employing agency. The leader needs to influence others in the work setting to want to implement the desired change. Directions for leadership skills can also be written but it is through experience that leadership skills can be truly developed. The practical/vocational nurse who has the skills of management *and* leadership will get the job done in the most efficient and effective manner. And the practical/vocational nurse manager and coworkers will enjoy the experience that much more! A manager is not automatically an effective leader. A leader is not automatically an effective manager. Your goal will be to develop skills of leadership *and* management.

Leaders cannot be appointed. Leadership is an informal role that is given to a person by a group of workers. You become a leader when your team members decide to follow you.

What Kind of Leader Are You?

There are several different ways to lead. What is your predominant leadership style? Each of the following statements of "A Short Test of Leadership Style" is an extreme. The responses are not positive or negative. One answer does not have value over another answer. They just are.

Leadership Activity III: Discovering Your Personal Leadership Style

Make a check next to the statement that *best* describes the way you *might be* at work, not how you want to be.

A Short Test of Leadership Style

1. My primary goal at work is to
   A. Get the job done
   B. Get along with the people with whom I work
   C. Do the job correctly
   D. Hope the work I do is noticed
2. My clinical coworkers would say I am
   A. Domineering in my relationships
   B. Friendly and personable in my relationships
   C. Likely to attend to details of the resident care plan
   D. Creative and energetic in giving care
3. At work, I feel like I have to be
   A. In control of the resident situation
   B. Liked by my coworkers
   C. Correct in giving care
   D. Recognized and praised for my care
4. When I communicate on the nursing unit,
   A. I am usually direct and to the point.
   B. I am more considerate of the person to whom I am talking rather than strongly getting my point across.
   C. I usually give detailed information.
   D. I usually elaborate on the point at hand.
5. My coworkers would say I am a person who
   A. Gets the job done regardless of what shift I work

   B. Is very likable and patient
   C. Is precise and accurate in giving nursing care
   D. Is optimistic and has good verbal skills
6. My charge nurse might describe my behavior while on my shift by
   A. *Sometimes* I alienate people.
   B. *Sometimes* I waste time and fall for excuses others may give.
   C. *Sometimes* I can be stubborn with coworkers.
   D. *Sometimes* I appear like a flake to my coworkers.
7. I react to a stressful incident on the nursing unit
   A. By being rude, blaming other departments, yelling at coworkers
   B. By being accommodating to the person in charge and passive in behavior
   C. By becoming silent and withdrawing from the situation
   D. By talking faster and louder
8. When I deal with my coworkers on the nursing unit regarding client matters, I like them to
   A. Get to the point and be business-like in their behavior
   B. Be casual and sincere in their behavior
   C. Use the facts of the matter and go step-by-step when explaining a resident-care situation
   D. Be enthusiastic about the situation and use demonstrations to explain their points

---

Count up your A and C answers. These answers are more characteristic of a task-oriented person. In leadership terms, this person is called an *autocratic* leader. Add up your B and D responses. These are more characteristic of a people-oriented person. In leadership terms, this person is called a *laissez-*

faire* leader. Your score can give you a rough estimate of the tendency of your leadership style.

Leadership Styles

The literature abounds with examples of leadership styles. Figure 13–3 illustrates a **continuum** (a line with extreme opposites at each end) of leadership styles. Table 13–1 compares and contrasts the leadership styles found on this continuum.

---

* *French:* Noninterference in the affairs of others.

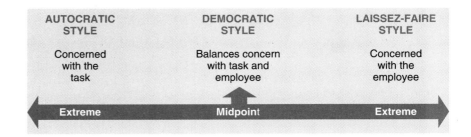

FIGURE 13–3. Extremes of leadership styles on a continuum.

Benefits and Disadvantages of Leadership Styles

To adopt the autocratic or laissez-faire style in Table 13–1 to use consistently as a leadership style is unrealistic and could be disastrous. As you can see, there is room for an autocratic leadership style—for example, in times of emergency. A purely task-centered leadership style (autocratic style) thrives on power. It involves telling someone what to do with little regard for the employee as a person who may have ideas about how to improve

resident care or reach the goals of the employer. List below two additional examples of situations that might require the autocratic style of leadership.

1. _____

_____

2. _____

_____

TABLE 13–1: Comparing Autocratic, Democratic, and Laissez-Faire Styles of Leadership			
	Autocratic	**Democratic**	**Laissez-faire**
General description	Does not share responsibility and authority with employees	Shares responsibility and authority with employees	Gives away responsibility and authority to employees
Importance of agency's policies	Emphasis on policies	Enforces policies but with concern for employees	Puts employees before policies
How leader gets the job done	Tells employees what tasks to do. Does not seek input from employees	Seeks input from employees and encourages problem solving	Tries to please everyone
What gets done	May reach goals	Because of involvement of employees, goals may be achieved with positive staff feelings	Maybe nothing
When style can be used	Crisis situations, code situations, emergencies	Daily nursing care situations, meetings, committees, review of care plans	When agency goals/policies are not a consideration

A purely people-oriented style (laissez-faire) focuses on people's feelings but ignores the task at hand and allows employees to act without any direction. The goals of the employer will be compromised when the laissez-faire leadership style is used. At times, persons in leadership roles may feel the need to be liked by all team members and use this leadership style, but the task of accomplishing goals will be seriously compromised.

Situational Leadership

A popular system of leadership for the twenty-first century is called *situational leadership*. Situational leadership involves varying your leadership style to meet the demands of the situation in the work environment. According to this system, the practical/vocational nurse needs to pick a leadership style that fits the work situation at hand.

Using the Leadership Continuum as a Guide

The value of a continuum, as shown in Figure 13–3, is that as you move along the continuum from each extreme toward the center or midpoint, the two extremes begin to blend together. You have some of each style, depending on where you are on the continuum. A blend to some degree of the two extremes in the appropriate work situation would be the leadership style needed at the moment.

Leadership Activity IV: Plotting My Leadership Style Score

Using your Leadership Style Score from Activity III, place an X on the continuum in Figure 13–3 to indicate where you are at this point in general leadership style tendencies.

Remember, this score is your tendency. If your X is far to the left or right, it may benefit you to be aware of this tendency and to avoid using this style consistently. Remember the continuum and the need to be flexible in your style. Balance task- and people-orientation as needed. Knowing what your predominant style of leadership is will be helpful in your evaluation of work situations and the style needed at that time. Some situations require a supportive style whereas others require a more directive approach

Core Knowledge and Skills Needed for Leadership

To function well in your expanded role as LP/VN charge nurse, you will strive to be a good leader. The scenario at the beginning of this chapter is an example of what not to do as a nurse leader. Much research in learning about the business of leading others and the theories that go with leading are available in the literature. *Core knowledge and skills lay the foundation for leadership.* They will help you develop other necessary knowledge and skills for your leadership role. We identify five **core areas** of knowledge and skills that are necessary for the LP/VN charge nurse to be an effective leader:

1. The ability to motivate team members to accomplish team goals
2. The ability to communicate assertively
3. The ability to problem solve effectively
4. The ability to build a team of cooperative workers
5. The ability to manage stress effectively

Understanding Motivation and Human Needs

As a leader, you will have the task of getting your team members to meet goals set by your employer. Getting people to do what needs to be done is a complex task. What motivates one person does not necessarily motivate another. However, generally understanding motivation and human needs will help you get started.

Motivation

Motivation is a drive that causes individuals to set personal goals and behave in a way that will allow them to reach those goals. The motivation drive comes from within an individual and thus is said to be *intrinsic*. Because motivation is intrinsic, an LP/VN manager, or anyone else for that matter, cannot motivate another person to do something.

Human Needs

All individuals have needs that must be filled in order to meet goals. Individuals are internally motivated to engage in various activities to meet these needs. The activity they engage in is called behavior and can be observed. Abraham Maslow, a psychologist, presented a pyramid of human needs that can assist the learner in understanding self and ranking human needs. You have studied Maslow's hierarchy of needs in your nursing courses.

The human needs theory developed by Maslow in 1962 outlines our basic needs in a hierarchy (Fig. 13–4). Meeting needs on one level of the pyramid acts as a motivator for meeting needs on the next higher level. However, progression through these levels is not clear-cut. In reality, as most of your needs are met on one level, you are already beginning to check out the next level. When faced with overwhelming difficulties, physical or emotional, some regression takes place. For example,

1. Physiologic needs become a priority if you have lost your job or housing.
2. Safety and security needs become a major issue if you are facing a serious illness or move into an unsafe neighborhood.

Once these issues have been dealt with or resolved, higher needs will emerge once more.

Adapting Maslow's Hierarchy

Maslow's hierarchy of needs can be adapted to help the first-line LP/VN leader understand motivation of team members in a health care setting based on needs (see Figure 13–5). Remember, all behavior is internally motivated. All levels of the pyramid in Figure 13–5, the **Howlett hierarchy** of work motivators, are considered to be needs of employees in an employment situation. With some exceptions, the opportunity to meet these needs can be encouraged or discouraged by the employer and the work

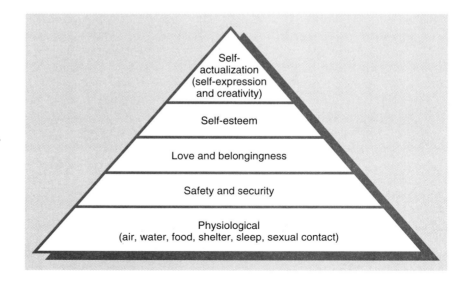

FIGURE 13–4. Maslow's hierarchy of needs.

Self-actualization (self-expression and creativity)

Self-esteem

Love and belongingness

Safety and security

Physiological (air, water, food, shelter, sleep, sexual contact)

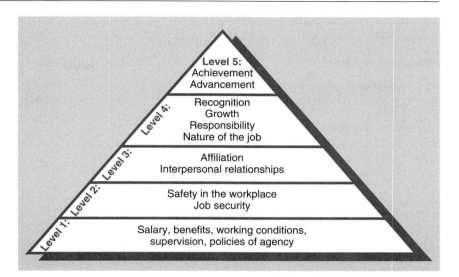

FIGURE 13–5. Howlett hierarchy of work motivators.

Level 5:
Achievement
Advancement

Level 4:
Recognition
Growth
Responsibility
Nature of the job

Level 3:
Affiliation
Interpersonal relationships

Level 2:
Safety in the workplace
Job security

Level 1:
Salary, benefits, working conditions,
supervision, policies of agency

environment, including the charge nurse (*extrinsic motivators*). If these needs are met, the person can proceed to the next higher level of the pyramid. If these needs are not met, a person may become dissatisfied with the work situation.

At a time when it is difficult to find and keep quality nursing assistants to work in a long-term care facility, keeping staff is very important. As an LP/VN manager, you can influence what nursing assistants might be motivated to do. You can provide encouragement for the motivation your nursing assistants already possess. If nursing assistants can see that doing a good job is in their best interest and helps them meet personal needs, they will work hard to meet the goals of their employing agency.

Meeting needs of employees on the Howlett hierarchy can help LP/VN managers influence and direct employees to act in certain ways to benefit the employer, as well as meet personal needs. It is a challenge for the leader to channel the motives of team members to meet the goals of the employer. As you go up the Howlett hierarchy in Figure 13–5, begin identifying strategies that could be carried out to encourage meeting needs of nursing assistants at each level. Also, identify whether the

employer needs to initiate the strategy or whether the strategy could be initiated by the first-line practical/vocational nursing leader. As needs are met on one level, movement can then be encouraged to the next level of the Howlett hierarchy. Strategies for Levels 3 and 4 can play an important role in motivation for team members at any level of the Howlett hierarchy. Praise, recognition, and rewards are extremely important tools for leaders. Research has shown that rewarding *desired behavior* of employees is instrumental in having that behavior repeated. Research also indicates that employees find personal recognition more motivating than money. See Leadership Activity V.

Applying Communication as an LP/VN Leader

One of the LP/VN leader's most productive tools is the effective use of verbal and nonverbal communication. The principles of communication in Chapter 8, Straightforward Communication Skills, and Chapter 11, Assertiveness as a Nursing Responsibility, are building blocks for the communication skills you will need as an LP/VN charge nurse. See Leadership Hints #1 and 2.

Leadership Activity V: Using the Howlett Hierarchy in Leadership Situations

Resources Needed:

Readings on motivation, the Howlett hierarchy, and your creativity to find ways to meet needs of nursing assistants.*

This learning activity encourages the nurse to be creative in finding ways to encourage motivation in nursing assistants. The activity gives you an opportunity to assume responsibility as an LP/VN leader. Examples of behaviors that encourage meeting needs at each level of the hierarchy are given. The person responsible for the behavior is listed in parentheses. Space is provided for you to fill in additional suggested behaviors at each level to show how you can meet needs of nursing assistants and therefore encourage their motivation.

Level 1: Salary, benefits, working conditions, supervision, policies of agency

Examples: Explanation of policies that affect employees (first-line PN/VN leader)
Cafeteria-style benefits—pick and choose benefits (employer)

_____

_____

_____

Level 2: Safety in the workplace, job security

Provision of adequate equipment to carry out standard precautions (employer and first-line PN/VN leader)
Establish policy for hostile clients (employer and first-line PN/VN leader)

_____

_____

_____

---

*Appendix G, The Howlett Style of Nursing Leadership, contains additional suggestions.

Level 3: Affiliation, interpersonal relationships

Plan monthly potluck dinners, pizza lunches, get-togethers (first-line PN/VN leader)

_____

_____

_____

Level 4: Recognition, growth, responsibility, nature of the job

Encourage attendance at continuing education seminars, in-service training, and so on (employer and first-line PN/VN leader)
Recognition for working short-staffed (employer and first-line PN/VN leader)

_____

_____

Level 5: Achievement, advancement

Recognition of successful completion of class, seminar (employer and first-line PN/VN leader)

_____

_____

Provide objective examples of how you can implement each of your suggested behaviors. For example, Level 5: Recognizing successful completion of classes and seminars, could be implemented by

1. A written account in the facility's newsletter
2. Posting an announcement on a special section of the bulletin board
3. A personal note of congratulations from the charge nurse

Leadership Hint #1: Communication of the LP/VN Charge Nurse

Verbal

1. In talking to nursing assistants, deliver your message with clear, specific language. Spell out objectively what has to be done for residents. You might be working with nursing assistants who do not have English as a first language. Until you determine their proficiency with English, verify that intended messages were received.
2. As an LP/VN charge nurse, you are a role model for the nursing assistants. Discourage profanity, personal criticisms, gossip, and rumors.
3. Use "I" instead of "You" messages. "I" messages indicate you take the responsibility for the message. For example, "I think you need to review how to apply a waist restraint." "You" messages imply you blame the person to whom you are speaking. For example, "You will not know how to restrain residents when the need arises." Take responsibility for your messages.
4. In talking with your supervisor, be valued for your input. Avoid being known as someone who just brings up problems. After objectively stating the problem, offer solutions.

Nonverbal

1. Be sure your body language and message are consistent and professional. For example, avoid smiling when you are delivering a needed reprimand, and face the person to whom you are speaking.
2. When delivering your message, appear sure of yourself. Have an attentive posture.

Written

1. Use language that all staff will understand.
2. Review your written messages to be sure the intent of the message is clear.
3. Provide written assignments that do not require the nursing assistant to make judgments.
4. Provide written reports of all meetings. If information is not restricted, a report from a meeting with management can dispel/prevent rumors about what "they" are doing now. The reports can be placed in a loose-leaf binder in an area that is accessible for the nursing assistant.

Telephone

1. Gather your thoughts, including the purpose for the call, before you make a call.
2. With a smile in your voice, greet the person called by name, identify yourself, and offer a brief inquiry as to their well-being if you know the person called. For example, "Hello, Mrs. Jones, this is Tricia Zak from The Home. How are things going?"
3. State the reason for the call. "I need to order a video and wanted to know if you had any specific needs."
4. You initiated the conversation. Terminate it when your business is completed. The exception is when the person you called brings up a work-related question.
5. Avoid long conversations about nonwork-related topics. This is what is considered allowing the telephone to extend into your time.
6. Arrange to have incoming calls answered quickly, by the second or third ring.
7. When you answer, identify the facility and give your name and title. "The Home, Tricia Zak, Charge Nurse."
8. Speak clearly in a moderate tone of voice. Most people talk too loudly on the phone.
9. Callers are "customers." Treat the caller respectfully and cordially.
10. If it is necessary to put the person on hold, ask permission to do so.
11. If necessary to put the person on hold, try to get back to her or him within 30 seconds. If you are still delayed, ask for a number so you can call back.
12. Provide information requested.

Leadership Hint #2: Encouraging Verbal Communication from Nursing Assistants

1. Actively listen to nursing assistants. Avoid distraction and inattention.
2. Stay focused on what the nursing assistant is saying.
3. Avoid forming a response while the nursing assistant is speaking.
4. Avoid judging the message or the nursing assistant.
5. Rephrase the message when the nursing assistant is done to verify that you understand the message.
6. Encourage comments. Your goal is to have the nursing assistant go back to the team and say, "She really listened to me!"
7. Encourage constructive evaluation. Create an environment in which nursing assistants are encouraged to give their input—positive or negative.
8. Respect all opinions. Nursing assistants need to feel safe to speak up, ask questions, identify problems, and suggest solutions to those problems.

Applying Problem-Solving as an LP/VN Leader

The basic hint for successful problem-solving is identify the real issue and solve it. What is the problem? Avoid spending precious time on finding solutions for what is not really the problem. Chapter 12 introduced you to the nursing process, an excellent problem-solving process. You have been using this problem-solving method throughout your LP/VN program. For problem solving, the nursing process can be used to solve resident problems as well as staff problems. The nursing process also works at home as well as the clinical area. See Leadership Hint #3.

Scenario: Late for Assigned Shift

Penny, a nursing assistant, is assigned to the day shift in a long-term care facility. Her shift begins at

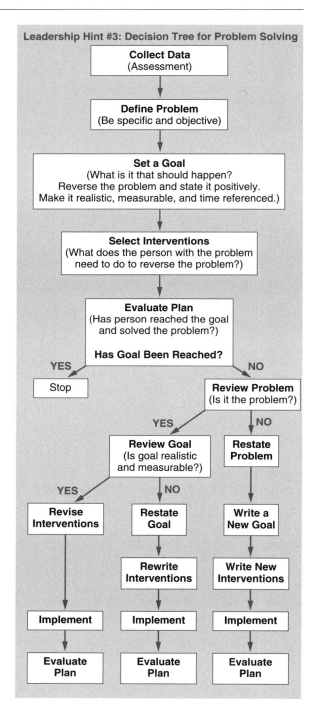

Leadership Hint #3: Decision Tree for Problem Solving

6:45 AM with a verbal report from the day LP/VN charge nurse for her wing. All nursing assistants are expected to attend this report and receive their assignments at this time.

Data Collection/Assessment

On May 8, 10, 15, 16, 23, and 24, Penny came to work either during the charge nurse report or after the charge nurse had finished. When questioned about this behavior, she states she has problems getting her teenagers up and started for school.

Problem

A record of Penny's tardiness indicates this is a recurring problem and not an isolated incident. A pattern has been established in being late for report.

Goal

Penny will be on time for the day charge nurse's report and will hear the entire report, starting immediately.

Interventions

As the LP/VN charge nurse, it is your responsibility to talk to Penny about this tardiness. This includes the times and days of her tardiness. Select a private spot for your discussion. Encourage Penny to figure out why this behavior is inconvenient for the staff and residents. Review the long-term care unit's policy on punctuality. Encourage Penny to come up with ideas that will allow her to be on time. Set limits with Penny. Identify that she needs to be on time for her assigned shifts. Plan to meet with her in one week to discuss her performance. At that time, if she has not improved her performance, a written reprimand will be given and included in her personal file. At the end of the meeting, compliment Penny on an area of her work that has been going well.

Evaluation

During the next week, continue to document Penny's arrival for her assigned shifts. If she complies, note and praise her change in performance.* If she continues to be late for her shift, issue a written reprimand. Place a copy in her file. Give a copy to your supervisor. Keep a copy in your file. Be sure the warning contains objective information such as the following:

1. Days and times late for shift
2. Date of oral warning
3. Seriousness of situation
4. The consequences

Team Building

Mission Statements

Mission Statement of The Home

■ The Home is a private, nonprofit, long-term care facility. The Home provides 24-hour nursing care in a manner and setting that maintain or improve each resident's quality of life, health, and safety. ■

The LP/VN charge nurse needs to be aware of the **mission statement** of the long-term care facility. A mission statement defines the purpose and goals of the organization. The foregoing mission statement contains what staff must do to meet the goals of The Home, a long-term care facility.

Each unit in the long-term care facility can write a specific statement of goals that spins off the facility mission statement. This will get the nursing assistants on your team thinking about what they believe and value in regard to resident care. One example of a unit mission statement that is a spin-off of The Home's mission statement follows.

---

*In the next week Penny actually arrived a few minutes before the other nursing assistants. The LP/VN charge nurse allowed her to choose her break and lunch time. Penny had never experienced this before and she was pleased.

The Home—Team A Goals

■ Nursing assistants of Team A of The Home are committed to providing competent, caring, safe, and personalized service to residents and their families. ■

The team you supervise has the goal to carry out the mission statement of the long-term care facility. As LP/VN charge nurse, you are in charge of creating the climate of the work environment that will motivate staff to meet this goal. In this situation, the goal is maintaining or improving quality of life, health, and safety of residents at The Home. You are a role model for attitudes and behavior. Your team will model the attitudes and behavior you expect of them. Suggested LP/VN charge nurse attitudes to convey while attempting team building include the beliefs that

1. Most employees want to do a good job at work.
2. Most employees want to reach their full potential. See Leadership Hints #4 and 5.

Stress Management

Stress is a part of all work environments. The long-term care area has its fair share because of in-

---

Leadership Hint #4: Utilizing Unit Mission Statements

1. Unit mission statements can be printed on small cards and carried in the pockets of nursing assistants.
2. Unit mission statements can be handed to residents when they are admitted and to their families. Nursing assistant's first name and title can be included on the card.
3. Unit mission statements need to be reviewed on a regular basis to refresh nursing assistants about their goals. These cards are a written reminder of common values in resident care.

Leadership Hint #5: LP/VN Charge Nurse Behaviors That Encourage Team Building

1. Review the mission statement of the facility with nursing assistants.
2. Using input from nursing assistants, develop a unit mission statement for your unit.
3. Use teamwork language, like "we" and "us." Convey the attitude, "We have common goals and together we will meet them."
4. Encourage politeness, cooperation, trust, and respect among nursing assistants.
5. Encourage honest feedback among nursing assistants.
6. Provide opportunity for sharing of ideas among nursing assistants.
7. Ask nursing assistants for ideas on how to do unit tasks more effectively.
8. Provide occasions for nursing assistants to spend time together.
9. Create a positive environment on the clinical area that nursing assistants will want to be a part of.
10. Provide positive reinforcement of behaviors that contribute to team goals by using rewards.
11. Reward group accomplishments.
12. TREAT NURSING ASSISTANTS ON YOUR TEAM AS YOU WOULD LIKE TO BE TREATED.

---

creased workloads (especially when a nursing assistant calls in sick . . . again) and conflicts with nursing assistants, physicians, families, and residents. Stress and anxiety in the clinical area can result in dysfunctional behavior on the job. Examples of dysfunctional job behaviors include:

1. Decreased performance of nursing assistants
2. Negative interactions with nursing assistants
3. Ineffective communication
4. Inappropriate body cues such as sharp tone of voice

5. High staff turnover
6. Unhappy residents, families, physicians, and nursing assistants

As the LP/VN charge nurse, you have the responsibility to be a stress manager and role model for the team. Your goal will be to:

1. Display the ability to cope with stress as it affects you.
2. Create a work environment with decreased stress levels.
3. Guide and support nursing assistants when they experience stress.

The LP/VN charge nurse needs to learn how to detect stress in the clinical environment. A good place to start is to be aware of stress in yourself. See Leadership Hints #6 and 7.

Leadership Hint #7: Creating a Less Stressful Work Environment

1. Your ability to organize your shift will help prevent some stressful situations.
2. Have available the equipment nursing assistants need to get their job done.
3. Encourage nursing assistants to take breaks.
4. Create a calm environment.
5. Treat nursing assistants with respect. Remember your communication skills, especially "please," "thank you," and "I sure appreciate _____."

Leadership Hint #6: Life Skills That Help Control Stress

1. The actual stress reduction/relaxation technique you choose is personal. Whatever works for you is the skill to choose.
2. Deep breathing.
3. Meditation, imagery, and other relaxation techniques.
4. Massage.
5. Daily exercise—walking is the easiest and least expensive form of exercise. No special equipment is required except good walking shoes.
6. Apply the principles you learned in nutrition and let the food pyramid be your guide for getting the fuel your body needs.
7. Get the amount of rest you need to function at your best.
8. Take your breaks when at work. You will be re-energized and increase your productivity.
9. Develop leisure activities you enjoy (or rediscover activities you put on the back burner during nursing school).

Leadership Activity VI: Identifying Signs of Stress

Resource Needed:

Any text identifying physical and emotional signs of stress

The next time you feel yourself getting stressed, identify how you are feeling and what you are thinking. List the physical and emotional symptoms you experience.

Additional Stress Control Skills for the LP/VN Charge Nurse

Controlling Stress by Altering How You Think

Stress is the body's reaction to the mind's analysis of a situation. It is not the situation, but your *reaction to* the situation, that creates stress. You have the only stress management tool you will ever need right inside your head. If you learn to manage how you think about the many interactions you have daily with nursing assistants, residents, and family members, you can control your reaction and therefore your stress level.

Thinking *Before* "Irrational Thinking" Class

Nursing Assistant (on phone): "I cannot come in today. I have a headache." LP/VN Charge Nurse *(thinking): I bet she has a headache. She probably spent half the night partying.* LP/VN becomes abrupt with the nursing assistant and hangs up. She feels angry and allows the incident to ruin her entire day. Nursing assistants can sense that the LP/VN charge nurse is upset and try to avoid any contact with her.

Ellis (1994) discusses rational versus **irrational thinking.** When we are in a situation, we engage in self-talk about what is happening. This self-talk is often irrational because it is based on judgments we make about the situation. Judgments are subjective and have no bearing on facts. The irrational thinking then causes negative emotions, and stress results. Ellis offers the A, B, C, D way of increasing awareness of irrational thinking and changing how we think to a more rational way. In learning to do so, we control our emotions, and therefore, the stress that results. Examples of how Ellis' A, B, C, D method of controlling irrational thinking applies to the LP/VN charge nurse follow.

A—Activating Event
   The nursing assistant called in sick with a headache.
B—Belief (Self-Talk) About the Situation
   The charge nurse thinks the nursing assistant must have been out partying.
C—Consequences
   The LP/VN nurse manager was abrupt with the nursing assistant on the phone. She allowed herself to feel angry about the absence. She allowed it to ruin her whole day. Nursing assistants avoided her like the plague.
D—Dispute Irrational Thoughts
   Choose a more rational, assertive response to the situation. Focus on the objective facts (nursing assistant has a headache). Avoid the subjective judgments that your beliefs

---

Leadership Hint #8: Avoiding Irrational Thinking

1. Be aware that beliefs about the situation are self-talk. Self-talk sometimes makes subjective judgments. These judgments, if negative, can cause an emotional reaction. The emotional reaction leads to stress.
2. See situations objectively. Rational thinking is based on facts. Objective facts do not cause emotion. The situation "just is."
3. Avoid thinking that nursing assistants *should, must,* or *always* do something. This is another example of irrational thinking and can lead to anger. When you use these words for yourself, they can lead to anxiety and guilt.
5. We do not have the power to make nursing assistants do anything. We can *encourage* or *prefer* that nursing assistants do something.
6. For yourself and team members, use the words *want, choose,* and *prefer* in your thinking.

(self-talk) call up (the nursing assistant was partying). You will avoid the anger over this incident and its effect on nursing assistants. Stress is avoided for all.

Thinking *After* "Irrational Thinking" Class

Nursing Assistant (on phone): "I cannot come in today. I have a headache." LP/VN Charge Nurse (tempted to use irrational thinking but remembers the A, B, C, D involved.): "I'm sorry to hear that. I hope you will feel better with rest." See Leadership Hint #8.

Specific Knowledge and Skills Needed for Leadership

To be a leader in long-term care, it is necessary to use the core areas of knowledge as a base and develop skills in three specific areas:

1. **Occupational (clinical) skills**—the knowledge and skills of nursing.
2. **Organizational skills**—skills necessary to function in the organization that delivers health care.
3. **Human relationship skills**—the ability to get along with and relate to people.

Occupational Skills for First-Line LP/VN Leaders

Nursing (Clinical) Skills, Including the Nursing Process

Solid clinical skills are a must to be a good nursing leader. Visible expertise in clinical skills is a plus with the nursing assistants and also gives you an informal power base. See the resident situation for yourself, assist in providing care, and demonstrate nursing skills to nursing assistants as needed. This conveys the attitude that resident care comes first. This action demonstrates that the facility mission statement and unit goals are not just a written exercise. It communicates that LP/VN charge nurses are there to support their staff.

Knowledge of your role in the nursing process is an important part of organizational skills. Your practical/vocational nursing program has started your skill development in this area. You will need to keep this area current and fresh. Refer to Chapter 12, The Practical/Vocational Nurse's Role in the Nursing Process.

Documentation

Utilize the guidelines in Chapter 18, Nursing Ethics and the Law, for all your charting. LP/VN charge nurses need to be aware of the documentation requirements of federal and state laws and accrediting agencies. Specific, objective documentation demonstrates whether or not the standard of care has been met. Effective nursing documentation is the basis for payment of resident fees or denial of payment. This is especially important when these agencies mandate patient outcomes. It cannot be emphasized often enough that you must make sure all your charting is specific, objective, and complete. Avoid subjective comments and personal judgments in your charting. Students sometimes find this area of charting difficult, especially if they see examples of general and subjective entries on charts by licensed staff in the clinical area. The following four situations are examples of **subjective as opposed to objective** charting.

Subjective as Opposed to Objective Charting

Subjective: Resident is drunk, confused, and uncooperative.
Objective: Odor of alcohol on breath, off balance, mistook nurse for a county sheriff, and refuses to stay in assigned room.

Subjective: Resident is noncompliant.
Objective: Found in room eating a large fastfood hamburger. Reminded of the need for restricted diet because of diabetes and receiving an intermediate-acting insulin.

Subjective: The family is nasty, abrasive, and difficult.
Objective: Resident's daughter yelled out when charge nurse entered room. Yelled that staff was out to get her Dad. Daughter refused to participate in health teaching regarding her Dad's diabetes.

Subjective: The decubitus area is healing.
Objective: Border of pressure ulcer area on right trochanter area is flat and pink. Area is 1 cm wide, 1.5 cm long, and 1.5 cm deep. Inner open area is reddish-pink. Small amount of clear, pink drainage on dressing.

Legal Aspects

The nursing assistants and you, as LP/VN charge nurse, are the people who have direct contact with residents and their families on a daily basis. You have the ability to ensure resident and family satisfaction with care and are a vehicle to voice concerns. This in turn will decrease the need for legal action to resolve disputes. Chapter 18, Nursing Ethics and the Law, provides you with information for being legally sound in your nursing career.

Be aware of your state nurse practice act, health care facility policies and procedures, state and federal regulations, and published standards of your nursing organizations and codes of conduct (NAPNES and NFLPN in Appendixes B and C). The standards and codes are guidelines to evaluate safe practice. Keep current and informed.

Federal Guidelines

Your facility must be in compliance with federal, state, and local laws. The impact of federal guidelines in your facility is most strongly felt in the **Omnibus Budget Reconciliation Act of 1987 (OBRA)** and the **Health Care Financing Administration (HCFA).** These guidelines will be reviewed in your orientation to the facility.

Omnibus Budget Reconciliation Act of 1987 (OBRA)

OBRA is major federal legislation that addresses the quality of life, health, and safety of residents. According to OBRA guidelines, long-term care units must provide care that maintains or improves each resident's quality of life, health, and safety. OBRA regulations will be reviewed with you at the time of your orientation. See Leadership Hint #9.

Health Care Financing Administration (HCFA)

HCFA is a federal agency that certifies nursing homes for Medicare and Medicaid reimbursement. To receive payment, facilities are required to meet conditions of participation. The long-term care unit

---

Leadership Hint #9: OBRA Provisions That Deal Specifically with Nursing Assistants

1. Nursing assistants require 75 hours of instruction before taking state-approved written and skills competency evaluation. This establishes a baseline proficiency and competence of nursing assistants.
2. Each state must have a nursing assistant directory. This directory is an official listing of persons who have successfully completed nursing assistant training and competency evaluation. To be listed in a state directory, the history of the nursing assistant must be free of incidents of abuse, neglect, or dishonest use of property.
3. Your state's directory must be notified before employment of nursing assistants. The directory of some states is online.
4. Nursing assistants' work must be evaluated "regularly."
5. Nursing assistants must have 12 hours of in-service training per year.
6. If two consecutive years have passed without a person being employed as a nursing assistant, training and competency evaluation must be repeated.

---

will have the conditions of participation in its policies. Current HCFA regulations will be presented at the time of your orientation.

Your State's Regulations

Long-term care units and nursing homes are licensed by the state in which they are located. Each state sets regulations that must be met in order to be licensed. Periodically, the facility will be visited by inspectors. At that visit it will be determined whether the facility has any deficiencies. Being cited for deficiencies can affect licensing. Your state's regulations will be reviewed at the time of orientation.

Leadership Hint #10: Applying the Nursing Process to Organize Your Shift

Assessment (Data Collection) of Tasks

1. Make a *"To Do" list* that reflects unit routines and schedules. When new to the job, listing unit routines and schedules is helpful until you experience the actual routine. This list includes break times, staff meal times, resident meals and nourishments, scheduled physician rounds, and routine times for vital signs, capillary blood testing, med administration, treatments, and so on.
2. Develop a *worksheet* to use during report. Develop a form with which you are comfortable. Some charge nurses develop a list according to a sequence of room numbers. Others list residents that need special assessments. Others list treatments, vital signs, and so on, by time.
3. *Prioritize* the list. To set priorities for residents, use Maslow's hierarchy. Remember, physiologic needs must be met before other needs are considered. *A's* are most important needs and *must* be done. They could be life-threatening or urgent resident needs. *B's* must be done but there is more leeway in the exact time they are accomplished. Some *C's* are necessary but not of urgent status. C's sometimes can be assigned to UAPs or postponed. Some C's might not need to be listed at all. Examples follow:

Tasks	Example	Comments
"A" tasks	STAT med, PRN med, q2 h neuro check after resident's fall on prior shift	"A" tasks always surface during the shift, requiring modification of the "To Do" list, these needs are unpredictable and cannot be planned
"B" tasks	Routine med administration, dressing changes, routine resident personal care, ambulation, activities, routine treatments, nourishments, meals	These needs are recurring and predictable
"C" tasks	Mail and flower delivery, chit-chat with family	Important but can be delayed

Planning Use of Time (Goal Setting)

1. Plan tasks within a time frame of 2 to 3 hours. Arrange blocks of time according to unit routine. Planning allows you to have the feeling you are in control of the situation. Take resident preferences into consideration when you are planning. For example, one resident prefers to eat breakfast at 6 AM, whereas breakfast is at 8 AM. Arrangements could be made for coffee and crackers at 6 AM.
2. Use the same guidelines for setting goals for planning time as with care plans or personal goals. Focus on goals as outcomes (the results expected after a given period of time). Using action verbs, make sure goals are realistic and measurable. A measurable goal states specifically and objectively what results are expected after a specified period of time. Set minigoals for timed tasks to keep you on task.
3. Planning involves having the equipment and supplies that the team needs for the shift and the shift that follows. As you make your assessment of residents when first starting your shift, check rooms and treatment closets for needed supplies. This includes linen, a well-stocked floor refrigerator, supplies for treatments, supplies for med administration kept on med cart, and so on.
4. Make sure you have your personal tools for the shift: your watch (working), a pen that writes, a bandage scissors, a stethoscope, and a small notebook. Use the notebook to jot down quickly equipment that is needed and results of assessments.

continued

Leadership Hint #10: continued

Implementing Your Plan

1. Remember, your plan is written in soft butter, not marble. Be flexible.
2. As you carry out your plan for the shift, expect interruptions of your planned activities. You know they *will* occur but not *when*. These include telephone calls, changes in residents' conditions, transfer of resident, staff injury.
3. When unexpected events occur, planning assists you to rearrange tasks. If you have a plan, you can return to the plan after interruptions. You can continue or revise the plan as needed.

Evaluating Your Use of Time

1. As nursing assistants give you reports for their assigned residents, seek input from them about the effectiveness and efficiency of the shift.
2. Ask for suggestions to improve staff and your use of time the next shift you work.
3. Keep a log of your shift activities. Look for a pattern of inefficient use of time. Examples of time wasters are putting things off, allowing unnecessary interruptions, socializing with staff, inability to say NO!, allowing telephone calls to exceed needed time for business.
4. At the end of your shift, take a few minutes to plan for the next day. This will allow you to leave work-related activities at work. And it will allow you to enjoy your much-needed leisure time.

The Joint Commission on Accreditation of Health Care Organizations (JCAHO)

The Joint Commission is an independent, not-for-profit organization whose purpose is to improve quality of care in hospitals, nursing centers, and home health agencies. Accreditation is a voluntary activity. If your facility participates in JCAHO accreditation, their requirements will be explained to you at the time of your orientation.

Organizational Skills for First-Line LP/VN Leaders

Organizational skills are an essential ingredient for leaders as well as team members. The emphasis on the personal and vocational issues/concepts course in your practical/vocational nursing program has given you the opportunity to learn and apply principles of time management (Chapter 4). Continuous quality improvement and conflict management are also necessary skills for the development of any nursing leader in today's health care organizations, including long-term care.

Time Management

Whether your dominance is on the left or right side of the brain, you have been given the opportunity this year to develop time management skills by applying the content of Chapter 4, For the Organizationally Challenged. Your school year has certainly provided the need to use your time effectively (doing the right thing) and efficiently (doing it the right way the first time and in the appropriate amount of time) for school and home. The step-by-step procedures learned in the nursing skills lab helped you prioritize your care for efficiency and the safety and comfort of the client. You have experience organizing work for one or two clients in the clinical area. As an LP/VN charge nurse, you will direct the care of approximately 30 residents and supervise a team of four to five nursing assistants.

Time management is more about management and less about time. Your ability to manage time will help you organize tasks and allow you to be successful as a charge nurse. Once again, the nursing process will be the tool to help you get organized. See Leadership Hint #10.

Continuous Quality Improvement

Continuous quality improvement (CQI) is a program found in all health care facilities. The principles of CQI found in health care are borrowed from those of the business world. The focus of CQI is quality of care. Quality is indicated by client outcomes. Client outcomes are observable, measurable results of nursing activities. The CQI program involves all departments of health care facilities, including long-term care. You will receive information about the CQI program at your facility during orientation. See Leadership Hint #11.

Leadership Hint #11: CQI Components That the LP/VN Charge Nurse Needs to Incorporate into the Leadership Role

1. Review job descriptions with your nursing assistants. Emphasize the role they have in achieving quality care and resident service for a reasonable price (do it right the first time).
2. Remember that CQI is a continuous, daily part of your unit.
3. Encourage nursing assistants to report inefficiencies in resident care and the work environment.
4. Encourage nursing assistants to offer suggestions to solve the problems in Numbers 2 and 3.
5. When inefficiencies are noted, initiate a plan for improvement.
6. Consider volunteering for a CQI committee. Policies and nursing procedures are revised based on the input you and your nursing assistants provide regarding resident care and the functioning of the unit. It is personally rewarding to be included in policy and procedure revision because revisions improve resident care.
7. Document resident information in an objective and specific manner. Your documentation will be used to measure the effectiveness of CQI efforts.

Example of CQI in Action

A nursing home in northeastern Wisconsin experienced a 100% incontinence rate on one resident unit. Nursing assistants were concerned about the team time that it took to wash residents and change linens, the risk for skin breakdown, and the cost of laundry to wash the mountains of bed linens, protective pads, and resident personal items. With the help of their LP/VN charge nurse and the director of nursing, the nursing assistants developed a plan to cut down on incontinence. They set a goal to decrease the amount of incontinence on the unit by 25%. Several months later, they were quite surprised and pleased to see the results of their planning. The rate of incontinence decreased to 0%. And the residents were pretty pleased about it, also.

Conflict Resolution

Conflict can occur whenever two or more persons interact. In long-term care, conflicts can arise with nursing assistants, staff, residents, families, and physicians. Conflict is not always a bad thing; sometimes it is an opportunity for growth and learning. Other times, the presence of conflict can point out the need for change in an organization. When conflicts are out in the open, the opportunity exists to settle issues. This is preferable to leaving conflicts unsettled. Unsettled, conflicts can act like cancer and slowly grow and grow into something much larger that may be more difficult or impossible to resolve. Tools to reduce conflicts include clear communication and the ability to work well as a team. Conflict resolution involves people settling their differences. Resolution of the conflict is an exercise in problem solving. See Leadership Hint #12.

Human Relationship Skills for First-Line LP/VN Leaders

LP/VN charge nurses can have excellent clinical skills, use the nursing process expertly, and document to the letter of the law. The LP/VN charge nurse can have a good understanding of federal and

Leadership Hint #12: Applying the Nursing Process for Conflict Resolution

Assessment/Data Collection—Obtain All the Facts

1. When a conflict arises, avoid pursuing it on the spot. Arrange for the involved parties to meet in an area that will provide privacy.
2. Separate the person from the problem. Attack the problem, and not each other.
3. Each party has its own perception and strong emotions about what happened. Unclear communication may result. Clarify subjective statements and generalizations. You need to get objective and specific facts. For example, clarify what is meant by "she always does that" and "they."
4. Actively listen to the person presenting the "facts."
5. Avoid formulating your response while the other party is giving the "facts."

State the Problem—Identify the Specific Issue

1. After hearing all sides, state in your own words what you understand is the conflict. Use "I" messages when presenting your perspective.
2. Ask parties for feedback as to the accuracy of your understanding of the conflict.

Interventions (Planning)

1. Convey the attitude of working side-by-side to settle the conflict. For example, sit side-by-side to work on the problem.
2. Involve all parties in identifying and discussing possible solutions to the conflict. The more alternatives the better. The goal is a solution that will be agreeable to everyone's interests.
3. *Avoid* bargaining over *positions (what you want)*. Egos are identified with positions. The parties involved will focus on defending their position. In the end, the parties need to save face.
4. *Focus* on *interests (why something is wanted)*. Behind a *position* is a *motivating interest*. Behind opposite *positions* lie shared and compatible *interests*. *Compromise* involves giving up aspects of an issue that are important to one of the parties. This is not a good intervention. *Collaborate* for a win-win solution that focuses on shared or compatible interests.

Implementation—Implement the Selected Solution

On a sunny, cool day in fall, two residents are sitting in the sun porch of a long-term care facility. Resident A's *position* is that he wants a window open and Resident B's *position* is that he wants the window shut. The LP/VN charge nurse asks Resident A *why* he wants a window open. He replies, "So I can get some fresh air." The charge nurse asks Resident B *why* he wants the window closed. He replies, "So it won't be drafty."

A solution built on *collaboration* would involve the charge nurse wrapping Resident B in a blanket and moving his wheelchair to the north end of the sun porch. She would move Resident A to the south end of the sun porch and open a window near him. This is a "win-win" solution. A solution built on *compromise* would involve the LP/VN charge nurse returning both residents to their rooms or returning one of the residents to his room and accommodating the other in the sun room. This is an "I win—you lose" solution.

Evaluation—Evaluate the Effectiveness of Interventions in Meeting the Goal

In the preceding situation, the LP/VN charge nurse returns 30 minutes later and finds both residents peacefully asleep in their wheelchairs.

state laws and requirements of accrediting agencies. LP/VN charge nurses can get the job done very efficiently. But perhaps human relationship skills are the most important skills for a practical/vocational nursing leader to have. Polly Practical *might* get the job done. Leaders with human relationship skills will get the job done with style and tact without sacrificing quality. Nursing assistants will value their leader's style a whole lot more and be more effective in reaching the goals of the unit. Since success depends on what is accomplished through others, the ability to relate well to others is crucial.

Practical/vocational nurses are well-versed in clinical skills. They risk bringing clinical problem-solving skills to the LP/VN charge nurse role when leadership/management skills are needed in this position.

Anger Management

Besides providing money on which to live, work provides you with the opportunity to be recognized for what you do, to belong to a group, and display your competence. (Review the Howlett hierarchy of work motivators.) When any of these needs are threatened in the course of the workday or you feel like a victim in the workplace with lack of control, you can get angry. Anger is not automatically bad. Anger gives you a cue that something is wrong. If your anger is justified, it can help you get your needs met by stimulating you to action. Harassment and discrimination are examples of situations in which anger is justified. If your anger is unjustified, or displayed inappropriately, it can get you and others in trouble. See Leadership Hints #13, 14, and 15.

Performance Evaluation of Nursing Assistant

The thought of **performance evaluation** can send shivers up the spine of the person doing the evaluating as well as of the person being evaluated. Perhaps this goes back to bad evaluation experiences in prior situations. Perhaps it even goes as far back as grade school. Perhaps you and the nursing

---

Leadership Hint #13: Preventing Anger in Nursing Assistants

1. Meet needs above level two on the Maslow and Howlett hierarchies, which include needs of belonging, affiliation, and recognition.
2. Use assertive communication, especially "I" messages. This will decrease the LP/VN charge nurse being perceived as a threat.
3. Actively listen, using direct eye contact and alert body posture, to convey to nursing assistants that you are interested in understanding their point of view.
4. Successful team building helps nursing assistants feel part of the group.
5. Seek input of nursing assistants to find solutions for unit problems. This provides a sense of control over one's work environment.
6. Utilize win-win strategies in conflict resolution to provide a feeling of having control over situations and being treated with respect.
7. Encourage nursing assistants to participate in objective evaluation of their clinical performance to maintain self-esteem, and give nursing assistants some control over what happens to them.
8. Encouraging self-evaluation also helps tone down an important but potentially volatile area, especially when areas for improvement are noted.
9. Attempts to help nursing assistants become self-confident, reach their full potential, and achieve the higher levels of the Maslow and Howlett hierarchies. When needs are met at these higher levels, nursing assistants are more satisfied in their work environment.

---

assistants have learned to associate evaluation with constructive criticism and weaknesses. Keep sight of the main purpose of evaluation which is *to encourage personal and professional growth.* Constructive evaluation gives you and team members a

Leadership Hint #14: Personal Anger Management Techniques for the LP/VN Charge Nurse

1. Learn your personal signs that communicate you are becoming angry. Pay attention to what you are thinking and feeling.
2. How you appraise events causes the anger response. Change irrational thoughts to rational thoughts.
3. If your heart is pounding, take deep breaths.
4. If you feel tension in a body area, rub the area for a few seconds.
5. When angry, speak slowly and in a lower tone of voice, acknowledge how you feel, take a time-out.
6. View a stimulus to anger as a problem. Use the problem-solving process to arrive at a solution.

As LP/VN charge nurse, your responsibilities in evaluating nursing assistants include:

1. Observing skill performance and attitudes of nursing assistants.
2. Providing daily oral/written feedback, including suggestions for improvement.
3. Documenting observations.
4. Presenting a final evaluation form.

Review the evaluation process and form for your facility. What you are evaluating is not subject to your personal judgment. You will be objectively evaluating skills and attitudes of nursing assistants. These work-related activities are expected of nursing assistants and are found in their job description and the facility's policy manual. If a checklist format is used for daily observations, be sure you understand the scale utilized by the long-term care facility. In observing nursing skills, you will be evaluating the application of nursing assistant

profile of strong behaviors and behaviors for improvement, along with a plan to improve. Evaluation encourages the development of employees who will meet the facility's objectives and fulfill the mission statement. See Leadership Hint #17.

Leadership Hint #15: Prevention of Workplace Violence

1. Suggest in-service education in anger management for all employees.
2. Create a work environment that is respectful and fun.
3. As LP/VN charge nurse, be a positive role model for anger management.
4. Take conflicts in the work environment seriously.
5. Refer/use your facility's employee assistance program (EAP).
6. If your facility does not have an EAP program, suggest that a program be developed.

Leadership Hint #16: Encouraging Nursing Assistants to Participate in the Evaluation Process

1. Provide nursing assistants with the evaluation form at the beginning of the evaluation experience. Tell them it contains the elements you will be evaluating. Encourage them to read it.
2. Encourage nursing assistants to evaluate themselves daily and record their evaluation on the form. This also gives them the opportunity to become familiar with the form.
3. Remind them to include their strong areas. People are good at identifying areas for improvement, but sometimes need reminders to acknowledge their strong points. Dispel the myth that to do so is egotistical or boastful. It is merely a statement of what is.
4. Encourage nursing assistants to include a plan on the evaluation form for improving areas that need improvement.

knowledge of a skill to actual skill performance. Attitudes are more difficult to evaluate. They are stated as observable behaviors and usually involve areas such as dress and grooming, attendance, functioning as a team member, and interpersonal skills.

The performance evaluation is written documentation of what you have been discussing and documenting throughout the period before the formal process of evaluation. Documentation is a time-consuming task. When you are used to the system for the long-term care facility, you will find it can be completed more quickly.

OBRA mandates regular evaluations for nursing assistants. In addition to scheduled performance evaluations, you will be giving spontaneous feedback to nursing assistants. Evaluation is the responsibility of the LP/VN charge nurse and the nursing assistant. No one needs ever to "give" another person an evaluation. Evaluation must be a joint proc-

ess. Evaluation is not a secret that you surprise team members with at the end of the evaluation period. It is a tool for personal and career growth. A team member has the right to be able to correct areas for improvement as time goes by. It is unfair to have your discrepancies loaded on you (okay, dumped) during the final evaluation interview. See Leadership Hints #16 and 18.

Your nonthreatening, objective approach to constructive evaluation will result in positive evaluation experiences for you and the nursing assistants on your team. Occasionally you may experience a situation in which a nursing assistant does feel threatened and becomes defensive during evaluation. If the defensiveness begins to escalate or the person displays anger, terminate the meeting. Set a new time for another meeting. Have your supervisor present at this time. Such experiences are the exception, not the rule.

Leadership Hint #17: Providing Feedback to Nursing Assistants

Positive Feedback Identifies Strong Behaviors to Be Encouraged

1. Most nursing assistants know what it is like to be caught doing something "wrong." Catch them doing something "right." This encourages them to repeat the behavior.
2. Let nursing assistants know you notice their efforts, believe in them, and feel good about their contributions to the long-term care facility.
3. Praise people in measurable terms (specific and objective) so that the behavior can be repeated. "You did a real thorough job disinfecting the shower."

Negative Feedback Identifies Behaviors That Need Improvement

1. Provide verbal feedback as close to the event as possible. The purpose of negative feedback is to point out behaviors that need to be modified. Focus on the behavior as one needing improvement. Avoid addressing the behavior as a criticism.
2. Without emotion, objectively point out what is wrong with the behavior and its consequences. You want the nursing assistant to remember the message and not the manner in which it was delivered. You also want the team member to know it is **performance** that is being evaluated.
3. Negative feedback needs to be accompanied by suggestions to correct the behavior. These suggestions need to be so specific that the nursing assistant will be able to correct behavior by following them.
4. Mention behaviors that need improvement first. Offer praise at the end of a reprimand. The message will be heard more clearly. The impact of the praising will not be ruined.

Ideas for feedback from Blanchard K, Lorber R. *Putting the One-Minute Manager to Work.* New York: Berkley Publishing, 1992.

Leadership Hint #18: Meeting for the Final Evaluation Interview

1. Remember that the goal of evaluation is to encourage personal and professional growth. In preparation for the evaluation, summarize strong behaviors of the nursing assistant and behaviors that need improvement. Develop a suggested plan for improvement. Attach this summary to the front of the evaluation. Remind nursing assistants to do the same and to bring their copy of the completed evaluation form to the meeting.
2. Schedule the interview for a private location.
3. Allow 10 to 20 minutes for the interview.
4. Conduct the interview in a neutral manner. Check your verbal and nonverbal messages.
5. Use "I" messages when discussing the summary sheet.
6. Start with strong behaviors and compare with the nursing assistant's list. This creates a good mood.
7. Compare behaviors for improvement.
   - Similar behaviors appearing on both lists can indicate insight into the problem. Both nursing assistant and LP/VN charge nurse have noted similar behaviors in the clinical area.
   - When the nursing assistant includes behaviors not noted by the LP/VN charge nurse, this can indicate the value of self-evaluation. The LP/VN charge nurse cannot observe everything.
   - If the LP/VN charge nurse includes behaviors not included by the nursing assistant, this can indicate lack of self-evaluation by the nursing assistant.
8. Finish the evaluation interview with the plan for improvement for any behaviors that need to be modified. The nursing assistant's plan is especially valuable because it indicates personal thinking through of interventions needed for improvement.
9. Check feedback throughout the interview to ensure clear communication. Have the nursing assistant rephrase feedback to see whether your intended message was heard. Some people may distort the message. Clarify messages given by the nursing assistant for information not understood. Encourage questions of any areas on the evaluation that are not understood.
10. Have the nursing assistant sign and date both evaluations. You do the same. The signature indicates the forms were discussed and all questions were answered.

Leadership Hint #19: Strategies to Increase Self-Confidence in Nursing Assistants

1. Provide opportunities to be successful in new situations.
2. Praise beginning successes in new situations.
3. On clinical evaluation forms, include positive statements as well as negative statements.
4. With administration's support, plan educational opportunities for nursing assistants (seminars, in-service programs, and so on).
5. Include nursing assistants in planning meetings, in-service ideas, and so on.
6. Stand up for and support nursing assistants.
7. Actively listen to problems involving the clinical area.
8. Teach nursing assistants a new skill and/or how to improve an old one.
9. Provide challenging assignments.

Leadership Hint #20: Strategies to Encourage Personal Growth in Nursing Assistants

1. Display a balanced interest in personal problems of nursing assistants.
2. Encourage nursing assistant to solve own problems.
3. Suggest referral when nursing assistant is unable to solve personal problems. Follow facility policies.
4. Think of nursing assistants as individuals. Clip and give pertinent cartoons, articles, and so on.
5. Be a mentor/coach/teacher.
6. Be a role model: display a positive work ethic; demonstrate good clinical skills; get out from behind the desk and see what is going on with residents; display good grooming; give objective, specific feedback; address problem, not people; actively listen.

Empower and Instill Confidence and Personal Growth in Team Members

It is rewarding to see the nursing assistants on your team increase their self-confidence and display career and personal growth. You can **empower** nursing assistants and encourage personal growth by your position as LP/VN charge nurse because of the leadership skills you have developed. See Leadership Hints #19 and 20.

Additional Resources for the LP/VN to Develop Organizational, Occupational, and Human Relationship Skills

There are various ways of adding occupational, organizational, and human relationship skills for survival in the workplace. Some of the following suggestions for additional learning for the LP/VN charge nurse offer continuing education credits. See Leadership Hint #21.

Leadership Hint #21: Sources of Learning Skills for LP/VN Charge Nurse Position

1. Check with your local vocational/technical school for a practical/vocational nursing leadership course.
2. Ask your boss to consider in-service programs on leadership techniques, as well as updates on nursing skills. Consider cosponsoring such in-services with the local technical college and making them available to a wide geographic area.
3. Form a network with other persons who fill first-line leadership positions. Be sure to go outside your institution as well as the discipline of nursing. You will find that the problems leaders have are very similar regardless of the discipline.
4. Attend seminars relating to leadership topics as well as nursing topics. Career Track is one example of companies that offer informative, interesting, fun, and affordable one-day seminars that could be of benefit to the first-line leader in nursing.
5. Read books and articles that offer hints for leaders. Be sure your nursing library is up to date.
6. Enroll for certification courses to enhance your knowledge and skills. See Chapter 17.

Summary

☐ When the state nurse practice act allows, practical/vocational nurses are used as first-line leaders, especially in the nursing home/long-term care unit as charge nurse.

☐ The practical/vocational nursing program itself offers students the opportunity to develop skills in nursing procedures, the nursing process, communication, time management, assertiveness, and stress control. These are skills needed for everyday practice as well as leadership positions.

☐ Development of a leadership style is important in guiding nursing assistants to meet the goals of the long-term care facility.

☐ Established leadership styles range from the extreme of autocratic, with a pure emphasis on the task, to laissez-faire, which solely emphasizes concern with the employee.

☐ Situational leadership adapts a leadership style to the environment and situation at hand. It is the suggested way of leading at the beginning of the twenty-first century.

☐ The five core skills of leadership are (1) the ability to motivate team members, (2) the ability to communicate, (3) the ability to problem solve effectively, (4) the ability to build a team of cooperative workers, and (5) the ability to manage stress effectively. These core skills lay the foundation for the development of other specific skills for leadership.

☐ Specific skill areas for nursing leadership include (1) occupational skills, (2) organizational skills, and (3) human relationship skills.

☐ No one chapter or course can teach you how to become a leader. The development of leadership skills is a process and evolves over time.

☐ In addition to training given by the institution, first-line practical/vocational nursing leaders need to educate and update themselves continually in the five core and three specific skill areas noted.

Review Questions

1. Select the strategy that will allow the practical/vocational nurse to practice situational leadership.
   A. Tell subordinates what to do.
   B. Put subordinates first before the policies of the nursing home.
   C. Seek input from employees for emergency situations during the actual situation.
   D. Evaluate the situation in the work environment and vary leadership style to meet the occasion.

2. Select the intervention that would help LP/VN charge nurses meet the affiliation needs of subordinates.
   A. Recognize nursing assistants when they attend a seminar as a group.
   B. Organize monthly potluck lunches for staff and provide the main food item.
   C. Encourage nursing assistants to attend in-service activities and seminars to gain skills that are lacking.

   D. Suggest that nursing assistants, as a group, develop in-service ideas for problem areas in the daily care of residents.

3. Which intervention needs to be used with a nursing assistant who is frequently late for work?
   A. Focus feedback on the behavior that needs improvement.
   B. Give feedback with a continual smile and downplay its importance to make nursing assistant feel better
   C. Avoid mentioning areas for improvement until evaluation time so as not to stress the nursing assistant more.
   D. Assume being present is something the nursing assistant cannot do because of home responsibilities and arrange for time management sessions.

4. Select the charting entry that is considered to be an objective entry describing the resident's response to the nursing intervention "force fluids."

A. Nursing assistant forced fluids all shift.
B. Resident drank a lot of fruit juice and soda from 3–9 PM.
C. Resident drank a total of 310 cc of liquid from 3 PM to 11 PM.
D. Resident loves 7-Up, Coca-Cola, and orange juice without the pulp.
5. To settle a conflict, it is suggested that the practical/vocational nurse focus on

A. Developing a compromise solution to solve the conflict.
B. Investigating what the conflicting parties want to achieve as an outcome.
C. Determining why parties in the conflict hold the positions that are in conflict.
D. Limiting the number of possible solutions to the conflict.

References

Blanchard K, Lorber R. *Putting the One Minute Manager to Work.* New York: Berkley Publishing, 1992.

Ellis A. *Reason and Emotion in Psychotherapy.* New York: Carol Publishing Group, 1994.

National Council completes 1997 job analysis of newly licensed practical/vocational nurses. Issues 18(4):1–2, 1997. Report also on Internet under National Council Publications.

Bibliography

Blanchard K, et al. *The One Minute Manager Builds High Performance Teams.* New York: Morrow, 1991

Blanchard K, Lorber R. *Putting the One Minute Manager to Work.* New York: Berkley Publishing, 1992.

Blanchard K, Johnson S. *The One Minute Manager.* New York: Berkley Publishing, 1993.

Davidhizer R, Dowd S. Benevolent power. Journal of Practical Nursing 49(1):24–33, 1999.

Farley V. *Nurses: Pulling Together to Make a Difference.* Orange, CA: Innovative Nursing Consultants, 1995.

Fisher R, Ury W. *Getting to Yes: Negotiating Agreement Without Giving In.* New York: Penguin Books, 1991.

Herzberg F. *The Motivation to Work.* New Brunswick, NJ: Transaction Pubs, 1993.

Howlett H. *The Howlett theory of management for nursing instructors* (unpublished paper). November, 1989.

Marrelli T. *The Nurse Manager's Survival Guide: Practical Answers to Everyday Problems.* St. Louis: C. V. Mosby, 1997.

Maslow A. *Maslow on Management.* New York: John Wiley and Sons, 1998.

Phillips D. *The Founding Fathers on Leadership: Classic Teamwork in Changing Times.* New York: Warner Books, 1997.

Porter-O'Grady T (ed.). *The Nurse Manager's Problem Solver.* St. Louis: C. V. Mosby, 1994.

Pugh J, Woodward-Smith M. *Nurse Manager: A Practical Guide to Better Human Relations,* 2nd ed. Philadelphia: W. B. Saunders, 1997.

Sorrentino S, Gorek B. *Mosby's Textbook for Long-Term Care Assistants.* St. Louis: C. V. Mosby, 1999.

Vision and Expertise: Nursing Education and the Future. Seminar presented by Venner Farley, RN, Lake Geneva, WI; April 24–25, 1995.

Wywialowski E. *Managing Client Care.* St. Louis: C. V. Mosby, 1997.

Yocum CJ, Lu D. *Job Analysis of Entry-level Practical/Vocational Nurses—1997.* Chicago: National Council of State Boards of Nursing, 1997.

Management, Supervision, and Charge Nurse Skills for Practical/Vocational Nurses

Outline

Key Terms

accountability
assigning

change-of-shift report
delegating

nurse practice act

Objectives

Upon completion of this chapter you will be able to:
1. Using your state's nurse practice act, identify the following as they apply to the charge nurse position for practical/vocational nurses:
   a. Requirements before assuming the LP/VN charge nurse position
   b. Site of employment
   c. Scope of practice

2. Review charge nurse job descriptions.
3. Identify specific institutional policies, regulations, and routines that the practical/vocational nurse needs to clarify when assuming a charge nurse position.
4. Describe elements that need to be focused on when receiving and giving a change-of-shift report as

charge nurse in the long-term care facility.
5. Discuss the assignment of tasks versus the delegation of duties with regard to the following factors:
   a. Your state's laws regarding the role of the practical/vocational nurse and the delegation of duties in the charge nurse position

b. Differences between assigning tasks and delegating duties

c. Examples of tasks that may be assigned and duties that may be delegated

d. Legal aspects of assigning tasks and delegating duties

e. Items that should be considered when assigning tasks and delegating duties

6. Gather a list of assessments that are needed before reporting a change of condition in a resident to a physician.

7. Discuss strategies for handling the following common LP/VN charge nurse problems:

a. When nursing assistants bring problems from home

b. Encouraging nursing assistants to be accountable for learning skills

c. Dealing with the demanding/complaining family

Tricia was always a "saver" as her several well-constructed scrapbooks and boxes of books and papers from nursing school testified. Tricia looked at the carefully clipped classified ad she had saved from five years ago when she had applied for her current position. Five years ago, her husband was transferred to the neighboring state of Oz. After three years of experience as an LVN in a nursing home, postgraduate courses at the local technical college, seminars, in-services programs, and workshops, Tricia thought that she was qualified for a charge nurse position.

Tricia smiled as she pictured herself going in for the interview. That navy blue blazer sure paid off! And all her preparation for the interview served her well. What a sage Mrs. Kelly had been in her Personal/Vocational (PV) course to recommend that a job applicant obtain a copy of the facility's mis-sion statement before the interview. She was sure her knowledge of the facility's emphasis and pride on providing quality care was a big plus in landing the job, even though she did not have LP/VN charge nurse experience. Not to mention the enthusiasm and positive attitude she displayed to the interviewer about being willing to learn and confidence that she would be able to do the job. Plus, the textbook suggestion that she purchase the state of Oz's Nurse Practice Act informed her of the ability of the LP/VN to delegate in that state and allowed her to ask questions in the interview about delegation.

Five whole years as LP/VN charge nurse! Tricia loved her job and smiled as she remembered many of the challenges she had faced early in her job as charge nurse. She began to page through that old fourth edition of her PV textbook . . . .

LPN

Full time position for an experienced LP/VN to join our long-term care facility as a charge nurse on the evening shift. Must have excellent communication and customer service skills. Needs to be team-oriented. Current State of Oz license. We offer a competitive salary and full benefit package. If you qualify, send resume and cover letter to: Quality Care Home, 982 Brick Lane, Wayback, Oz 00005 for further information, contact Claudette Radant, DON at 987-123-4516

Where to Begin? Job Description for Charge Nurse

Before continuing, review Leadership Activity II: Determining Your State's Requirements to Assume the Charge Nurse Position for Practical/Vocational Nurses, found in Chapter 13.

Tricia looked at the job description the director of nurses gave her during her job interview. Now it all seems so routine and a comfortable part of her job. But Tricia remembered how overwhelming it was to read the 12 areas of responsibility along with the 15 duties.

QUALITY CARE NURSING HOME EVENING CHARGE NURSE—LP/VN JOB DESCRIPTION

QUALIFICATIONS

Licensed practical/vocational nurse with a current license to practice in the state of Oz under Chapter 747. The LP/VN should have a certificate of successful completion of an approved course in Medication Administration.

STANDARDS

The job of the LP/VN charge nurse is to ensure that residents receive nursing care, treatments, and medications that have been ordered by their physicians. The LP/VN charge nurse shall help coordinate resident care services, e.g., physicians, dietitian, activity director, physical therapist, and social worker. The LP/VN charge nurse shall assist the Director of Nurses in the orientation of new employees. The LP/VN charge nurse shall evaluate work performance of nursing assistants.

RESPONSIBLE FOR

1. Knowledge of residents' condition at all times.
2. Assigning actual nursing care tasks to nursing assistants.
3. Providing nursing care according to physician's orders and in agreement with recognized nursing techniques and procedures, established standards of care as described in Oz state statutes, and administrative policies of this long-term care facility.
4. Recognizing symptoms; reporting residents' condition, including changes; and assisting with remedial measures for adverse developments.
5. Assisting physician in diagnostic and therapeutic measures.
6. Administering medications and treatments as prescribed.
7. Maintaining accurate and complete records of nursing assessments and interventions, including documentation on the residents' charts and Kardex records.
8. Efficiency of execution of work load, including neatness and orderliness.
9. Delegating duties, as appropriate, to nursing assistants.
10. Maintaining a safe and hazard-free environment.
11. Ensuring the residents' right to privacy.
12. Maintaining the dignity of residents.

DUTIES

1. Observes and reports symptoms and conditions of residents.
2. Administers medications as prescribed by physicians. Assesses therapeutic response and side effects of same.
3. Takes and records vital signs when appropriate.
4. Maintains charts and Kardexes, including residents' condition and medications and treatments received.
5. Calls physician when necessary. Receives and records telephone orders.
6. Calls pharmacist for prescription drugs as needed.
7. Assists in maintaining a physical, social, and psychological environment for residents that is conducive to the best interests and welfare of residents.
8. Receives report at beginning of shift from off-going personnel and assigns tasks to nursing assistants under the LP/VN charge nurse's supervision.
9. Delegates duties, as appropriate, to nursing assistants.
10. Evaluates the completion of nursing assistant assignments in a safe and timely manner.
11. Provides report to oncoming shift.
12. Evaluates nursing assistants in the performance of their job description and reports same to Director of Nursing.
13. Attends supervisory staff meetings.
14. Interprets state and federal guidelines to employees. Uses authority as LP/VN charge nurse to "follow code."
15. Participates in orientation of all new employees assigned to LP/VN charge nurse.

Management Tool #1: Reviewing LP/VN Charge Nurse Job Descriptions

Resources Needed:
LP/VN charge nurse job descriptions of long-term care facilities/nursing homes

Review LP/VN charge nurse job descriptions of nursing homes/long-term care facilities at sites at which you affiliate during your student year.

The charge nurse job description might seem overwhelming at first. But it illustrates the reason state laws require that practical/vocational charge nurses have education, training, or experience beyond the basic practical/vocational nursing curriculum and documentation of such. It is difficult to prepare health care workers in one year to be able to function in this position immediately after graduation. After additional education, training, and experience, many practical/vocational nurses become charge nurses, also called first-line managers, in long-term care units and nursing homes. And they are doing an excellent job in that role. When questioned about administrative responsibilities, 30% of practical/vocational nurses, in the latest job analysis to gather data for content areas for NCLEX-PN, stated they regularly had administrative responsibilities (Yocum, 1997).

How Long Will It Take Me to Prepare to Be a Charge Nurse?

You are probably thinking, "How long will it take for me to get to this point in my practical/vocational nursing career?" The answer to that question is individual to the person asking it. The law of some states specifically states that the charge nurse functions *in a nursing home* and under the direct supervision of a registered nurse. In such a state, the practical/vocational nurse could not function as a charge nurse in a medical clinic. Also, the practical/vocational nurse could not function under general supervision until after passing NCLEX-PN. *Be sure to check your state's **nurse practice act.*** Some practical/vocational nursing programs offer a postgraduate course preparing graduates for an expanded role. North Dakota has made practical/vocational nursing a two-year program and focuses on management in the second year.

The answer to "How long will it take for me to get to this point in my practical/vocational nursing career?" depends on your state nurse practice act, additional education, your motivation to learn the manager role, your ability to be a risk taker, and how you use your nursing experience. This book is unable to provide you with a concise cookbook of how to function in the role of charge nurse as a practical/vocational nurse. However, through active learning and an interactive format, this chapter presents 17 Management Tools. These tools inform you of the many areas that need to be considered, understood, and investigated when assuming an LP/VN charge nurse position. The chapter also discusses areas of problems/responsibilities/concerns that affect the LP/VN charge nurse in a long-term care unit or nursing home. This chapter builds on Chapter 13, Developing Leadership Skills.

You will be expected to be self-directed, to problem solve, and to think critically as you apply the information in Chapter 13. These are the very attributes employers expect of you as an LP/VN charge nurse. Reference is provided to specific resources needed to work through the Management Tools. You are encouraged to use the information from the entire book and your other classes as well as to work through the self-directed Management Tools. Your instructor is also a valuable resource. And remember the usefulness of peer group discussion.

At times we will flash back to Tricia as she reminisces about her beginning days in the LP/VN charge nurse position. Her initial experiences and adjustment to the charge nurse role will show you the challenges and opportunities the LP/VN charge nurse role provides.

Tricia thought back to the orientation phase of her job. It too seemed so overwhelming at the time.

The thought of going through those thick manuals of policies, regulations, and routines was enough to give her a headache. But they sure did contain valuable information. Here is the sample checklist Mrs. Kelly gave the class as a guide when reviewing these manuals.

A Checklist of Policies, Regulations, and Routines for the LP/VN Charge Nurse

Not all the areas included here are the responsibility of the LP/VN charge nurse in a nursing home/long-term care facility. But LP/VN charge nurses need to have information for all the areas included so they can carry out their management duties. Since the LP/VN charge nurse has the responsibility to supervise nursing assistants, information about policies and routines is also needed by these personnel. Orientation to your facility must include these items.

Personnel Policies

- Time sheets—location and interpretation
- Vacation, holiday, sick leave policy
- Special request for time off, leave of absence
- Communication—reporting: on and off duty, sickness, absence, and memos; bulletin board
- Meal "hours," coffee break
- Smoking regulations
- Use of facility telephones
- Uniform regulations
- Job descriptions and duties of unlicensed personnel
- Organizational chart

Federal, State, and Private Agency Regulations

- Inspection protocols
- Current federal and state regulations
- Regulations of the Omnibus Budget Reconciliation Act (OBRA) of 1987
- Regulations of the Health Care Financing Administration (HCFA)
- Regulations of The Joint Commission on Accreditation of Health Care Organizations (JCAHO)

Records and Unit Routines

- General shift routine for days, evenings, and nights
- Duties of each of the three shifts
- Methods of reporting
- Procedure manual
- Facility policy manual
- Procedures specific to each division of the facility
- Nursing Care Plan system
- Nursing Kardex and Medix systems
- Routine for care planning conferences
- Routine for physician's visits
- System of transcribing physician's orders
- Location of reference books

Unit Administration

- Admission, placement, transfer, and discharge of residents
- Care of clothing and valuables, including personal property list
- Routine for seriously ill residents
- Routine for death of a resident
- Autopsy permit
- Authorization procedure and forms for diagnostic tests and surgery
- Visiting hours
- Notary Public

Safety Policies

- Siderails
- Restraints
- Fire regulations: reporting, evacuation plan, fire exits, location of fire extinguishers, preventive measures
- Use of oxygen
- Transportation of residents by cart, wheelchair
- Body mechanics
- Door alarms

Housekeeping, Maintenance, and Supplies

- Linen—how supplied, extra linen
- Care of contaminated linens and dressings
- Unit cleaning procedure and responsibilities
- How to obtain supplies: drugs, sterile supplies, personal care items
- Kitchen items
- Maintenance and repairs
- Conservation of supplies, linen, and equipment

Equipment—How to Use and Where to Obtain

- Oxygen
- Suction equipment
- Therapeutic beds
- Respiratory therapy equipment and services

Food Service for Residents

- Ordering diets/diet changes
- Tray service
- Unit food stock items
- Special nourishments
- Policy for feeding residents
- Policy for dining room

Nursing Care Procedures/ Assisting Physician

- Bathing, mouth care
- Bedmaking
- Temperature (devices used), pulse, and respiration
- Blood pressure
- Catheterization
- Enemas
- Suppositories—rectal
- Recording intake and output
- Systems used for pressure ulcer care
- Collecting, delivering, and labeling specimens
- Assisting physicians with physical examinations, foot care
- Policies for sterile technique procedures

- Blood glucose monitoring
- Colostomy care
- Nasogastric and gastrostomy tubes: flushing, feeding, administration of medication
- Standard precautions
- Postmortem procedures

Medications

- Medication system
- Policy for reordering
- Unit stock
- Ordering from pharmacy
- Review of metric system, proportions, abbreviations
- Drug errors: reporting, incident reports
- Narcotic count
- Sources of drug administration

Charting

- Method of charting
- Forms used
- Flowsheets used
- Policy for phone orders
- Incident reports
- Lists for wanderers, hearing aid use, and so on
- Federal and state chart forms and requirements

Special Areas

- Emergency supplies
- Central supply area
- Physical therapy
- Occupational therapy
- Laundry
- Maintenance
- Break room
- Dining room
- Kitchen
- Business offices
- Social services
- Director of nurses
- Staff educator
- Administrator of facility
- Conference rooms
- Activity department

Miscellaneous

- Paging system
- Call-light system
- Disaster plan
- Routine for residents who desire cardiopulmonary resuscitation
- Chaplain service
- Volunteer services
- On-call schedule
- Handling of wanderers
- Procedure for signing resident in and out of facility
- Hair care services

See Management Tool #2.

Tricia kept paging through her PV text and notes. What memories they brought back! All those shifts of taking report and focusing on important aspects of each client or resident on the clinical area had a purpose. Tricia remembered the first time she had taken report as an LP/VN charge nurse. Her new position of responsibility gave her a heightened sense of awareness of the data being given.

Reporting

Reports in long-term care units and nursing homes, as in other health care agencies, are a way to pass pertinent information to the oncoming shift. In this way, the residents are guaranteed continuity in their care.

Report When Coming on Your Shift

The report you receive when you are coming on your shift will be your basis for assessing resident needs. This is legally necessary so that you can adequately assign nursing assistants to provide care for specific patients. Report can be taped or oral, depending on agency policy.

When report is taped, off-going personnel usually are still on duty, answering call lights and attending to residents' needs, while the oncoming charge nurse listens to report. This will enable you to question unclear information after report. Nurses develop personal ways of gathering data when they

 Management Tool #2: Reviewing Policies and Routines

Resources needed:

- Above checklist of policies, regulations, and routines for the LP/VN.
- Your opinion and reasons (rationale)

All policies, regulations, and routines of a health care facility are important. After reading the checklist, complete the following.

a. List the five items from *Records and Unit Routines* that you think are most necessary for effective running of the resident wings of the long-term care unit. Provide the reason (rationale) for your choice.

Item	*Rationale*
1. _____	_____
2. _____	_____
3. _____	_____
4. _____	_____
5. _____	_____

b. List the five items from *Unit Administration* you think are most necessary for effective running of the resident wings of the long-term care unit. Provide your reason (rationale) for your choice.

Item	*Rationale*
1. _____	_____
2. _____	_____
3. _____	_____
4. _____	_____
5. _____	_____

are taking report, including use of symbols and abbreviations.

Management Tool #3: Developing Your Personal Tool for Gathering Data During Report

Resources Needed:

- Method of gathering data during report that you have developed during the clinical year
- Your creativity

Develop a form that will help you gather the pertinent information needed to assume responsibility of taking charge of your assigned residents. Include format, symbols, and abbreviations you find helpful and will allow you quickly and accurately to gather the information. Compare your form with forms of classmates.

Reporting at the End of Your Shift

Giving report at the end of your shift requires planning. As LP/VN charge nurse, nursing assistants need to report to you before you can tape or give report. This is where the concise, clear directions that you gave to these team members during assignment of tasks will pay off. Be sure to personally assess residents who have changes in condition, current ongoing problems, new orders (and resident response to those new orders), and suspected side effects to medications. You will need to set priorities in deciding pertinent information to give to the next shift.

Use the same sequence of data for each resident. This will make it easier for the oncoming charge nurse to take notes from your report. An example of a suggested sequence of data for residents in a long-term care unit follows:

1. Resident name, room number, and physician
2. New problems/concerns
3. Contact with physician and new orders
4. Progress of current, established problems

5. PRN medication—name of drug, time given, and reason for PRN medication; time follow-up is required.
6. **Briefly** describe resident's behavior during shift. Include any changes in resident's physical and mental status.
7. Resident's voiding, bowel movement (continent vs. incontinent)

Things to avoid during report include:

1. Meaningless chatter that has nothing to do with residents' nursing care and goals
2. Routine nursing care, unless it has a bearing on current nursing problems
3. Personal opinions about residents' conditions
4. Value judgments about residents' life styles, behavior, or families

Management Tool #4: Reporting When Starting and Ending Your Shift

Resources Needed:
Reading: Report when coming on your shift
Reading: Reporting at the end of your shift

Whatever your current site of clinical affiliation, focus on information that is given to you when you report on duty. This can be a formal report or informal passing of information in acute-care, long-term care, or the community.

1. Identify unnecessary information that may have been passed on to you.
2. Using suggestions under *Report When Coming on Your Shift* on page 243, list ways you could improve the way information was passed on.
3. Using the suggestions under *Reporting at the End of Your Shift* on page 243, provide the appropriate person with the appropriate data before you leave the clinical site.

Tricia stopped at the topic of Assigning Tasks to Nursing Assistants. She remembered her early struggles in assigning the right task to the right person.

Assigning Tasks to Nursing Assistants

Assigning Tasks in the Long-Term Care Unit

Assigning unlicensed personnel, such as nursing assistants, to care for specific residents follows change-of-shift report. When practical/vocational nurses make assignments to nursing assistants, they are allotting tasks that are in the job description of these health care workers. The assigned tasks are tasks nursing assistants are hired and paid to perform. The tasks are in *their* job description. These unlicensed personnel have the responsibility to complete the assignment in a safe and timely manner. The LP/VN charge nurse shares responsibility with unlicensed personnel for the quality of the care delivered. In this situation, the LP/VN charge nurse needs to evaluate the quality and effectiveness of the care that was assigned.

Assigning the Right Task

A crucial legal consideration in assigning tasks to nursing assistants is nursing judgment. The LP/VN charge nurse needs to avoid real and/or potential harm to residents when assigning tasks to unlicensed personnel. You are *legally liable* for improper assigning of tasks. Change-of-shift report gives you the opportunity, as LP/VN charge nurse, to assess the specific nursing needs of the residents for your shift and the complexity of those needs. Specific suggestions of tasks to assign to nursing assistants include routine bathing, feeding, ambulating; vital signs, weight, assistance with elimination, and maintaining safety factors. Actual tasks assigned depend on needs of the residents on your unit, the training of nursing assistants, and policies of the long-term care unit. More complex skills to assign depend on what is allowed by law in your state, unit need, and further training of nursing assistants.

Management Tool #5: Reviewing Nursing Assistant Job Descriptions

Resources Needed:
Job descriptions of nursing assistants.

Obtain job descriptions of nursing assistants of health care agencies where you affiliate. Make a list of the tasks nursing assistants can perform at these sites.

Assigning Tasks to the Right Person

Legally, you need to know the job descriptions of nursing assistants to whom you assign tasks. Be sure to check these job descriptions of the facility in which you are employed. Know the level of clinical competence of nursing assistants whom you supervise. What are their strengths? What are their weaknesses? How much training have they had? What skills did they learn in their training program? Have they had orientation to your unit? See Management Tool #5.

Once you work consistently with nursing assistants, they will prove their dependability and ability to pursue assigned tasks. If the nursing assistant has had the proper training but is new to your long-term care facility, make sure this person has completed orientation. Assign another nursing assistant who has proved dependable to work with this person until comfortable with the job.

Tricia chuckled as she thought about the time she asked a nursing assistant to force fluids on a resident. When the nursing assistant was approached during the shift, she kept reporting that she was forcing fluids. At the end of the shift, when asked for the volume of fluid taken by the resident during the shift, the aide replied that although she had forced fluids every hour, the resident took only 80 cc on the day shift. Tricia thought that served her right for not explaining the assignment objectively as taught by Mrs. Kelly.

Management Tool #6: Assigning Residents in Long-Term Care

Resources Needed:
Personal judgment and reason (rationale) for choices you make

Tasks for Day Shift of Wing 1 of Nursing Home

4 showers. Each of these residents transfers with the help of two. Each of these residents needs to be weighed, have BP checks, and complete linen change on shower day. One resident scheduled for a shower states she feels dizzy today and has a congested-sounding cough.

16 partial baths. Ten residents are able to wash own face and hands when set up. Of the remaining six, one has developed a rash over his entire body, one needs glucose-monitoring × 2 on day shift, and four are confused and incontinent of urine and feces. Each of these residents needs one assistant to transfer and ambulate.

1 complex dressing change for a resident on a Clinitron bed (this resident is transferred by a client-lifting device and requires total care).

1 PEG tube intermittent feeding with commercial tube feeding formula × 2 and drug administration × 2 on day shift (this resident is confused and requires two persons to ambulate).

Staff Available

2 student practical/vocational nurses who have completed half of their nursing program. Instructor makes assignments.

1 nursing assistant who has worked at the facility for 10 years (on state directory).

1 nursing assistant who has 7 years' experience and has worked at your facility for 6 months (on state directory).

1 nursing assistant who was sent from a temp agency to fill the position of a nursing assistant who has the flu. She completed a nursing assistant–advanced course two months ago (on state directory).

1. As LP/VN charge nurse, how would you make assignments for the day shift for Wing 1? Include the reason (rationale) for your assignment decisions.
2. You have just completed assigning team members when one of the nursing assistants states she feels warm and faints. Turns out she has a temperature of 104.2°F and needs to be sent home. Reassign the residents on Wing 1.

Using the Right Communication to Assign a Task

The objective in assigning a task is to have a task completed safely. Give clear, concise, objective directions to nursing assistants when you are assigning a task. Be specific about the results you are expecting. Make sure your directions are complete.

Clarify the message by asking nursing assistants to tell you what it is you expect them to do. Consider writing assignments in a concise, objective manner on a master assignment sheet. Explain what is expected at the nursing assistant's level of understanding. A "please" and "thank you" are in order as part of common courtesy.

Using the right communication and motivating

techniques is an excellent example of the leadership skills that are needed by LP/VN charge nurses. The LP/VN charge nurse's ability to motivate nursing assistants to carry out tasks to meet goals depends on these skills. These skills need to be learned by studying and using the techniques. Refer to Chapter 13 for hints that can be used to motivate team members and also review Leadership Activity V, using the Howlett Hierarchy in Leadership Situations. See Management Tools #7 and #8.

Management Tool #7: Communicating Assignments Objectively

Resources Needed:
Chapter 12. Reading: The Practical/Vocational Nurse's Role in the Nursing Process (Goal Setting)
Chapter 13. Reading: "Subjective as Opposed to Objective Charting"
Signs and Symptoms list on page 252
Any med/surg or geriatric text

Write the following tasks/observations to be assigned to nursing assistants in objective terms. The tasks need to be realistic, measurable, and time-references.

1. Be sure to clean up the resident.
2. Make sure this resident drinks today.
3. The resident MUST get up today.
4. If Mr. Jones does not pass any urine, let me know.
5. Have this resident ready for his doctor's appointment.

After Assigned Tasks Are Completed

When nursing assistants accept an assignment, they accept the primary responsibility for safely and efficiently completing that assignment. LP/VN charge nurses have the responsibility to verify the nursing

Management Tool #8: Providing Nursing Assistants with Pertinent Data (Assessments) About Medical Conditions of Assigned Residents

Resources Needed:
Medical-surgical textbook
Chapter 13. Reading: "Subjective as Opposed to Objective Charting"
Problem-solving ability

This is your first month as charge nurse at Quality Care Home. Provide objective data (assessments) for the nursing assistant to collect while giving care in the following resident situations.

1. Resident has compensated right-sided congestive heart failure.
2. Resident is a poorly controlled diabetic on Humulin each morning.
3. Resident has lost five pounds in the past two weeks.
4. Resident has an order for a cathed urine for residual.

assistant's ability and success in performing the task that was assigned. Check the completed task that was assigned. *Legally, the LP/VN charge nurse may not assign a task without checking the outcome of that assignment.* Was the task completed? Was the task done safely? Have resident goals been met?

Sometimes nursing assistants to whom you have assigned a task are not functioning at their highest level of competence. General suggestions for reporting this type of situation follow but *be sure to check the facility policy.* Document the unsafe care you observe. Describe the incident *objectively.* Include date, time, place, and resident involved. Inform your supervisor in writing and provide this information. Request in your documentation that the team member involved receive additional training in the specific area of observed unsafe care. See Management Tool #9.

Tricia remembered well the confusion she experi-

Management Tool #9: Documenting Unsafe Care by a Nursing Assistant

Resources Needed:
Reading: "After Assigned Tasks Are Completed" on page 246
Reading: Chapter 13—"Subjective as Opposed to Objective Charting"

You assigned a nursing assistant the task of giving a resident a shower. You observed that this team member "unsafely" showered the resident. Using the preceding suggestions, compose a mock letter to your supervisor to report unsafe care.

Management Tool #10: Reviewing Your Nurse Practice Act for Authority to Delegate

Resources Needed:
Your state's nurse practice act

1. Locate the section of your nurse practice act that discusses your ability (or not) to delegate nursing duties as an LP/VN charge nurse.
2. In your own words, write that position here.

_____

_____

_____

_____

enced in her basic VN program in trying to understand the difference between assigning and delegating to nursing assistants. The fact that she went to school in a state that did not allow her to delegate to nursing assistants compounded her difficulty. In her present role as charge nurse in a state that allows delegation, this area was very important. She began to read the coverage of delegating tasks from her PV textbook. This area still perplexes nurses at all levels. Although Tricia has gained much experience in delegating tasks, sometimes she still has questions and concerns. But learning to delegate duties generally has given her more time for duties that cannot be delegated.

Assigning Versus Delegating Tasks

Delegating Tasks

■ At this time, not every state in the United States allows practical/vocational nurses to participate in delegating in their charge nurse positions. It is crucial that you check your state's nurse practice act to determine whether you may delegate as an LP/VN charge nurse in your state. If you cannot clearly find an answer, contact your state's board of nursing. ■

When allowed by your state's nurse practice act and facility policies, **delegating** duties in the long-term care unit involves entrusting duties that are in the job description of the LP/VN charge nurse (the person doing the delegating) to nursing assistants. The duties being delegated are in *your* job description. The primary responsibility for the outcome of delegated acts rests with the registered nurse with whom the LP/VN charge nurse functions under general supervision. *Duties can be delegated but the responsibility that goes with those duties can never be delegated to another.* See Table 14–1 for a comparison of assigning tasks and delegating duties.

Delegating Duties

If your state's nurse practice act allows LP/VN charge nurses to delegate duties, you will have the opportunity to delegate duties to nursing assistants. In addition to your state's nurse practice act, be sure to review

1. Rules and regulations of your state's board of nursing
2. Interpretations developed by your state board of nursing regarding delegation

TABLE 14–1: Comparison of Assigning Versus Delegating by the Practical/Vocational Charge Nurse

	Assigning Tasks	Delegating Duties
To whom may tasks or duties be assigned or delegated?	Nursing assistants and other unlicensed personnel	Nursing assistants and other unlicensed personnel
Are tasks or duties in nursing assistant's job description?	Yes	No. Specific tasks are not listed. Tasks depend on the situation
May nursing assistant refuse?	No, unless staff person thinks he or she is unqualified for the assignment	Yes. In addition, staff person must voluntarily accept delegation
Who has primary responsibility for the completion of care?	Nursing assistant	LP/VN charge nurse

3. Standards of your nursing organizations that apply to delegation of duties
4. Facility policy regarding delegation of nursing duties by LP/VN charge nurse

Learning to delegate duties from your job description to nursing assistants, when allowed by your nurse practice act and facility policies, can increase your effectiveness and efficiency as an LP/VN charge nurse. Delegating to nursing assistants also helps these team members increase and improve their job skills. The suggestions in this chapter that were given for assigning tasks apply also to delegating duties. But delegating is a complex skill. There are some important differences. See Management Tool #12.

Differences Between Assigning and Delegating

The word assignment in this chapter is used in its traditional sense. Assigning tasks is done before and during your shift as a regular part of *your* job. Assigning tasks is in *your* job description. Since assignments involve allocating the nursing care that is to be done by nursing assistants within *their* job description, these team members cannot refuse the assignment (Wywialowski, 1997, p. 181). The ex-

ception is when nursing assistants receiving the assignment decide they are unqualified to carry it out. The nursing assistant would then be reassigned. Arrangements would be made for this team member to receive the training necessary to do the task(s) he or she felt unqualified to do. Nursing assistants assume primary responsibility for completing tasks safely when they are assigned to them. See Management Tool #11.

Delegating duties is written in the job description of the LP/VN charge nurse at Quality Care Home. When allowed by your state's nurse practice act, delegating is a voluntary function. When delegating duties, you decide to ask nursing assistants (unlicensed personnel) to do part of *your* job. You are not asking them to do duties that you dislike doing. You are asking them to help you perform some of your job description so that you may get to other responsibilities with the ultimate goal of improving resident care. Because you are delegating part of your job, the nursing assistants must give approval to the assignment. They must voluntarily accept the delegation—they cannot be forced. Delegation involves the ability to share power with another team member. When delegating duties, the LP/VN charge nurse needs to provide the nursing assistant with the authority and equipment to carry out the delegated duty.

Management Tool #11: Handling Refusal of Assignment by Nursing Assistants

Resources Needed:
Reading: Differences Between Assigning and Delegating, preceding section

A nursing assistant on the team has refused your assignment to give a resident a whirlpool bath because she does not feel qualified to do the job safely. List two actions you as LP/VN charge nurse would carry out in this situation.

1. _____

2. _____

_____

Legal Aspects of Delegating

In 1994, the president of the National Council of State Boards of Nursing stated that "Boards of nursing must clearly define delegation in regulation, promulgate clear rules for its use, and follow through with disciplinary action when there is evidence that the rules are violated" (Rachels, 1994). Check with the board of nursing in your state for their interpretation of delegation.

To be legally sound when delegating duties, keep the following criteria in mind:

1. Delegate functions only if allowed by your state's nurse practice act and facility policies.
2. Never delegate what is in your legal scope of practice. See p. 250.
3. Delegate duties for which nursing assistants have had the educational preparation and demonstrated ability. See Management Tool #13.
4. Provide clear, objective directions to nursing assistants for delegated duties.
5. Provide assistance to nursing assistants when you delegate a duty.
6. Monitor the activities of nursing assistants when they carry out delegated duties.

Management Tool #12: Locating Positions of Nursing Groups on Delegation Function of LP/VN Charge Nurse

Resources Needed:

- Rules and regulations and interpretations of delegation of your state's board of nursing
- Standards of NAPNES and NFLPN; see Appendixes B and C
- Standards of the NLN; see Appendix D
- National Council of State Boards of Nursing (NCSBN).* See Appendix A.
- Policies on delegation of affiliating agencies

Review the position papers/standards of the following agencies in regard to delegation of nursing tasks:

1. Rules and regulations of your board of nursing
2. Interpretations of your board of nursing
3. Standards of nursing organizations: NAPNES, NFLPN, NLN, and NCSBN
4. Policy of health care facility

---

*Includes *Delegation: Concepts and Decision-Making Process,* which was prepared by the National Council of State Boards of Nursing as a resource for licensed nurses in all types of health care settings. It provides a decision-making process to facilitate the provision of quality care for licensed nurses to delegate nursing tasks in accord with their legal scope of practice.

---

7. Evaluate the safety and effectiveness of duties delegated to nursing assistants.

When the registered nurse delegates a duty to an LP/VN or a nursing assistant, the legal principle of *respondeat superior* comes into play. By that principle, the nursing act delegated is the act of the supervising nurse, the RN, the person who delegated the act. In the long-term care facility, the LP/VN as charge nurse is managing and directing the activities of nursing assistants under the *general* supervision of a registered nurse. The registered nurse is *ultimately* responsible for the supervision of nursing assistants. But the LP/VN first-line manager assists in the supervision of these health care workers and shares accountability with the RN for their actions.

Duties That Might Be Delegated

A concise, across-the-board list of what nursing duties to delegate and what not to delegate does not exist. A specific list of duties to delegate has the following drawbacks.

1. Duty lists for unlicensed assistive personnel (UAP), such as the nursing assistant, eliminate assessment of the needs of each client of health care. A duty could be on a list of acceptable duties to delegate to a UAP, but the client situation might be such that the duty would be dangerous or inappropriate for an unlicensed person. For example, a tub bath for a resident who has had a change in condition requiring continual nursing assessment during movement, turning, and so on.
2. A duty list for UAPs puts the control of nursing care into the hands of persons who have had minimal training for client care. Your board of nursing has the responsibility to protect the client of health care. Licensed nursing personnel carry out this responsibility.

The exact duties delegated to unlicensed personnel are interpreted by each state's board of nursing and by each client situation. Within this framework, employers may suggest that certain duties be delegated. But the person doing the delegating is ultimately responsible for the following:

1. Deciding to delegate a duty.
2. Deciding to whom to delegate the duty.
3. Deciding under what circumstances to delegate the duty.

Generally, necessary, routine, repetitive duties for stable clients that do not require frequent, repeated assessments during the nursing activity can be delegated. Duties that are part of your legal scope of practice may never be delegated. Do not assume that simpler duties may be automatically delegated. Examples of what *not* to delegate *might* include:

1. Complex sterile technique procedures
2. Crisis situations (you be there)
3. Initial patient education by an RN

See Management Tool #13. **It is your license that is at stake in the matter of delegating nursing duties.**

The review of delegation in her old PV text proved demanding for Tricia. She decided to break for a snack. She felt good with how far she had come since those beginning days of feeling insecure. At least by now, she knew what to question and where to find the answers. It felt good to have a grasp of her LP/VN charge nurse position. While relaxing, she remembered the emphasis her PN/VN program put on the practical/vocational nurse's role in data collection (assessment). Actually being on the job would prove the value of this nursing skill. Data collection (assessment) and what you did with that data really separated the licensed from the unlicensed in a resident situation. Mrs. Kelly had provided a list of signs and symptoms and stressed it would not be a complete list but would be something to get you started. It had been some time since Tricia had updated that list, and she quickly finished her snack and got back to her treasured boxes of books and papers.

Collecting Data (Assessing) as an LP/VN Charge Nurse

As LP/VN charge nurse, you need to do an initial assessment of residents for whom you have charge immediately after report. You will also assess periodically during your shift. The frequency of data collecting (assessment) depends on patient conditions. The following is a list of signs and symptoms that may indicate illness, exacerbation of a previous disease condition, injury, or decline in prior functioning.

Be observant with each resident interaction. When nursing assistants report that "something does

Management Tool #13: Deciding to Delegate

Resource Needed:
Chapter 14. Reading: "Tasks That May Be Delegated"

You practice in a health care facility that allows the LP/VN charge nurse to delegate nursing duties to nursing assistants. List two additional things to consider before actually delegating:

1. _____

2. _____

Refer to the job description for the Quality Care Nursing Home at the beginning of this chapter. Examples of LP/VN charge nurse duties that *could* be delegated if allowed in this state, based on this job description, are

1. "Administers medications" (Item 2)—federal and some state regulations allow nursing assistants to administer medications after successful completion of a drug administration course. Giving selected medications could be delegated to nursing assistants *if* they have successfully completed requirements of the state in which they are employed.
2. "Takes and records vital signs when appropriate" (Item 3)—this duty refers to other than routine vital signs. In this situation, the resident has probably had a change in condition. The LP/VN charge nurse may decide to delegate the duty of taking frequent vital signs to a nursing assistant who has proved competence and reliability with vital signs skills and quickly reports results to the LP/VN charge nurse. This would allow the LP/VN charge nurse to report to the physician via phone, assess/collect data for other residents with changes in condition, and perform treatments that cannot be delegated.
3. "Participates in orientation of all new employees" (Item 15)—the LP/VN charge nurse would assume the primary responsibility for orientation of new nursing assistants. An experienced nursing assistant can be delegated to conduct orientation of specific aspects of the routine of the shift to which a new employee is assigned.

Remember, even though the above tasks *could* be delegated if permitted by this state's nurse practice act, the final determination to delegate rests on

1. The policy of the facility regarding delegation.
2. The decision of the nurse to delegate.
3. The condition of the resident.

Examples of LP/VN charge nurse duties in the Quality Care Nursing Home job description that would not be delegated would be:

1. Calls physician when necessary (Item 5)
2. Evaluates nursing assistants (Item 12)
3. Interprets state and federal guidelines (Item 14)

If your state's nurse practice act allows delegation, discuss LP/VN charge nurse duties that could be delegated, depending on the client's condition and agency policy.

not seem right," visit the resident to assess/collect your own data. After collecting the data, record it on the proper form and report all abnormal observations according to agency policy. The actual assessment parameters given here are guidelines. Follow specific parameters given for assigned resident.

Signs and Symptoms

1. Weight: Increase or decrease of 5 to 10 pounds in one week.
2. Temperature: Elevation over 100° F orally or 100.6° F rectally. Temperature under 96.6° F orally.
3. Upper respiratory: Head congestion, headache, sore throat, ear pain, runny nose, postnasal drip.
4. Lower respiratory: Acute onset or worsening of: shortness of breath, dyspnea with exertion, orthopnea, cough (productive or nonproductive), wheezing or other abnormal sounds on inhalation or exhalation.
5. Cardiac: Blood pressure over 140/90 (new symptom); blood pressure below 80/50; irregular pulse (new symptom); chest, neck, shoulder, or arm pain; fatigue; increased frequency of angina; shortness of breath; orthopnea; peripheral edema; sacral edema; or distended neck veins.
6. Breast: Lump found on palpation, discharge from nipple.
7. Abdomen: Localized or generalized pain, especially of acute onset; epigastric burning or discomfort; constipation; diarrhea; nausea; vomiting; bloody or tarry stools; loss of appetite.
8. Musculoskeletal: Swollen and tender joints, loss of strength in limbs, pain, loss of motion, ecchymosis, edema.
9. Reproductive system: Vaginal discharge, abnormal vaginal bleeding.
10. Genitourinary: Urgency, frequency, dysuria, nocturia, hematuria, incontinence. Male: Dribbling, inability to start or stop stream.
11. Sleep and rest patterns: Changes from nor-

mal routine, requirement of medication for sleep, nightmares or dreams.
12. Appearance of skin: Changes in color, turgor, contusions, abrasions, lacerations, rashes.
13. Mobility and exercise: Need for support in ambulation, changes in posture, weakness of extremities, changes in coordination, vertigo.
14. Hygiene status: Mouth: Condition of mucous membranes, gums, teeth, tongue, mouth odor. Body: Cleanliness, odor. Hair: Grooming, distribution, scalp scaling, presence of disease. Nails: Color, texture, grooming.
15. Communication: Verbal and nonverbal expression, aphasia, level of understanding.
16. Sensory-perceptual: Ability to hear, condition of hearing aid; ability to see, condition of glasses; ability to feel in all extremities; ability to discriminate odors; ability to distinguish tastes.
17. Cultural/religious: Food preferences, wellness/illness beliefs, religious practices (rosary, Bible, medals, icons, communion, clergy visits, confession, sacrament of the sick).
18. Psychological status: Level of consciousness, disorientation, intelligence, attention span, vocabulary level, interests, memory.

Tricia remembered how Mrs. Kelly stressed the importance of getting to a room and personally assessing clients, especially when there was a change of condition. She found the example Mrs. Kelly gave so that the same situation could be avoided by members of the class.

The Report That Wasn't

An aide reported to the LP/VN charge nurse (CN) that Mr. Jones "doesn't look too good to me." The charge nurse immediately called the physician.

Doctor Grimm: What seems to be the trouble?
CN to Aide: What seems to be the trouble?

Aide to CN: I don't know. He just doesn't look right.

CN to Doctor: He just doesn't look right.

Doctor: How long has he looked like this?

CN: I don't know. We just noticed.

Doctor: What's his temperature?

CN: Just a minute. I'll find out.

CN to Aide: Take Mr. Jones' temperature.

Doctor: What's his other vital signs?

CN: I don't know. The aide is going to check them.

Doctor: How much fluid has he had?

CN: Just a minute. (She puts the phone down and goes to check Mr. Jones' IV.)

CN: He's getting an IV now.

Doctor (with sarcasm in his voice): Is he breathing? Never mind, don't send anyone to check. I will be over and check myself. (The doctor slams the phone down. The charge nurse says to the aide, "I don't know why he gets so upset every time I call him. What am I supposed to do?")

Management Tool #14: Reporting Change of Condition to the Physician

Resources Needed:

- A checklist of signs and symptoms from this chapter
- A med-surg textbook

List the assessments you would perform and any other pertinent information you would gather before notifying the physician of a "change of condition" in the following residents:

1. Resident has history of compensated left-sided congestive heart failure.
2. Resident has cancer of the esophagus and uses a Duragesic patch for pain control.

Tricia began to think of the "people problems" she continually experiences in her job as LP/VN charge nurse. Mrs. Kelly was not kidding when she said that figuring out delegation would be the least of her concerns as LP/VN charge nurse. But with each day that passes, handling these problems becomes easier and easier. Mrs. Kelly's basic advice, "Treat people as you would like to be treated," has saved the day on many occasions. That was good advice even for reporting change of condition to the doctor . . . "What information would I need if I were the physician and my resident had a change of condition? As for dealing with doctors, residents, staff, and families, I sure remember situations that arose as clearly as if they happened yesterday."

Common Problems of LP/VN Charge Nurse

Tricia remembered one morning the second week of work after orientation to the charge nurse position. The nursing assistants were all tied up in knots. The babysitter for the three young children of Jenny, one of the nursing assistants, had quit the evening before, and when Jenny got up the next morning for work, her car would not start. All the nursing assistants were talking about Jenny's problems from the time they hung up their coats straight through lunch and beyond. It was only the week before that Jenny found out she was overdrawn at the bank because she wrote checks before her paycheck was deposited by Quality Care Home. It seemed as though "things always happened to Jenny and she was such a nice girl . . . it just was not right." All the nursing assistants were feeling guilty because all this stuff happened to Jenny. Everyone was involved with how to get Jenny out of her current mess. Several of the nursing assistants forgot to do some of their cares, and Jenny needed a lot of assistance to get her assignment completed. At the time, a picture flew through Tricia's mind. It was Mrs. Kelly standing in the front of the class with a stuffed toy monkey on her back.

When Nursing Assistants Bring Problems from Home

As an LP/VN charge nurse, it is important that you do not fall into the "monkey trap," as described by Blanchard, Oncken, and Burrows in *The One Minute Manager Meets the Monkey* (1989). You fall into the trap each time you take on a responsibility (monkey) that belongs to an employee. And as you know, once monkeys are adopted, they take a lot of time in their care and upkeep. LP/VN charge nurses can help nursing assistants become aware of this trap and be a role model for avoiding it.

Realize that you do not own any problems that nursing assistants experience. The nursing assistant owns the problem. Avoid feeling guilty because you cannot solve the problems of team members. Be supportive and express genuine concern and empathy, but realize that you do not have a license to counsel nursing assistants. Team members need to solve their own problems. Follow facility policies when personal problems interfere with work performance. Report the situation to your supervisor. Professional counseling in the community may be necessary.

Management Tool #15: When Nursing Assistants Bring Problems from Home

Resources Needed:

* Reading: "When Nursing Assistants Bring Problems from Home" (just preceding)
* Creative thinking

You are LP/VN charge nurse the morning Jenny comes to work with her problems. Identify a way to handle the situation.

Tricia remembered Wendy, a nursing assistant who had been employed at Quality Care Home for six months when she told Kay, a nursing assistant on her wing, that she did not know how to use the new patient-lifting device. Kay stated she did not

really have time but Wendy coaxed Kay to take the time to get the resident out of bed for her. Tricia had suggested to Kay a way of handling the situation that she had learned in PV class that would help Wendy be more accountable. See Management Tool #15.

Encouraging Personal Responsibility in Nursing Assistants

When nursing assistants can't do something that is in their job description—for example, transferring residents by a lifting device—it is their problem. Staff persons need to avoid assuming it is a staff problem. Be sure to follow the policy of the facility. For safety reasons, encourage nursing assistants to report to the charge nurse when they are having problems with mechanical devices. This gives the charge nurse the opportunity to determine what staff member is skilled and available to assist in the situation. Encourage the nursing assistant to offer suggestions for learning to do the part of their job that they do not know how to do. Praise them for coming up with a plan. Add to the plan if necessary. Write a note to your supervisor explaining the situation objectively and how you proceeded to remedy the situation. Request additional training for the nursing assistant if necessary. Learning who owns problems will help you control a large part of the stress you experience as an LP/VN charge nurse and help improve resident care.

Management Tool #16: Encouraging Nursing Assistants to be Accountable for Learning Skills

Resources Needed:
Reading: "Encouraging Personal Responsibility in Nursing Assistants" (above)

Develop a plan to encourage Wendy to approach the lifting-device situation in a more accountable manner.

Tricia remembered instances in her student days and throughout her career when families had complained about care given to their relatives. This was a troubling area for Tricia, who had high standards and prided herself on the quality of her nursing care. She would take the complaints seriously and investigate each criticism thoroughly. But sometimes nothing could be found out of order. Sometimes she began doubting her ability to self-evaluate. Once again, Mrs. Kelly offered insight into this common problem that Tricia uses down to today.

Dealing with Demanding/ Complaining Families

A common problem in the nursing home is dealing with complaints of family members regarding care of their relatives. A common complaint involves

---

TABLE 14–2: Interventions to Use for the Demanding/Complaining Family

See Bauer B, Hill S. *Mental Health Nursing*, Philadelphia: W. B. Saunders, 2000, for interventions for additional specific behaviors.

1. Develop a sincere, nonpunitive relationship with the family.
2. Encourage the family to ventilate feelings about resident's placement in a nursing home, aging, and behavior.
3. Try to identify the unconscious issue and address it.
4. Determine needs the family is trying to fulfill through their demands, criticism, and complaints.
5. Spend time with family when demands are not being made or complaints are not being made.
6. Establish rapport with the resident's family to provide emotional support during this difficult time.
7. Explain the resident's disease and expected behavior.
8. Suggest joining a support group. These groups offer explanations for diseases, as well as a place to share feelings and frustrations.
9. Encourage family to stay involved with resident and continue care giving and visiting.

---

physical care. Sometimes the family members become verbally aggressive, express concerns in an angry manner, and are very critical of the charge nurse. Others will be nonassertive and sarcastic. Remember the problem-solving process. First in importance is to gather data to determine the real problem. If there is a problem with physical care, identify it and correct it. Sometimes when the problem is identified and solved, the complaints continue. Sometimes when no problem with physical care is identified, the family may continue the attack.

It is necessary to consider the situation the family finds itself in. They are in a position of seeing their loved one progressively aging and deteriorating. This is a time of loss for the family. They may feel guilty about placing a relative in a nursing home or about not being able to continue care giving. They may have grieving issues to contend with. Lashing out may be their attempt at relief. To avoid personal issues, family members may unconsciously project blame onto nursing assistants and

 Management Tool #17: Dealing with the Demanding/Complaining Family

Resources Needed:
Reading: Chapter 13: Leadership Hint #3: Decision-Making Tree for Problem Solving

Mrs. Duffy, age 82, was admitted two weeks ago to Quality Care Home. You are LP/VN charge nurse on her wing on the evening shift. Mrs. Duffy has osteoarthritis, short-term memory loss, and Parkinson's disease. In the past few days, her family has been complaining about her hair care, mouth care, appearance, and missing items in her laundry.

1. Develop a plan with specific interventions to investigate and alleviate these complaints.

Despite modifications in Mrs. Duffy's care plan, the complaints continue.

2. Plan specific interventions to handle the continuing specific complaints.

other members of the nursing staff. It is like looking at skeletons in other people's closets so you do
not have to look at those in your own closets. This
behavior can make a family feel better. It is important for staff to understand these issues and avoid
hurt feelings. Avoid personalizing the situation.
Suggested interventions to deal with the demanding
or complaining family are included in Table 14–2.
When family complaints surface, investigate them,
but remember to keep broad shoulders.

*Tricia was very tired and began to put her books
and scrapbook away. It had been very pleasant
reminiscing about her school days and early years
as an LP/VN. It was good to realize how far she
had come in her career. Later, as Tricia was relax-*
*ing in a warm tub, a big smile came over her face.
Tomorrow would be a big day in her life. Mrs.
Kelly had strongly recommended membership in
professional organizations. Tricia had been a member of the National Federation of Licensed Practical Nurses at the national, state and local level
since graduation. Over the years she had assumed
various committee assignments and officer positions
at the local level of the organization. But tomorrow
she would be installed as the first president of the
organization at the state level from her local district! Tricia was proud to be of service to her career and looked forward to promoting and having a
say in the direction practical/vocational nursing
would take in the twenty-first century.*

Summary

- [ ] State nurse practice acts specify requirements needed by practical/vocational nurses in order to assume first-line manager positions. A common first-line manager position is charge nurse in long-term care units/nursing homes.
- [ ] Oncoming shift report gives the charge nurse the opportunity to assess resident needs and to assign unlicensed personnel duties for resident care from *their* job description. The charge nurse shares responsibility with unlicensed personnel for the quality of care that is given.
- [ ] Practical/vocational charge nurses routinely assign care to unlicensed personnel. Charge nurses, as part of their jobs, evaluate the thoroughness and safety of all tasks they assign.
- [ ] *If allowed in your state's nurse practice act,* the practical/vocational nurse as charge nurse may elect to delegate duties from the *practical/vocational nurse's* job description to unlicensed personnel. Delegation gives the charge nurse time to focus on tasks that cannot be delegated.
- [ ] Tasks can be delegated, but the responsibility that goes with those tasks remains with the registered nurse under whom the charge nurse functions under general supervision. 'The practical/vocational charge nurse shares accountability in these situations.
- [ ] The charge nurse position is a complex role for practical/vocational nurses. With addi-tional education and experience, many practical/vocational nurses are doing an excellent job in this expanded role position.
- [ ] Common charge nurse problems include nursing assistants who bring problems from home to work, the need for nursing assistants to be accountable for learning new job skills, and dealing with demanding/complaining family members.
- [ ] *It is your license that is at stake in the matter of assuming the charge nurse position. Know your state laws regulating nursing.*

Review Questions

1. Select the best response for an LP/VN with 2 months' experience in a nursing home who is approached to perform nursing duties within the expanded role of the practical/vocational nurse in her state but has not had a leadership component in her educational program.
   A. "I am unable by law to do this."
   B. "I will not function in the expanded role because I did not study this in my one-year program."
   C. "I need some time to contact my Board of Nursing and clarify state statutes in this matter."
   D. "I am willing to assume this role if you will train me for the duties I was not taught to carry out and document them in my file."

2. Select the statement that indicates the correct meaning of delegation.
   A. The nursing assistant cannot refuse a delegated task.
   B. LP/VNs delegate tasks to nursing assistants that are in the job description of the person to whom they are delegating.
   C. LP/VNs delegate specific job duties that are in their job description to unlicensed personnel.
   D. LP/VNs delegate their practical/vocational nursing role to unlicensed personnel who have proved they are capable of assuming the role.

3. Select the statement that applies to LP/VNs working in a state that allows LP/VNs to function in their expanded role but does not allow delegation of nursing tasks to unlicensed personnel.
   A. The LP/VN may not assume the charge nurse role.
   B. The LP/VN will not be able to practice in a management role.
   C. The LP/VN may assign tasks to unlicensed personnel that are in their job description.
   D. If a state does not allow practical/vocational nurses to delegate tasks to unlicensed personnel, then they may not assign any task to nursing assistants.

4. Select the defense mechanism that may be present in a family member who continually finds fault and criticizes the care given to a relative by nursing assistants.
   A. Projection
   B. Rationalization
   C. Introjection
   D. Conversion

5. When LP/VNs are accountable it means that they are functioning
   A. Applicably
   B. Responsibly
   C. Appropriately
   D. Befittingly

References

Blanchard K, Oncken W, Burrows H. *The One Minute Manager Meets the Monkey.* New York: William Morrow, 1989.

Entry Level Competencies of Graduates of Educational Programs in Practical Nursing. New York: National League for Nursing, 1999.

Rachels M, President of the National Council of State Boards of Nursing, Inc. Letter. August 24, 1994.

Wywialowski E. *Managing Client Care.* St. Louis: C. V. Mosby, 1997.

Yocum C. *1997 Job Analysis of Newly Licensed Practical/Vocational Nurses.* Chicago: National Council of State Boards of Nursing, Inc., 1997.

Bibliography

Boucher M. Delegation alert. Am J Nurs 98(2):26, 28–32, 1998.

Cummings J, Nugent L. Integrating management concepts into licensed practical nurse and associate degree in nursing student clinical experiences. Nurse Educator 22(4):41–43, 1997.

Eyles M. *Mosby's Review for Long-Term Care Certification for Practical and Vocational Nurses.* St. Louis: C. V. Mosby, 1996. Copyright by National Council of State Board of Nursing, Inc.

Harris T. Educating tomorrow's nurses. *Practical Nursing Today* 2(2):18–20, 1999.

Howlett H. *The Howlett theory of management for nursing instructors* (unpublished paper). November 1989.

Marrelli T. *The Nurse Manager's Survival Guide: Practical Answers to Everyday Problems.* St. Louis: Mosby–Year Book, 1997.

McGuffin J. *The Nurse's Guide to Successful Management.* St. Louis: C. V. Mosby, 1999.

Neumann Update on legal matters in the State of Wisconsin. Fall Conference of Wisconsin Association of Licensed Practical Nurses. Wisconsin Dells, WI, Nov. 3, 1995.

Porter-O'Grady T. *The Nurse Manager's Problem Solver.* St. Louis: Mosby–Year Book, 1994.

Pugh J, Woodward-Smith R. *Nurse Manager: A Practical Guide to Better Employee Relations,* 2nd ed. Philadelphia: W. B. Saunders, 1997.

Sheehan J. Directing UAPs—safely. RN 61(6):53, 55, 1998.

Spitzer-Lehmann J. *Nursing Management Desk Reference: Concepts, Skills and Strategies.* Philadelphia: W. B. Saunders, 1994.

Ventura M. Staffing issues. RN 62(2):26–27, 1999.

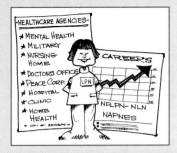

PART **FIVE**

Where You Are Going

Chapter **15**

Health Care Settings

Outline

Public Versus Private Health Care
  Agencies
    Public Health Care Agencies

Private Health Care Agencies
Examples of Public Health Care
  Agencies

Examples of Voluntary Health
  Care Agencies
Examples of Private Health Care
  Agencies

Key Terms

acute care
assisted care
domiciliary care
free-standing
intermediate care

long-term residential care
official (government) health care
  agencies
primary care

private health care agencies
sheltered housing
skilled care
voluntary health care agencies

Objectives

Upon completing this chapter you will
be able to:
1. Compare public and private health
   care agencies according to the following criteria:
   a. Source of funding
   b. Services provided

c. Examples of agencies in your
   geographic area
d. Possible places of employment
   for practical/vocational nurses
2. Discuss the difference between
   community nursing services, public health, and home health service.

3. Identify four levels of long-term
   care.
4. Name the two purposes of rehabilitation regardless of the setting.

The purpose of this chapter is to provide information about health care agencies. Financing issues
and trends are discussed in Chapter 16. The various
health care settings described could also be a potential source of employment for practical/vocational
nurses in health care, especially in the community.

Public Versus Private Health Care Agencies

For ease of understanding, the various health care services in the United States can be grouped into two general categories: (1) services delivered by the *public* sector, and (2) those delivered by the *private* sector.

Public Health Care Agencies

There are two types of public health care agencies—official and voluntary. Official health care agencies are government agencies that are supported by tax money and are accountable to the taxpayers and the government. The primary emphasis of government (official) agencies is the delivery of programs of disease prevention and wellness promotion, but direct health care services are sometimes provided.

Voluntary health care agencies are supported by voluntary contributions and sometimes by a fee for service. Although they are tuned in to public opinion, voluntary agencies are accountable to their supporters, and their activities are determined by supporter interest, not legal mandate. The primary emphasis of these agencies is research and education. They may also offer direct health services to the client. Some official and voluntary health care agencies operate at the local, state, federal, and international levels.

Private Health Care Agencies

You may be most familiar with private health care agencies. Entrance to the health care delivery system in the United States is generally gained through private health care agencies. Although some voluntary or nonprofit agencies are found in the private sector, private health care agencies are generally proprietary, or for profit. They charge a fee for their services. Their primary emphasis has been on curing disease and illness, but a change in emphasis to include disease prevention and wellness promotion has occurred. Table 15–1 outlines the major differences between public and private health care agencies. As you read about public and private health care agencies, think of them as potential sources of employment for the practical nurse.

TABLE 15–1: A Comparison of Health Care Agencies in the Public and Private Sectors			
	Public		Private
	Official (Government)	*Nonofficial (Voluntary)*	
Support	Tax money	Voluntary contributions and fees for service	Fees for service
Primary service	Programs of disease prevention and wellness promotion	Research and education	Curing disease and illness
Additional services	Sometimes direct service of health care	Offer direct health services	Disease prevention and wellness promotion
Accountability	Taxpayers and government	Supporters, boards, etc.	Owners
How programs determined	Mandated and nonmandated	Supporter interest	Defined goals of the organization

Examples of Public Health Care Agencies

Official Government Agencies

LOCAL. The official health agency at the local level is the city or county health department. This agency is funded by local tax money as well as by subsidies from the state and federal levels of government. The local health department carries out state laws concerning community health. It also carries out nonmandated programs such as health promotion programs.

STATE. Each state has a state health department. This official health agency is funded by state tax money and sometimes receives money from the federal government.

FEDERAL (NATIONAL). The official health agency at the federal level in the United States is the Department of Health and Human Services (DHHS). It is funded by federal taxes and is headed by a person appointed by the President of the United States. This person advises the President in health matters. The division of the Department of Health and Human Services that is concerned primarily with health is the U.S. Public Health Service (USPHS). The six agencies that make up the USPHS are

- Food and Drug Administration (FDA)
- Centers for Disease Control and Prevention (CDC)
- National Institutes of Health (NIH)
- Health Services Administration (HSA)
- Health Resources Administration (HRA)
- Alcohol, Drug Abuse, and Mental Health Administration

INTERNATIONAL. Health activities take place at the international level through the World Health Organization (WHO), an agency of the United Nations. The WHO is located in Geneva, Switzerland. The major objective of the WHO is the highest possible level of health for people all over the world. This organization defines health as a state of complete physical, mental, and social well-being and not merely as the absence of disease or infirmity. The WHO is funded through fees paid by member nations of the United Nations.

Examples of Voluntary Health Care Agencies

Voluntary or nonofficial health care agencies are so named because they are not for profit. The health services they provide are complementary to official health agencies and often meet the needs of persons with specific diseases (for example, heart disease) and certain segments of the population (for example, the handicapped). Although paid personnel work in voluntary health agencies, volunteers form a major part of their support system. Voluntary organizations are sites of volunteer service for practical/vocational nurses. A few examples of voluntary health agencies follow. Refer to your local telephone directory for additional names and numbers of voluntary health care agencies.

Community Hospitals

These nonprofit hospitals are operated by community associations or religious organizations. They provide short-term inpatient care for people with acute illnesses and injuries.

Visiting Nurse Association (VNA)

This public voluntary agency provides home nursing care for those with acute and chronic diseases. Staff of this agency visit mothers with newborn infants. Visiting nurses are engaged in health teaching. They frequently involve the family in the care of its own members. Visiting nurses assist with referrals for clients to other community services. Nurses with a bachelor of science in nursing are employed in public health agencies.

American Cancer Society (ACS)

This voluntary agency is a national organization with regional and local units. It is involved in extensive cancer research and education of the public about cancer. ACS is a source of up-to-date information for health professionals, family, and clients. A "one-stop shopping" phone line or web site is available 24 hours a day for any information.

Toll-free phone: 1-800-ACS-2345
Web site: www.cancer.org

A phone call will provide a seamless transfer to a local office if needed (Carlson, 2000).

American Lung Association (ALA)

This voluntary agency works for healthy lungs, healthy people, and healthy air. This includes advocating for increased adult influenza/pneumococcus immunization rates, easing costs of prescriptions for persons with debilitating lung disease, asthma management, smoking prevention, and clean outdoor and indoor air choices. The ALA is involved in professional education and research and provides programs, events, and educational resources for both professionals and the public. The ALA strengthens its reach through alliances with organizations that share similar goals. For information, call 1-800-LUNG-USA or visit the web site at www.lungusa.org (McKone, 2000).

American Heart Association (AHA)

The AHA is involved in research and education about heart disease and stroke. Their web site provides up-to-date information on warning signs, risk factors, heart and stroke guidelines, family health, research, and more. Contact: AHA at 1-800-242-8721 or www.amheart.org and American Stroke Association at 1-800-553-6321 or www.strokeassociation.org (Levy, 2000).

Alcoholics Anonymous (AA)

If assistance is desired, this voluntary agency provides rehabilitation help for alcoholics and their families. Look in your local phone book for information on available programs.

ALS Society of America

This voluntary organization gathers information about clients with amyotrophic lateral sclerosis (Lou Gehrig's disease) for research purposes. It provides information about this rare disease to lay persons and health care workers. This agency also gives client care tips to nursing personnel. For information, contact the National Office of ALS at 1-800-782-4747.

Easter Seals National Headquarters

This voluntary organization conducts research and provides rehabilitative services for disabled children and adults. Treatment services are individualized. Contact: 1-800-221-6827 or www.easterseals.org.

National Multiple Sclerosis Society

This voluntary organization conducts ongoing research with the aim of finding a cure for multiple sclerosis. It also provides education about this disease to clients, nursing students, and health care workers.

LaLeche League

This voluntary organization provides information and support for breastfeeding mothers. The League provides breast milk for infants who must have this form of nourishment but lack a source. For information, call 1-800-LaLeche.

United Ostomy Association (UOA)

This voluntary organization provides education, information, and advocacy for clients who are undergoing intestinal or urinary diversion procedures. For information, call 1-800-826-0826.

American Diabetes Association (ADA)

This voluntary agency provides information on Type I and Type II diabetes, nutritional information, referrals to doctors, and educational programs. For information, call 1-800-342-2383. Web site: www.diabetes.org.

Examples of Private Health Care Agencies

Private health care agencies also complement and supplement government agencies. Compared with public health services, the greatest changes in health care services have been noted in this area.

Family Practice Physicians

Primary care is a term used to describe the point at which an individual enters the health care system. Family practice physicians are a source of primary care. These physicians provide diagnosis and treatment. The client is billed a fee for the services. If further diagnostic evaluation is needed, the client is referred to a specialist. Medical doctors function within the medical practice acts of their respective states.

Private Practice Nurses

Specializing in primary health care, advanced practice nurses (see Chapter 2) provide consulting and counseling services to groups of individuals. These nurses practice in all areas of health care. Private practice nurses fill an especially acute need in rural areas where physician services are sometimes difficult to obtain. These nurses function within the nurse practice acts of their respective states.

Proprietary Hospitals

For-profit hospitals are operated for the financial benefit (profit) of the owner of the hospital. The owner may be an individual, a partnership, or a corporation. By using good management techniques, the hospital can be run efficiently, and a profit can be realized. When clients are admitted to the hospital today, they are more acutely ill and require more skilled nursing care. This setting for health care is called **acute care.**

Ambulatory Services

The continual rise in cost of inpatient care has resulted in the rapid development of a variety of ambulatory services. As a consequence, the number of inpatient days and the length of stay in acute care facilities have decreased. Ambulatory services offer less expensive care because admission to an acute care facility is avoided.

These settings are generally used by persons who live at home, do their own care, or have care provided by family members. They come to ambulatory settings for assessment, advice, monitoring, teaching, treatment, evaluation, and care coordination. The major settings in the *private sector* are located in university hospital outpatient departments, community hospital outpatient departments, physician group practices, health maintenance organizations (HMOs), physicians' offices, free-standing ambulatory centers, and nursing care centers. *Public sector settings* include community health clinics, Indian Health Service, and community and migrant worker health centers. Examples of ambulatory services follow.

OUTPATIENT CLINICS. Outpatient clinics provide follow-up care to clients after hospitalization, and these clinics manage disease on an ambulatory basis for those who do not need to be hospitalized. Outpatient clinics may be part of health care facilities or **free-standing.** These clinics function by appointment only. They include specialty areas such as diabetes, neurology, allergy, and oncology. The number of specialized clinics depends on the population of the area. A full-time staff is employed.

AMBULATORY CARE FACILITIES (URGENT CARE CENTERS). Services are available in ambulatory care facilities for walk-in clients who do not have an appointment. These clinics make available primary health care as an alternative to care by a family physician or care offered in the more expensive emergency room. Ambulatory care clinics are used by persons who do not have a family physician. These clinics are also used by clients who desire quick service outside of regular office hours. The names given to ambulatory care services reflect the type of care they provide: convenience clinics, express care, quick care, and so on.

AMBULATORY SURGERY CENTERS (OUTPATIENT SURGERY). One-day surgical care centers perform surgery at a scheduled date and time. Clients are discharged when they have recovered from anesthesia and are considered to be in stable condition. This eliminates the need and the monetary charge for being hospitalized overnight. These services are also known as outpatient surgery within an established hospital. Free-standing outpatient surgery centers provide outpatient surgery as their only service. Approximately 80% of surgical procedures are performed in this type of setting.

Free Clinics

Some communities have established free clinics as an alternative means of providing primary health care. These clinics are used by persons who cannot afford traditional health services or are reluctant to use more traditional services. The fee is minimal. The environment is as free of red tape as possible.

Rehabilitation Services

After a client has been stabilized following an acute illness or injury, a rehabilitation phase lasting from days to years may follow. Rehabilitation may take place in rehabilitation centers, long-term care facilities, outpatient facilities, group residential homes, or the client's home base. The focus, regardless of the setting, is the return of function and prevention of

further disability. Nurses play an important role in the rehabilitation team.

Long-Term Care Facilities

Currently, **long-term residential care** consists of (1) domiciliary care, (2) sheltered housing, (3) intermediate care, (4) skilled care, and (5) assisted care. A single facility may offer more than one level of care, depending on state approval.

Domiciliary Care. The resident is provided with room, board, and supervision. Twenty-four-hour care is not available, and the residents come and go as they choose to.

Sheltered Housing. In addition to what is provided in domiciliary care, there is some modification in care for frail elderly people, such as community dining facilities. Twenty-four-hour care is not provided.

Intermediate Care. Custodial care, such as is usually associated with nursing homes, is provided. Residents usually need assistance with two or three activities of daily living (ADLs). Twenty-four-hour-a-day personnel are on duty. An RN serves as Director of Nursing. An LP/VN is required to be on duty at least 8 hours a day.

Skilled Care. Skilled professionals are on duty 24 hours a day. Care is supervised by a physician. A registered nurse, physical therapist, and speech therapist are required on the staff.

Assisted Care. Connected to skilled nursing facilities, these apartments are utilized by older adults who want to remain as independent as possible but cannot manage all of their ADLs. The apartments are handicap accessible and planned to accommodate the changing needs as residents age. Individual support services are available 24 hours a day, as needed. These services include bathing, dressing, daily activities, and health maintenance. The facilities are family oriented, have activities, and assist the client with travel to outside appointments. The fee for one- or two-bedroom apartments includes utilities, weekly house cleaning, linen changes, and so on. An additional fee is charged for meals. The client can be moved into the skilled nursing facility if that level of care becomes necessary.

All long-term care focuses on promotion of independence, maintenance of function, and autonomy.

Community Health Nursing Services

Nurses have always been at the forefront of community health nursing activity. The major focus of community health nursing is to (1) improve the health status of communities or groups of people through public education, (2) screen for early detection of disease, and (3) provide services for people who need care outside the acute care setting. Community health nurses work with many different people and groups on prevention and modification of health issues. Among the many possible roles are advocate, caregiver, case finder, health planner, occupational health nurse, school nurse, teacher, and so on (Linton et al., 2000, p. 15). Community health nursing services may exist as a part of an outpatient clinic service, a service attached to an HMO, or a free-standing private service.

Home Health Agencies

Home health agencies differ from community nursing services and public health by providing more direct care to clients. They differ from hospital and nursing home care by increased focus on the family and the client's environment. An important role is to teach the client and family self-care. Home health agencies exist as a part of hospital extension services, as HMO clinic services, and as private agencies. "The primary skilled services in home health care are (1) nursing, (2) physical therapy, and (3) speech therapy. Secondary services include occupational therapy (which may be primary under certain conditions), social work services, and home health aide services" (Linton et al., 2000, p. 17).

Skilled nursing includes skilled observation and assessment, teaching, and performing skilled procedures. Specialty home care includes intravenous therapy and ventilator therapy.

Adult Day Care Centers

Hospital-based and free-standing adult day care centers provide services for individuals who need supervision because of physical or safety needs, yet are not candidates for nursing home placement. Some clients and families prefer adult day care instead of nursing home placement.

Wellness Centers

An emphasis on promoting wellness continues to result in a multitude of services being offered in this area of health care. Not only have hospitals developed programs to detect disease in early stages, they also have developed programs to promote wellness. These programs include nutritional counseling, exercise programs, stress reduction, and weight control. The private sector continues to be active in the wellness area. People have developed an interest in exercise and fitness clubs, weight-reduction programs such as Weight Watchers, smoking cessation classes, stress control, and parenting classes.

 Learning Exercise: Identify Private Health Care Agencies

Identify specific private health care agencies in your community. These agencies are a growing source of employment for practical/vocational nurses.

Summary

☐ Health care services are delivered in the public and private sectors. Public health care agencies are classified as official and voluntary. Official public health care agencies are supported by taxes. Voluntary health care agencies are supported by contributions. Private health care agencies are generally proprietary or for profit. In addition to providing direct care, both public and private health care agencies are interested in preventing disease and promoting wellness.

☐ Community health, public health, and home health share many responsibilities. A major difference in home health involvement is providing direct client care.

☐ Rehabilitation services take place in a variety of settings, depending on the level of rehabilitation required.

☐ With changes in the health care system, the responsibilities of care agencies continue to be modified.

Review Questions

1. How does an official public health care agency differ from a voluntary health care agency?
   A. Entry into the health care system is usually through a public health care agency.
   B. The primary emphasis of public health care agencies is on curing disease and illness.
   C. The primary emphasis of public health care agencies is disease prevention and wellness promotion.
   D. The voluntary health care agencies are tax supported and responsible to taxpayers and the government.

2. Which of the following is an international official health agency funded by the United Nations?
   A. WHO
   B. CDC
   C. NIH
   D. FDA

3. What is the major purpose of most national voluntary health agencies?
   A. Provide specialized home care
   B. Be politically active
   C. Research and education
   D. Provide mandated programs

4. What is the major difference between the levels of residential care?
   A. Domiciliary care provides 24-hour per day supervision, with permission to leave as desired.
   B. Sheltered care provides custodial care and assistance with ADLs.
   C. Intermediate care provides room and board with supervision and no 24-hour care.
   D. Skilled care provides 24-hour per day professional staff supervised by a physician.

5. Which service do persons need if they live in a high-rise building and want their blood pressure measured monthly?
   A. Public health
   B. Community health
   C. Home health
   D. Rehabilitation services

References

Carlson F. *American Cancer Society: Midwest Division.* Duluth, Minnesota. January, 2000.

Levy L. *American Heart Association; Northland Affiliate.* Duluth, MN, January, 2000.

Linton AD, Matteson MA, Maebius NK. Patient care settings. In *Introductory Nursing Care of Adults,* 2nd ed. Philadelphia: W. B. Saunders, 2000, Chapter 2.

McClosky JC, Grace HK. Health Care Systems. In *Current Issues in Nursing,* 5th ed. St. Louis: C. V. Mosby, 1997.

McKone P. *Healthy Lungs, Healthy People, Healthy Air.* Duluth, MN: American Lung Association of Minnesota, January, 2000.

Bibliography

Alter, J. Washington washes its hands. Newsweek 128(7): 42–44, 1996.

Baer E. Money managers are unraveling the tapestry of nursing. Am J Nurs 94(1):38–40, 1994.

Davidhizer R. Health care reform: What every practical nurse should know. J Pract Nurs 45:49, 52–55, 1995.

Hastings K. Health care reform: We need it but do we have the national will to shape our future? Nurse Practitioner 20(1):52–54, 1995.

Ignatavicius DD, Workman ML, Mishler MA. *Medical-Surgical Nursing Across the Health Care Continuum,* 3rd ed. Philadelphia: W. B. Saunders, 1999.

Leahy JM, Kizilay PE. *Foundations of Nursing Practice.* Philadelphia: W. B. Saunders, 1998.

Lindeman CA, McAthie M. *Fundamentals of Contemporary Nursing Practice.* Philadelphia: W. B. Saunders, 1997.

Manion J. Understanding the seven stages of change. Am J Nurs 95(4):41–43, 1995.

Chapter 16

Health Care System Financing and Trends

Outline

Financing of Health Care Costs
  Fee-for-Service
  Capitation
How Your Clients Pay for Health Care
  Services
  Personal Payment (Private Pay)
  Private Group and Individual
    (Nongovernment) Health In-
    surance
  Government-Sponsored Health
    Insurance Plans

Issues and Trends in Health Care Fi-
  nancing
  Need for Cost Containment
  Private Health Insurance
  Government Health Insurance
  The Uninsured
  Effect of Lack of Health Insur-
    ance Coverage

Incremental Changes in Health Care
Restructuring of the Health Care Sys-
  tem
  Changes in Health Care Facilities
  Methods of Delivering Health
    Care
  Quality Improvement
Dealing with Change

Key Terms

alliances
ambulatory service (outpatient)
capitation
catastrophic illness
charting by exception
continuous quality improvement (CQI)
copayments
cost containment
critical pathways
cross-trained
decentralized
deductibles

diagnosis-related group (DRG)
downsizing (rightsizing)
fee-for-service
group health insurance
health maintenance organization
incremental method
Joint Commission on Accreditation of
  Healthcare Organizations (JCAHO)
managed care
Medicaid
Medicare
paradigm shift

patient-focused care
political activism
preferred provider organizations
  (PPOs)
private pay
restructuring
"seamless" systems
service, quality, and cost control
third-party coverage
total quality management (TQM)
universal coverage
unlicensed assistive personnel

Objectives

Upon completing this chapter you will
be able to:
1. Describe two general methods of
   financing health care costs:
   a. Fee-for-service
   b. Capitation
2. Explain method of payment options for clients of health care:
   a. Personal payment (private pay)
   b. Nongovernmental health insurance
      plans

c. Government-sponsored health
   insurance plans
3. Discuss issues and trends affecting financing of health care:
   a. Need for cost containment
   b. Private health insurance limita-
      tions
   c. Medicare and Medicaid regu-
      lations
   d. The uninsured
4. Discuss the effect of restructuring

of the health care system on health
care.
5. Explain how the practical/voca-
   tional nurse participates in quality
   improvement.
6. Identify your reaction to change
   involving your nursing career and
   personal life.
7. Develop a personal plan to help
   you adapt to change in your nursing career and personal life.

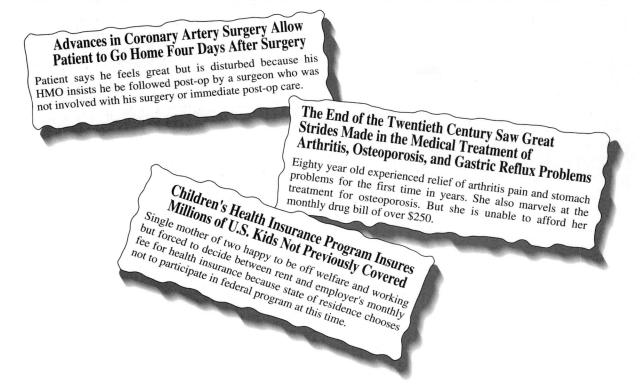

Advances in Coronary Artery Surgery Allow
Patient to Go Home Four Days After Surgery

Patient says he feels great but is disturbed because his
HMO insists he be followed post-op by a surgeon who was
not involved with his surgery or immediate post-op care.

The End of the Twentieth Century Saw Great
Strides Made in the Medical Treatment of
Arthritis, Osteoporosis, and Gastric Reflux Problems

Eighty year old experienced relief of arthritis pain and stomach
problems for the first time in years. She also marvels at the
treatment for osteoporosis. But she is unable to afford her
monthly drug bill of over $250.

Children's Health Insurance Program Insures
Millions of U.S. Kids Not Previously Covered

Single mother of two happy to be off welfare and working
but forced to decide between rent and employer's monthly
fee for health insurance because state of residence chooses
not to participate in federal program at this time.

Over 44 million people in the United States do not have a health insurance plan. Many are unable to afford individual health insurance premiums. Some individuals covered by some sort of health insurance plan find themselves unable to have access to all technology available, are unable to afford deductibles, and/or complain of a decreasing quality in health care. Canadian citizens who have National Health Insurance report increased waiting time in emergency departments, longer waiting time for elective surgery, decreased availability of nurses in hospitals, increased waiting time for diagnostic tests, decreased access to specialists, and a decrease in federal funds for health care. It is clear that even when people have access to health care through some type of health insurance plan, problems of **quality, service, and cost** arise.

The purpose of this chapter is twofold. One is to provide information about how your clients pay for their health care services. The second is to identify and discuss current issues and trends that affect the health care system. The basic information about agencies that deliver health care services (Chapter 15) and the contents of this chapter will help you have a better understanding of the health care system that employs you.

Financing of Health Care Costs

There are two major ways of financing health care service: fee-for-service and capitation. A knowledge of health care financing can encourage the need for practical/vocational nurses to avoid waste in the workplace. It also can lead to an appreciation of the value of health insurance as a fringe benefit of employment for a practical/vocational nurse.

Fee-for-Service

The traditional method of paying health care bills is the system called **fee-for-service.** In this method, physicians are paid a fee by the client for each service they provide. Under the fee-for-service system, if the attending physician has an agreement with the health insurance company of the client, he or she is directly reimbursed for most diagnostic tests and treatments for illness that were ordered. If the physician does not have an agreement with the issuer of health insurance, the client is reimbursed by the insurance company and then pays the physician. The tests and treatments that could keep clients healthy or could identify illnesses in the early stages when they are less expensive to treat are in some instances not reimbursed by insurance companies under the fee-for-service system. Over the years, insurance premiums soared under this type of fee system. To improve their margins of profit, insurance companies began charging **deductibles** (the amount the subscriber must pay before health insurance will begin to pay the bills) and **copayments** (the percentage of the bill paid by the subscriber).

Capitation

Capitation is an alternative to the traditional fee-for-service method of payment. Capitation involves a set monthly fee charged by the provider of health care services for each member of the insurance group for a specific set of services. At the end of the year, if any money is left over, the health care provider keeps it as a profit. Suddenly, if a provider of health care services can keep a member of the insurance group healthy, the provider will make a profit! Study Table 16–1 for a comparison of the fee-for-service and capitation methods of payment for health care services.

TABLE 16–1: Comparison of Methods of Payment for Health Care Services

	Fee-For-Service	Capitation
Services covered	Each service claimed by the physician (e.g., diagnostic tests, treatments)	Services in group contract
Are preventive tests or treatments covered?	Depends on the plan	Yes. Wellness practices covered
Cost	Set fee per member of group	Set fee per member of group
Advantages	All tests and treatments for illness covered	Wellness encouraged. No deductibles and copayments
Disadvantages	Emphasis on illness. Deductibles and copayments keep patient from reporting illness in early stages	To realize a profit, needed tests may not be ordered

How Your Clients Pay for Health Care Services

Personal Payment (Private Pay)

Payment directly by the client (**private pay**) was the primary method of payment of health care costs prior to the 1940s. Some clients use this method of payment today, but the cost of health care services discourages this method by most of the 44 million people in the United States who do not have health care insurance. Some negotiate with a health care provider for a lesser fee by paying the fee in cash.

Private Group and Individual (Nongovernment) Health Insurance

Group health insurance is a method of pooling individual contributions for a common group goal—protection from financial disaster due to health care bills. When insured, an individual is said to have **third-party coverage,** that is, a fiscal middleman. This fiscal middleman pays the individual's health care bills. Three examples of private group health insurance are:

- Blue Cross and Blue Shield: Blue Cross covers hospital inpatient costs and Blue Shield covers inpatient physician costs. A major medical plan is available to include the cost of outpatient services. Individuals can purchase coverage from Blue Cross and Blue Shield, but the cost for individuals is higher than for group plans. This is an example of fee-for-service coverage.
- Health policies offered through commercial or independent insurance companies: Many major insurance companies offer health insurance to individuals and groups.
- A health plan issued through a health maintenance organization (HMO). Regardless of how many services the HMO provides, it is paid an annual fee to maintain the health of each

of its members (capitation). The healthier clients are kept, the fewer treatments the HMO needs to deliver and the larger the profit margin for the HMO. For a fee, clients seek medical care at the first sign of symptoms. This is the time when health care is least expensive to deliver.

Government-Sponsored Health Insurance Plans

Medicare

Some older persons generally find themselves ineligible for group insurance plans because they are not employed. Many are unable to afford individual private plans. This inability to get insurance occurs at the very time when individuals are likely to encounter more medical costs because of chronic disease. In 1965, **Medicare** was added to the Social Security Act. This federally sponsored and supervised health insurance plan finances health care for all persons over age 65 years (or their spouses), who have at least a 10-year record in Medicare-covered employment and are a citizen or permanent resident of the United States.

Basic Components of Medicare

PART A provides inpatient hospital benefits. Part A is available without cost to those who meet eligibility requirements. Part A includes a deductible and coinsurance. The deductible for 1999 was $768.

1. Part A also provides coverage to persons under age 65 years who are permanently and totally disabled.
2. Part A also provides coverage to victims of end-stage renal disease.
3. Part A coverage includes post-hospitalization skilled nursing facility care for rehabilitation services. A coinsurance charge is applied.
4. Under certain conditions, home health care services are provided with coinsurance charges for medical equipment.

5. Part A helps pay for hospice care for terminally ill beneficiaries who select this benefit.
6. Part A does not pay for telephones or televisions provided by hospitals or skilled nursing facilities or private rooms.
7. Part A does not pay for nursing home custodial services.

PART B is similar to a major medical plan. Part B required a $100 deductible in 1999. Part B pays 80% of most covered charges. The 1999 monthly premium for Part B was $45.50. The premium is deducted from the monthly social security check.

1. Examples of services Part B helps pay for are doctor's services, outpatient hospital services (including emergency room visits), ambulance transportation, diagnostic tests, laboratory services, and mammography and Pap smear screenings.
2. Part B does not pay for most prescription drugs, routine physicals, services not related to treatment of illness or injury, dental care, dentures, cosmetic surgery, routine foot care, hearing aids, eye examinations, or glasses.

Because of the items Medicare does not cover, persons over age 65 years who can afford to also carry private supplemental coverage in addition to Medicare to cover deductibles, coinsurance, and limited-coverage situations that exist in the federal program. A Medigap plan is an example of a health insurance plan that fills in for the original Medicare plan coverage for health care. Medigap plans are available in all states. Each plan has a different set of benefits. Medigap plans exist in the fee-for-service and capitation forms of financing health care costs. As a government information site on the Internet states, shopping for health insurance is a complicated matter!

Diagnosis-Related Groups (DRGs)

Payment for Medicare is a major item in the federal budget. Because the federal deficit (caused by less money coming in than is going out to run all government programs) was consistently growing larger,

the federal government was the first group to try to stop the skyrocketing cost of health care. On October 1, 1983, the Health Care Financing Administration adopted a system of paying hospitals a set fee for Medicare services by telling them in advance how much the hospitals would be reimbursed. Because the government announces to a hospital in advance what it will pay for health care costs, this system is called the *prospective payment system.* Prior to 1983, hospitals submitted a bill to the government for the total charges they incurred for Medicare clients and were reimbursed for this amount. This was called a *retrospective payment system.*

Under the **diagnosis-related group (DRG)** system, hospitals have an incentive to treat clients and discharge them as quickly as possible. Hospitals receive a flat fee for each client regardless of the client's length of stay. If the hospital keeps the client longer than the government's fee will cover, and the client cannot be reclassified in the DRG system, the hospital has to make up the difference in costs. If the acute care facility can treat the Medicare client for less than the guaranteed reimbursement, the facility can keep the difference as profit.

Because Medicare clients, as all clients, are discharged sooner from hospitals than they were in the past (because of the DRG system of reimbursement), extended care units are frequently used to continue convalescence.

Medicaid (Medical Assistance)

Poor people generally find themselves ineligible for private health insurance coverage because they are unable to afford the cost of premiums. Another provision that was added to the Social Security Act in 1965 was the **Medicaid** program. This program expanded the financial assistance provided by the federal government to states and counties to pay for medical services for the eligible poor. The Medicaid system developed out of the welfare system that serviced low-income families. Medicaid also is a major item in the federal budget. Three more recent acts of Congress have reformed the Medicaid system:

1. In August, 1996, *The Personal Responsibility and Work Opportunity Reconciliation Act* reformed the nation's welfare laws. This act created a mechanism for temporary assistance for families in need. One of the primary goals of current federal welfare policies is to move people from welfare to work.
2. *The Balanced Budget Act of 1997* authorized welfare-to-work grants to states to create additional job opportunities for the hardest-to-employ of the recipients of the 1996 act. The goal is for successful progression of recipients into long-term unsubsidized employment. Once employed, employees are eligible for employer health insurance benefits if the employer offers these benefits.
3. Also in 1997, Congress passed the *Children's Health Insurance Program (CHIP)*. This act provides health insurance coverage to uninsured children up to 200% of the federal poverty level. If they choose to participate, states are provided grants to provide this coverage by expanding Medicaid or by expanding or creating a children's health program.

Issues and Trends in Health Care Financing

One of the competency requirements in The National League for Nursing's *Entry Level Competencies of Graduates of Educational Programs in Practical Nursing* (1999) is "**Political activism**— the practical nurse, through political, economic, and societal activities, can affect nursing and health." Practical/vocational nurses can help shape health policy by educating their clients and state and federal legislators about issues in health care. To do this, the practical/vocational nurse needs to understand the many trends and issues affecting health care.

Need for Cost Containment

Today, the driving force in all public and private health care agencies continues to be **cost contain-**

ment (the need to hold costs to within fixed limits) while remaining competitive in the health care marketplace. In 1960, health care was a $27 billion dollar a year industry. In 1999, the yearly cost of health care exceeded 1 trillion dollars. However, in 1999, after several years of modest cost containment, the rate of inflation for health care again exceeded the general inflation rate of the economy.

 Learning Exercise: What Is a Trillion Dollars?

If you spent $1,000,000 an hour, 24 hours a day, 365 days a year, it would take you 171 years to spend 1.5 trillion dollars. The U.S. government spends 1.5 trillion dollars a year (Pintar, 1995).

Pressure continues to be felt from the federal government, the insurance industry, and consumers to reduce the cost of health care while maintaining high-quality care and service. The practical/vocational nurse needs to remember that health care agencies are interested in improving their "bottom line" by reducing waste and inefficiency. Practical/vocational nurses who identify wasteful practices and inefficient routines in their work settings while maintaining quality may be saving their very jobs.

Private Health Insurance

There are several concerns in the area of private health insurance as health care costs continue to rise. Some subscribers have been refused coverage for **catastrophic illness.** Examples include cancer treatment and transplant surgery. In August, 1996, the issue of *guaranteed coverage* (the inability of an insurance company to drop a subscriber for any reason) was addressed when President Clinton signed into law *The Health Insurance Portability and Accountability Act.* Provisions of this law include:

1. Required renewal of a health insurance policy regardless of the health status of any member of a group.
2. Guaranteed access to health insurance for small businesses, regardless of the health status of an individual or family.
3. Guaranteed access to individual coverage for those who lose their job or change jobs. This coverage is without regard to health status. Renewal is guaranteed.

However, the bill did not address the cost of this coverage, and some persons find the cost of obtaining health insurance prohibitive. Other insurance issues include (1) increasing amounts of coinsurance and deductibles, and (2) the rising cost of health insurance premiums. For employers paying health insurance premiums, 1999 was a high-cost, high-increase year. Depending on the size of the company, premium increases of from 8% to 85% were reported, with coverage reduced.

The government's DRG system has encouraged private insurers to adopt cost-cutting measures. Many health insurance plans now require second opinions for surgery and clearance for hospitalizations and emergency care. Some offer reduced premiums for selected wellness practices. Hospitalized clients with health insurance are discharged sooner than they expected to be discharged. Clients who are privately insured face higher deductibles and copayments.

Government Health Insurance

Medicare and Medicaid continue to be major issues at the state and federal levels because of the increasing cost of health care. There is continued debate about possible changes in future Medicare and Medicaid benefits. Including the cost of prescription medications under Medicare is being discussed. The 1998–1999 U.S. Congress focused on the impeachment process of President Bill Clinton; therefore health care reform and issues were not addressed. In 1999 Congress debated on what to do with an anticipated future federal budget surplus. Some con-

gresspersons suggested a tax cut, and others suggested putting part of the surplus toward assuring the viability of future Social Security and Medicare programs. Higher monthly premiums and deductibles for Medicare are being considered. The Social Security trust fund is predicted by some to become depleted in 2032 while others continue to debate this prediction.

In 1999, Congress picked up the issue of the *Patient's Bill of Rights* and introduced the *Managed Care Improvement Act.* A form of the Patient's Bill of Rights has been introduced in both houses of Congress. Changes in health insurance for those already with coverage (the Health Insurance Portability and Accountability Act) have taken place. The Children's Health Insurance Program (CHIP) is in place. Because of these efforts, changes in health care are occurring in a piecemeal fashion.

In 1999, a *National Bipartisan Commission on the Future of Medicare* adopted a plan to introduce more competition and consumer choice into the Medicare program. The commission failed to get the two thirds majority necessary to send the recommendations to Congress. In mid-November, 1999, two senators who were on the national bipartisan commission introduced to the Senate a broad reform to modernize Medicare and add a prescription drug benefit. Since Congress was preparing to adjourn for the year, the proposed legislation was shelved. Health care issues continue to be debated in Congress and by presidential candidates for the 2000 election.

Critical Thinking Exercise

What changes in legislation at the federal level and at your state level have affected Medicare and Medicaid since the fourth edition of *Success in Practical/ Vocational Nursing* was published? Review the resources listed in Chapter 7 for suggestions that can be used in obtaining up-to-date information for your nursing courses.

The Uninsured

Despite the various methods of paying for health care services and the 1997 Health Insurance Portability and Accountability Act, approximately 44 million Americans lack health insurance coverage. These numbers are growing. Two major ways to accomplish health care reform are (1) to enact comprehensive changes at the federal level, and (2) to allow incremental changes in the marketplace.

At the federal level, the 1993 health care reform debate included the issue of **universal coverage,** which is coverage of all Americans. Suggested ways of increasing coverage of Americans include creating a system of national health insurance and mandating employers to provide health insurance benefits for all employees. Some persons opposed to universal coverage object to the idea of tax money being used to insure all Americans. Persons who favor universal coverage think it would be a more efficient and effective use of tax money that is already being used for health care but in an inefficient manner.

Effect of Lack of Health Insurance Coverage

Lack of access to health care prevents individuals from seeking treatment when a health problem is developing. These individuals may seek treatment during the later stages of illness, usually at greater expense. For example, the most cost-effective means of diagnosing and treating a sinus infection would be an assessment by a family physician or nurse practitioner. However, this solution is not realistic if (1) you do not have a family physician or nurse practitioner, (2) your insurance company does not cover this type of office visit, or (3) you do not have the money to pay for a visit even if you do have a family physician or nurse practitioner. The individual with a sinus infection might seek treatment at the local emergency department when the problem reaches the stage when it can no longer be tolerated. Emergency department treatment is ex-

pensive for any condition. Such treatment is intended for seriously ill or injured persons and not for less serious illnesses.

Critical Thinking Exercise

If the client in the above scenario does not have health insurance or the ability to pay the emergency department fee, who pays the bill?

Incremental Changes in Health Care

Although there is currently no organized attempt at the federal level to achieve comprehensive health care reform, health care agencies, insurance companies, and individual states continue to initiate their own changes to attempt to control the cost of health care. This method of solving health care problems is called the **incremental method.** In this method, changes occur here and there without affecting the system as a whole. Some states have devised plans to help persons obtain health insurance who cannot afford traditional health insurance programs. Incremental changes have not solved the problem of access to care for millions of uninsured persons. (See Private Health Insurance issues, on pp. 273–274.) And the rate of inflation in health care still outpaces the general inflation rate. Some predict a return to double-digit inflation. The escalating cost of health care continues. The "person" who pays for health care is calling the shots.

The single word that describes health care in the United States continues to be *change.* The changes are dramatic, staggering, and continual. Some persons see the changes as chaos. Those who will survive see the changes as opportunities to improve the delivery of health care (*service*), increase the *quality* of that care, and decrease the *cost* of care.

Restructuring of the Health Care System

A major change that continues to take place in health care services today is the **restructuring** of the health care system in response to escalating costs. Strategies designed to decrease the cost of health care require a radical shift in viewing how health care services are delivered, especially for those used to doing things the old way. These strategies require a "new lens" in the nurse's eye (called a **paradigm shift**). They do not reflect business as usual. And the word business is used intentionally. Practical/vocational nurses need to look at health care services from a business point of view. Business principles are running health care services. **Service, quality, and cost control** are attributes of health care that need to be understood and brought to all clinical situations by the practical/vocational nurse.

Changes in Health Care Facilities

The number of hospital inpatient days continues to decline. Fewer inpatients spend less time in the hospital. The acuity level of these inpatients is higher. More clients receive care in **ambulatory service (outpatient)** settings. Hospitals continue to engage in **downsizing** (some hospitals call it **rightsizing**) both staff and services. Regional nurse layoffs continue while at the same time acute care agencies are experiencing shortages of nurses, especially in specialty areas. In the late 1990s, new federal regulations cut into the revenue of hospitals and skilled nursing facilities and some were forced to close down or decrease services. The 2000 federal budget restored some of these cuts. Some critics say "too little, too late." When staff resign or retire, some of their positions are not filled. Other staff assume the responsibilities of these staff persons. The mid-1990s saw a decline in nursing school enrollments. The average age of registered nurses was calculated

to be in the midforties. As these nurses approach retirement, a shortage of nurses is projected well into the future.

One survival strategy for acute care facilities is the use of **unlicensed assistive personnel (UAPs)** (see Chapter 2 for a review). These workers are known as nurse extenders, multiskilled workers, patient-care extenders, patient-care assistants, and externs. They can be found as patient care team members in all patient care units. Some business managers claim that many services and skills of highly educated persons can be delivered by less trained personnel without sacrificing quality. These skills include those performed by the practical/vocational nurse.

This assumption is being challenged. Nursing research has demonstrated the financial benefit and positive clinical outcomes of care delivered by licensed nurses. Current staff are being **cross-trained** to perform specific tasks of other health care team members. Examples of this role shifting include nurses drawing blood and respiratory therapists bathing and feeding clients.

In October, 1999, California passed landmark legislation in safe staffing. When implemented in 2002, the law requires the state health department to set minimum nurse-patient ratios on all hospital units. In the fall of 1999, New York lawmakers introduced legislation to establish minimum staffing ratios in nursing homes to maintain shift-specific levels of RNs, LPNs, and CNAs. Changes in health care continue to come fast and furiously.

What changes in staffing levels for hospitals and nursing homes in your state have occurred since the publication of the fourth edition of *Success in Practical/Vocational Nursing?*

Methods of Delivering Health Care

Patient-Focused Care

The most dramatic change in the way health care is delivered has been a shift toward **patient-focused care**. Delivery of health care through separate (centralized) departments in acute care facilities was inefficient. The client had to travel to different departments to be admitted and often to be diagnosed and treated. Separate departments discouraged the professional relationships necessary to deliver health care effectively.

In patient-focused care, service departments, including equipment and supplies, are **decentralized**. Health care providers in this method of health care delivery are located in client care units instead of being scattered throughout the agency. Functions once performed by centralized departments are shifted to the unit level. Instead of asking the client to go to different departments for diagnostic tests and treatments, the client stays on the unit. The professional nurse is the coordinator of the team and is accountable for all client care under this system.

Procedures are simplified and made more efficient. One example is the charting method called **charting by exception** (CBE). In this charting system, normal events are charted merely by placing a check mark on a flowsheet. Only abnormal events or changes are charted in narrative form.

Another example of efficient health care is the use of **critical pathways** (CPs), also called care maps and care guides. CPs are plans of care that show a sequence of care that is to be delivered within a definite time frame. Critical pathways also include potential problems and expected outcomes. They form a picture of the expected course of recovery for the client that all members of the health care team can follow. This method helps the client reach discharge in the fastest time possible. See Figure 16–1 for an example of a CP for a client experiencing nausea and vomiting during chemotherapy for cancer. Some facilities use multidisciplinary action plans (MAPs) or clinical guidelines instead of CPs.

Managed Care

Health Maintenance Organizations (HMOs)

Managed care is a health care delivery system developed to provide quality health care with cost controls. An example of managed care is the **health maintenance organization** (HMO). The HMO discourages physicians from ordering excessive diagnostic studies and treatments and encourages prevention of disease by the practice of preventive medicine. In an HMO, the client may not have the option of choosing her physician each time treatment is needed. Depending on the HMO, a member may go outside the HMO to see a desired physician with a *point of service* (POS) option. With the POS option, the member pays an extra fee.

The National Committee for Quality Assurance (NCQA) provides objective nationwide assessment of HMOs. This group issues report cards similar to "*Consumer Reports*" guides so that potential subscribers can evaluate an HMO before they join it

Preferred Provider Organizations

Preferred provider organizations (PPOs) are similar to HMOs. Whereas HMOs are located in buildings that are used solely for HMO business and all physicians working in the HMO are hired specifically for the HMO, family physicians may be hired as members of a PPO. These physicians remain in the same office in which their practice is located and continue to belong to the same physician group. Part of their day is spent treating clients in their own general practice. However, part of the day is spent treating clients who are enrolled in the PPO under the rules of the PPO. Think of airline travel today. The person sitting next to you probably paid a different ticket price for the same service you paid for. The same may be true for the client sitting next to you in the waiting room of the fam-

1 - 7-3
2 - 3-11
3 - 11-7

LAST ☐ Chemotherapy Date _____
     ☐ Radiation Date _____

CARE NEED	DAY 1 ADMIT DAY date ___	DAY 2 date ___	DAY 3 date ___	DAY 4 date ___
ASSESSMENTS/ TREATMENTS	Postural BP on admission & prn Weight documented I&O Baseline vital signs documented Vital signs q shift and prn Review old chart Previous admit for n/v/d date: ___ Safety/fall assessment	AM weight I&O Vital signs q shift — stable Evaluate lab results	AM weight I&O Vital signs ONLY 7-3 and 3-11 if stable	
FLUIDS/ NUTRITIONS	Start IV hydration @ admit 1000cc D_5 ½ NS 20 KCL @ 100 IV antiemetics Adjust IV fluids based on lab results within 8° of admit Clear liquids as tolerated	IV fluids continue Start PO or PR antiemetics q 6° around-the-clock Cont. IV antiemetics for BREAKTHROUGH Clear liquids-Intake: 7-3 500; 3-11 400; 11-7 100 Advance to full liquid dinner or as tolerated	DC or HL IV by noon Antiemetics AC and HS PO only Advance to regular diet for lunch Fluid Intake: 7-3 600; 3-11 500; 11-7 100	
LAB/ DIAGNOSTICS	CBC—if not available from MD office SMA 20-SMA 7 stat	SMA-7		
ACTIVITY	Up to BR Ambulate in room 1x day/evenings	Up to BR Ambulate ½ length of hallway TID	Ambulate full length of hallway TID	
SELF-CARE	Mouth care Face/hand washing Feeding	Mouth care Self bath @ bedside Feeding	Mouth care Shower	
DISCHARGE PLANNING	Evaluate home care support Refer to Social Services if: Social Work intervention needed	Document discharge plan: Social Services or Nursing	Finalize home care needs	Discharge by 11:00 AM
TEACHING	___ Assess current knowledge of antiemetics; document on kardex	___ Medication instruction ___ Dietary consult evaluate need for diet counseling	___ Review/reinforce med instruction ___ Review/reinforce diet instruction	___ Verbalizes understanding of meds for home care and diet
	RN ___	RN ___	RN ___	RN ___
	D E N	D E N	D E N	D E N
	Initial Signature	Initial Signature	Initial Signature	Initial Signature

Good Samaritan Hospital
A division of Good Samaritan Community Healthcare
407-14th Ave SE, PO Box 1247, Puyallup, WA 98371-0192 (206) 848-6661

Oncology
Clinical Pathway
Nausea/Vomiting/Dehydration

FIGURE 16–1. Oncology clinical pathway. Nausea, vomiting, and dehydration in clients with cancer (Karen Graybeal, MS, RN: Cynthia Marion, RN, OCN; Margaret Brown, MN, RN, OCN; Patty Patch, RN, OCN; Deanna Kruckenberg, RN, OCN; courtesy of Good Samaritan Hospital, Puyallup, WA. In Ignatavicius DD, Workman ML, Mishler MA. *Medical-Surgical Nursing: A Nursing Process Approach.* 3rd ed. Philadelphia: W.B. Saunders, 1999, p. 507.)

ily physician who has added a PPO service to her or his practice.

Open Access Plan

A newer plan being offered by some managed care plans is the *open access plan.* This plan allows members to see specialist physicians within the network for treatment without need of a referral as in traditional HMOs. This option may affect the subscriber's copayment.

Reaction to Managed Care and HMOs

Some people were pleased with their treatment by HMOs. However, by 1999, there was a backlash of anger and frustration by subscribers directed to managed care and HMOs. HMOs originally came into existence to improve health care by allowing consumers to shape their own health plans with an emphasis on preventive care. Dissatisfaction with HMOs includes allegations and instances of delay in receiving needed diagnostic services and refusal of HMOs to approve procedures for various diseases and illness situations. By 1999, some HMOs were reporting large losses in profits. In the fall of 1999, UnitedHealth Group, a large HMO in the United States, announced it would no longer require its physicians to obtain prior authorization from the insurance company for most procedures. The HMO could save millions of dollars a year by this change in policy. The decision also addressed the concern of consumers that HMOs were making decisions that doctors alone should be making. In June 2000, over 700,000 Medicare and Medicaid subscribers were dropped by HMOs because of federal reimbursement policies.

Critical Thinking Exercise

Identify consumer-friendly changes in policy of HMOs that have occurred since the publishing of the fourth edition of *Success in Practical/Vocational Nursing.*

Health Care Alliances and Regional Alliances

Changes in the delivery of health care in the community involve new partnerships (**alliances**) among hospitals, clinics, laboratories, health care systems, and physicians. By joining together or networking, these alliances can coordinate the delivery of care and contain costs via partnerships among providers. This system is a way to deliver health care services in a climate of shrinking resources. All members of an alliance can buy supplies in quantity. They can share a computer system. Duplication of services and equipment is avoided. Client records can be more readily available on referral to another health care provider within the *network.* For this reason, alliances are called **"seamless" systems.** Alliances allow small rural hospitals to continue to exist in a competitive market. Public-private partnerships continue to emerge. For example, public health agencies contract for services from private community nursing agencies. Such services control costs and continue to deliver quality care.

Critical Thinking Exercise

Identify alliances or networks that have occurred in your area of the country.

Quality Improvement

The emphasis on quality assurance has been replaced by an emphasis on **continuous quality improvement (CQI)** and **total quality management (TQM)**. Quality assurance stressed the identification of care that needed to be given to clients and evaluation of the results of that care. Quality improvement stresses the need to search continually for new ways to improve the process of client care, prevent errors, and identify and fix problems. This makes the search for approaches to nursing problems a never-ending quest. Total quality management is the method by which CQI is carried out.

A major way of improving the process of client care has been the formulation of nursing care plans by the RN, assisted by the practical/vocational nurse. The **Joint Commission on Accreditation of Healthcare Organizations (JCAHO)** has removed the requirement for a separate nursing care plan for each client. However, JCAHO encourages quality improvement. Whatever method replaces the nursing care plan in health care situations, practical/vocational nurses still have a responsibility to assist the RN with problem solving in client care situations.

In the twenty-first century, practical/vocational nurses need to define their role as more than the list of nursing tasks they perform. These nursing tasks are also being performed by less trained, unlicensed persons on the health care team. Practical/vocational nurses need to define their role in light of their assisting role in the nursing process. Practical/vocational nurses are effective in noting new client problems and collaborating with RNs in setting client goals, performing nursing interventions, and evaluating the results of planning. It is this problem-solving and critical-thinking aspect of nursing that makes practical/vocational nurses valuable members of the health care team.

An important component of quality health care is that the providers of that care be able to demonstrate competency throughout their careers. The present method of licensing considers a practical/vocational nurse competent upon receiving the initial license, and continued competence is assumed throughout a career. Clients, lawmakers, employers, and professional organizations are questioning this assumption. As this matter is debated and a method is devised to assure clients that their health care providers are competent and qualified, practical/vocational nurses need to update themselves continually in their area of practice.

Critical Thinking Exercise

Identify ways practical/vocational nurses can remain current in their areas of employment.

Dealing with Change

If you have had no prior experience in health care before entering the practical/vocational nursing program, you may not be aware of the changes taking place in the workplace. If you have had prior experience in the health care field, some of the changes you now observe in health care services may be obvious while others may be more subtle. Even new workers in a health career will see changes as their program of study progresses. How do you react to changes in your life? Whether changes occur in your personal life or career, it is important for you to remember that you have choices. Shuman (1995) describes how you can be a victim, a survivor, or a navigator of change.

Victims look at change in a negative way. Victims fear the worst will happen because of the proposed change and feel helpless in the situation. Victims do not willingly participate in the change process, allowing change to control them. Survivors resist change but go along for the ride. Survivors claim the change will never work, and if their prediction comes true they will be heard to say, "I told you so." Navigators of change feel in control of the situation. They feel confident and excited about the possibility of being part of the solution to a problem. Navigators believe they have some control over change rather than being controlled by the change. When change is in the wind, are you a victim, a survivor, or a navigator?

Practical/vocational nurses need to present themselves in clinical situations as invaluable to the health care agency. Be self-directed, motivated, positive, and a problem solver in your daily work. Avoid being known as the staff person who always asks what needs to be done next. Identify what needs to be done and do it. Respond flexibly to changes that are presented. Identify tasks or proto-cols that could be done more efficiently. Use the critical thinking skills that were encouraged in nursing school to devise innovative suggestions to make these areas more efficient and effective. Be a role model for practical/vocational nurses.

Summary

☐ The cost of health care has dramatically increased in past years. Cost is the driving force for change in the health care system. Traditional fee-for-service as a means of financing health care is being replaced by capitation. Insurance plans, both private and government-sponsored, are the major third-party payment systems in existence today.

☐ Comprehensive health care reform at the federal level has not occurred. Incremental health care changes in the marketplace center around decreasing the cost of health care while improving service and quality of care.

☐ Changes in health care delivery, including patient-focused care, HMOs, PPOs, open access plans, health care alliances, and quality improvement, address the issues of quality, service, and the cost of health care.

☐ Practical/vocational nurses need to be self-directed, motivated, and positive problem solvers in their areas of employment. Change needs to be approached with flexibility and viewed as an opportunity to improve the quality of client care.

☐ Practical/vocational nurses need to ensure quality of client care by keeping updated and current in their areas of employment.

Review Questions

1. Select the one word that best describes the health care system in the United States to-day.
   A. Change
   B. Stability
   C. Equitable
   D. Problem-free
2. The driving force in health care today is
   A. Cost control
   B. Client expectations
   C. Explosion of technology
   D. Increase in population
3. Select the statement that best explains Medicare as a prospective payment system.
   A. Hospitals like the prospect of being paid by the federal government for health care services for elderly people.
   B. When the patient is discharged, the hospital totals up the bill and sends it to the federal government for reimbursement.
   C. Because of diagnosis-related groups (DRGs), the federal government tells the hospital in advance how much the government will pay for an illness.
   D. The benefits covered by Medicare are changing rapidly because of new legislation.
4. Select the act of Congress that protects workers in the United States from loss of health insurance coverage, regardless of health status, if they should lose a job or change jobs.
   A. The Balanced Budget Act
   B. The Children's Health Insurance Program (CHIP)
   C. The Health Insurance Portability and Accountability Act

(Continued)

D. The Personal Responsibility and Work Opportunity Reconciliation Act
5. Select the statement that describes a health maintenance organization (HMO).
    A. Each time the client visits an HMO, the care provided is paid for out-of-pocket and the client sends the bills to the HMO for reimbursement.
    B. The doctors hired by the HMO give clients their care and the HMO pays the bills automatically.
    C. Clients go to their family doctor, receive care, pay for it, and send the bills to the HMO.
    D. Permission must be requested for each doctor visit prior to receiving care.

References

Entry Level Competencies of Graduates of Educational Programs in Practical Nursing. New York: NLN Council of Practical Nursing Programs, 1999.

Ignatavicius DD, Workman ML, Mishler MA. *Medical-Surgical Nursing: A Nursing Process Approach,* 3rd ed. Philadelphia: W. B. Saunders, 1999.

Nursing Data Source, 1994. Vol. III: *Focus on Practical/Vocational Nursing.* New York: NLN Division of Nursing, 1994.

Pintar L. What does Medicare cover? Do I need supplemental insurance? What about gaps in my insurance? Professional Development Seminar, Northeast Wisconsin Technical College, Green Bay, WI, December 22, 1995.

Shuman J. Navigating the white waters of change. Am J Nurs 95(pt 1 of 2):15–17; 1995.

Bibliography

Davidhizer R. Health care reform: What every practical nurse should know. J Pract Nurs 45:49, 52–55, 1995.

deVries C. Continued competence: Assuring quality health care. Am J Nurs 99(10):60–61, 1999.

Elder K, et al. Managed care: The value you bring. Am J Nurs 98(6):34–39, 1998.

Farley V. *Nurses: Pulling Together to Make a Difference.* Orange, CA: Innovative Nursing Consultants, 1995.

Franklin K. Social Security: Nurses work to protect the future. Am J Nurs 99(4):24, 1999.

Gratz, N. Hospitals get limited relief from new Medicare legislation. Nursing Matters, Madison, WI: Madison Newspapers, Inc. 11(2):1, 15, 2000.

Gross L, Reed S. ANA calls for Medicare reform. Am J Nurs 99(11):50, 52, 1999.

Manion J. Understanding the seven stages of change. Am J Nurs 95(4):41–43, 1995.

Shindul-Rothschild J. Nurses Week tribute: A nursing call to action. Am J Nurs 98(5):36, 1998.

Watson R. HMOs go under the knife. Newsweek, pp. 62–65, Nov. 8, 1999.

Yocum C. *Job Analysis: Newly Licensed Practical/Vocational Nurses.* Chicago: National Council of State Boards of Nursing.

Chapter 17

Career Mobility

Outline

Employment Opportunities
Job Outlook
Work Sites and Nursing Characteristics
    Extended Care Facilities
    Home Health Care
    Mental Health Nursing
    Military Service
    Hospital Nursing

Operating Room Nurse
Outpatient Clinics, Doctors' Offices, and Chiropractic Offices
Subway Nurses
Other Job Opportunities
Continuing Education
    Orientation to the Facility
    Inservice Training
    Workshops

Continuing Education Units
    (CEUs)
Certification Opportunities
Moving Up
    Educational Mobility for Nurses
    ADN Advanced Standing for
      LP/VNs
    No-Credit RN Programs

Key Terms

career ladder programs
certification in addiction

certification in long-term care
certification in managed care

certification in pharmacology
progression programs

Objectives

Upon completing this chapter you will be able to:
1. Identify areas of LP/VN employment currently available in your community.

2. Contact a postgraduate certification organization of your choice for current information.

3. Describe your postgraduate career goals (review your answer periodically).

Introductory courses in nursing are meant to excite you about the process of nursing education, the careers available in practical/vocational nursing, and how you can be a part of it all. The formal educational process opens up new doors of knowledge and skill as well as responsibility for you. Many of the things you see and learn throughout your course of study will create a sense of awe and excitement.

Careers in practical/vocational nursing are varied. Some of you have already made career decisions in advance, such as serving in the Peace Corps, working in a skilled care facility, or perhaps entering the military services. Both usual and atypical careers await you as a practical/vocational nurse.

Employment Opportunities

The 1997 Job Analysis of Newly Licensed Practical/Vocational Nurses revealed the following from a study of 1662 entry level nurses (National Council, 1998).

■ The majority of LP/VNs work in long-term care facilities or hospital-based medical units on either the day or evening shift. They care primarily for adults or aging clients with acute, chronic (stable or unstable), or terminal illness. The majority of their time is spent providing direct client care. Thirty percent indicated they regularly have administrative responsibilities. There is no important difference since the 1994 job analysis in the work setting or work characteristics for the LP/VN. They continue to work with clients of all ages, although a majority work in long-term care settings. ■

Job Outlook

The 1998–1999 Occupational Outlook Handbook (Bureau of Labor Statistics, 1999) reports that the employment of LP/VNs is expected to increase faster than the average for all occupations through the year 2006. This is in response to long-term care needs of the growing number of elderly people and the general growth of health care. The number of hospital jobs is expected to go down, with replacement jobs as the major source of job openings. There is speculation, however, that hospital jobs for practical/vocational nurses will increase.

During 1996, LP/VNs held about 699,000 jobs. Thirty-two percent worked in hospitals, 27% in nursing homes, and 13% in doctors' offices and clinics. Others worked for temporary help agencies, home health care services, or government agencies. Atypical jobs were not identified. Almost one third of the LP/VNs worked part-time.

The 1997 distribution by wage range for 32,505 LP/VNs who cared for the ill, injured, convalescent, and handicapped persons, in hospitals, clinics, private homes, sanitariums, and similar institutions appears in Table 17–1. Note that the largest (29%) salary range was $11.25 to $13.24 per hour, with

an annual income of $23,400 to $27,600 (Bureau of Labor Statistics, 1998).

The British Columbia (Canada) Ministry of Advanced Education, Training, and Technology describes licensed practical nursing as a fairly large occupation. Employment rates in 2001 are estimated to be 2680 LP/VNs. This includes 390 new positions and 400 replacement openings. Employment is expected to grow as fast as average. Cutbacks in hospitals will decrease hospital employment opportunities. However, the increased need for elder care will continue long-term (Bright job future, 1999, p. 18).

Work Sites and Nursing Characteristics

The LP/VN entry level role is to provide nursing care for clients with common, well-defined health problems in structured health care settings, under the guidance of an RN or licensed physician or dentist. LP/VNs must be caring and have an empathetic nature. Emotional stability is essential because work with sick and injured clients can be stressful. LP/VNs work as part of a team and must be able to follow orders and work under supervision.

Extended Care Facilities

The growing number of persons aged 65 years and over has a positive impact on the availability of

TABLE 17–1: Wage Ranges for 32,505 LP/VNs									
Hourly	Under $5.75	$5.75– 8.49	$8.50– 9.99	$10.00– 11.24	$11.25– 13.24	$13.25– 15.74	$15.75– 19.24	$19.25– 24.24	$24.25– 43.24
Annual	Under $11,960	$11,960– 17,659	$17,660– 20,779	$20,780– 23,399	$23,400– 27,559	$27,560– 32,759	$32,760– 40,039	$40,040– 50,439	$50,440– 89,959
Percent of Employment	*	3	11	18	29	23	12	3	*

*, Less than 3% of employment. Percentages may not sum to 100 due to rounding.
From *1998–1999 Occupational Outlook Handbook,* Bureau of Labor Statistics, Washington, D.C.

jobs for practical nurses. The Omnibus Budget Reconciliation Act (OBRA) of 1987 mandates that as of October 1, 1990, all skilled nursing facilities (SNF) and intermediate care facilities (ICF) provide 24-hour licensed practical nurse care 7 days a week, with at least one RN employed 7 days a week, 8 hours a day, although this requirement can be waived if personnel are unavailable. If you enjoy longer-term contact with people, this employment option is certainly available and may be the area for you.

The nursing home population is made up of residents who are (1) completing recovery from surgery or trauma and are too well for the hospital but not well enough to go home; (2) elderly people who are unable to care for themselves because of medical or psychological impairment; (3) mentally retarded people who are unable to live independently or in group homes; (4) young to middle-aged victims of chronic debilitating disease or accidents; and (5) young, chronically mentally ill persons who need continuing supervision and are not candidates for independent living or halfway houses.

The special qualities needed for this kind of nursing include patience, ability to see below the surface, willingness to listen, maturity, ability to determine priorities, ability to set limits, interest in working with people with disabilities, willingness to work with other health care givers, communication skills, acute observation skills of physical change, and a sense of security in regard to your own value system. Practical/vocational nurses who work in nursing homes are challenged to assist in providing a homelike atmosphere while dealing with the immediate, long-term, and terminal health problems of the residents.

The level of responsibility is great in that the LP/VN frequently works in a charge nurse role, and although supervision is available from an RN, at some times during the day supervision may be general, meaning at the other end of the telephone. Consequently, a solid knowledge and skill base is essential to know when to seek help and from whom. Nursing process is the basis for good care.

The charge nurse role also means that the practical/vocational nurse is responsible for managing care given by other LP/VNs and nursing assistants. (Refer to Chapters 13 and 14 for more specific details.)

As the LP/VN in a nursing home facility, much of your work ultimately relates to assisting the residents to attain or maintain whatever capabilities they have in all areas of health. Through your efforts residents who are recuperating from surgery or trauma can realize their goal of discharge. For other residents, your role includes supporting them through the final step of the growth process—a dignified death.

Home Health Care

According to the Bureau of Labor Statistics (1999), faster than average growth is expected in home health centers. This is in response to the number of elderly with functional disabilities, preference for home care, and technology advances to take into the home.

Because of shorter hospital stays, clients are receiving increased care in the home. The actual care given is under the supervision of an RN, who makes the initial assessment and the nursing diagnosis and develops the plan of care. The postdischarge (subacute) level of care fits in well with the LP/VN's basic education, thereby making the LP/VN invaluable in implementing the plan of care. The LP/VN's background allows additions to the continuing data collection and evaluation of the plan of care. Because of difficulty in receiving payment from nonprivate sources, some home health agencies use LP/VNs for private-pay clients only. Others employ LP/VNs as home health aides to avoid the restrictions. This is an unfortunate practice because the pay is lower and you are always held to the requirements of your highest license in legal situations.

Helpful qualities for home health nurses include

1. Flexibility—you will have to improvise in the home yet practice sound nursing principles;
2. Communications skills—you will be working in the client's domain. You have to un-

derstand the client's expression of needs and also make sure that you express yourself clearly (and tactfully);

3. Self-confidence—an air of insecurity or uncertainty will be picked up by the client, resulting in a lack of confidence in the LP/VN on the client's part. This does not imply that you should fake it. Rather, you must have knowledge and basic nursing skills that enable you to perform tasks efficiently. Do not ask for unnecessary reassurance when performing basic skills. Question what you do not know, but do it away from the client unless an emergency exists;

4. Sensitivity to physical and emotional changes—once the initial assessment is completed by the RN, it will be up to you to be alert to any changes of which the RN must be made aware. The RN must be able to depend on your observational skills for safety's sake;

5. Ability to deal with emergencies—staying calm and following the agency protocol is essential; and

6. Nonjudgmental attitude—a must, because you work right in the client's home.

Remember at all times that you are providing a service. If you are comfortable with your own values, different values are not personally threatening.

Mental Health Nursing

Mental health nursing includes both community mental health centers and group homes for the recovering mentally ill. Many community mental health centers are staffed primarily with LP/VN and nursing assistants, with RNs in a supervisory role. Yet many practical/vocational nursing programs have dropped the mental health nursing theory class and related clinical experience. This is a questionable practice since the 1999 NCLEX-PN may include up to 24% of questions in the psychosocial category.

In this area of work, LP/VNs are involved in performing treatments, administering medications, and tending to activities of daily living. Furthermore, LP/VNs perform a significant role in developing a therapeutic relationship with the client and following through with the appropriate interventions according to the client's care plan. A solid knowledge of mental health concepts and nursing process is essential.

Helpful qualities include

1. An ability to deal with stress;
2. Empathetic rather than sympathetic approach to clients;
3. Good communication skills;
4. Nonjudgmental attitude;
5. Sound mental health;
6. Alertness to physical and emotional changes in clients;
7. Ability to set client-centered limits;
8. Ability to differentiate between personal and client goals;
9. Willingness to function as a team member; and
10. Ability to avoid getting involved in promises of client secrets, which may be damaging therapeutically.

Fortunately, some mental health facilities offer orientation and continuing inservice programs. If this is an area of interest for you, we recommend Bauer and Hill's *Mental Health Nursing, An Introductory Text* (2000). This book is useful both as a basic textbook and as a continuing reference book.

Military Services

As a practical/vocational nurse, if you volunteer for military service in the reserves or active duty, you will have to take basic training. If you are interested, contact recruiters for all branches of the military services. Compare the differences to determine which branch best fits your needs.

Desirable qualities for military service nursing include (1) interest in teamwork; (2) a strong ego; (3) ability to cope with changing situations; (4) emotional stability; (5) good communication skills;

(6) self-direction; and (7) a desire for adventure. Certainly, a desire for a challenging career and an ability to adjust quickly to new situations are handy prerequisites for this kind of nursing.

Hospital Nursing

The acute care experience in most practical/vocational nursing programs is found in the medical and surgical units of hospitals. This is an area of employment when available. The number of hospital-based jobs is expected to decrease and to be available primarily to replace nurses who leave.

If you do consider specialty areas, they should be areas in which you have had both theory classes and clinical experience. Areas with complex nursing duties mean that additional postgraduate education and experience are required.

Refer to the nurse practice act for your state to see how performance of nursing acts beyond basic nursing care is handled. These acts are referred to as the expanded role of the practical/vocational nurse or performance of acts in complex client situations. See Chapters 13 and 14.

Desirable qualities in hospital nursing include (1) attention to detail in performing technical skills; (2) organizational skills; (3) nursing process skills; (4) strong ego; (5) ability to cope with stressful situations; (6) teamwork; (7) flexibility; (8) ability to prioritize; and (9) ability to think critically and solve problems.

The anticipated pay scale is approximately two thirds that of the RN pay scale. Other benefits vary according to agency policy.

Operating Room Nurse

Technicians hired as operating room (OR) nurses for cost-cutting reasons *are not nurses, are not licensed, and lack the extensive training that is required of licensed practical nurses and licensed vocational nurses* (Gilmore, 1998, p. 9). LP/VNs who have worked in ORs for years describe their work as assisting the surgeon with instruments and equipment, providing nursing assessments (collecting data), and preop and postop client care and education. They strongly urge that if you are interested in this line of work, stress your education and clinical skills as an LP/VN to your future employer. Helpful personal attributes include good personal stress management skills, ability to separate personal and professional feedback from physicians and supervisors, strong math skills, self-worth, ability to accept direction, reliable and strong knowledge of nursing process, empathy, consistent practice of standard precautions, and good personal health.

Outpatient Clinics, Doctors' Offices, and Chiropractic Offices

Outpatient clinics and doctors' offices continue to provide jobs for many LP/VNs. Most clinics and offices are open Monday to Friday. The day begins later and consequently runs a little later. Assigned work varies. It generally includes checking supplies, greeting the client, measuring vital signs, weighing the client, limited data collection (assessment) about the purpose for being there, giving the client directions on preparing for the examination, assisting the doctor with the examination, and performing additional duties delegated by the physician. If you are working as a private nurse for a physician, you can also expect to accompany the physician on hospital rounds, assisting with examinations and treatments as needed. Because the clientele remains essentially the same, these nurses develop rapport with the clients, which is an asset to both the client and the physician.

Desirable qualities include (1) good communication skills, (2) attention to detail, (3) enjoyment of routine, (4) organizational skills, and (5) self-sufficiency, because work expectations will vary with the number and type of clientele. Previous work experience in a medical-surgical unit is advised.

Subway Nurses

A unique system of providing health care to ill and injured subway users, on site, has been developed by the New York Metro Transit Authority. The health team includes LPNs, registered nurses, and emergency medical technicians. Passenger illness has become the number two reason for train back-ups. As of March, 1998, health providers have been placed at five strategically located subway stations. The conductor is notified if a passenger becomes ill, and he radios the command center. The dispatcher calls the emergency medical center, from which a transit authority health team member is dispatched to meet the train. Within three minutes, the ill person receives assistance. The program started out with two supervisors and eight LPNs and EMTs.

Other Job Opportunities

Critical Thinking Exercise

You decide that you wish to apply for an atypical nursing job. What arguments can you provide to have the employer consider hiring you?

Other job opportunities to consider are

- Residential treatment centers
- Medical management companies
- State, federal, or private prison systems
- Corporate short- or long-term disability benefit administration
- Day care centers for adults and children
- Weight loss clinics
- Social service agencies
- Ambulance and emergency medicine
- VISTA or the Peace Corps
- Occupational health in manufacturing and industry: Some LP/VNs have found excellent support in this area and work under the general supervision of a doctor.
- Veterans Administration hospitals and homes for retired veterans

- Hospices—care of terminally ill clients in institutional settings or in their homes
- Insurance companies: Companies provide in-depth orientation for the work required, and some prefer to hire practical/vocational nurses immediately upon graduation.
- Veterinary clinics and hospitals: An opportunity to combine your love of nursing with a love of animals. In some states you may work as an assistant to the veterinarian in the care and treatment of animals. Other states, such as California, require a special training program and a passing grade in a state test to assist veterinarians.
- Pharmaceutical/medical equipment sales: Some pharmacies, for example, select LP/VNs to staff this particular area. One such nurse has become the colostomy care expert in her city and gives seminars on the topic to agencies, clients, and health professionals. She enjoys the backing of the drugstore management and a pharmaceutical company.
- Coroner's nurse: A former student practical nurse doing this work commented, "I never saw myself as doing this, but it is so interesting. I've learned a lot about myself, people, pain, compassion. The doctor I work with is a born teacher."
- Private duty nurse: LP/VNs have been employed for years as private duty nurses. This is frequently a long-term commitment on the part of an LP/VN. The most common responsibility is for ill, elderly individuals who wish to be cared for in their home rather than in an institution. The LP/VN may be part of an around-the-clock care system with nurses on opposing shifts. Responsibilities vary according to the shift involved and will include basic nursing skills. The LP/VN works under the general supervision of the client's physician.
- Parish nurse: Some parishes employ their own nurse to take care of basic health needs of their congregation. This will include basic nursing skills such as measuring blood pressure, temperature, pulse, and respirations and contacting a physician as needed. Foot care

under the supervision of a podiatrist is sometimes included.

Continuing Education

Historically, practical/vocational nurses have a reputation for being apathetic in pursuing continuing education classes. This is difficult to believe because many LP/VNs have gone on to learn complex nursing skills after graduation. Continuing education classes are available in many formats and through many agencies. Often the agency you work for is willing to pick up part or all of the fee if the education benefits the agency. Some agency courses are free and are part of continuing service within the agency. Initial licensure is being questioned as providing competency for life. Your continued course of study will help ensure your competency as an LP/VN. Continuing education includes the following.

Orientation to the Facility

This provides an opportunity to learn about policies, regulations, routines, nursing care procedures, and variations in routine plus a review of selected previously learned information and skills. Learning all this information is going to take a period of time. Facilities generally have an education/inservice director who is in charge of orientation for new employees.

Inservice Training

Inservice training is information chosen to meet specific needs within a facility. Attendance at some inservice programs, such as a yearly update on bloodborne pathogens, is required. You can offer employers suggestions for content. Usually a specified amount of time is required for inservice programs, such as one hour per month or three times per year, according to the agency policy. Depending on the credentials of the instructor, continuing education credits may be available.

Workshops

Workshops present information and an opportunity to practice what is being taught. Workshops provide excellent opportunities to learn new skills. The length varies according to the content. Some agencies pay the workshop fee or expenses if the topic is specific to and enhances your nursing skills. Workshops are also a major source of continuing education credits required by many states as a part of relicensure.

Continuing Education Units (CEUs)

Classes are often taught on complex nursing skills such as intravenous therapy, physical assessment, LPN or LVN charge nurse, mental health concepts, nursing process for LP/VNs, and so on. Actually, many vocational schools and community colleges will provide any course you are interested in if you request it and enough people are available to make up the required minimum enrollment. Many of these classes provide continuing education units as opposed to course credit. You receive a certificate if you have completed course work satisfactorily.

One of the most valuable benefits of continuing education classes is the opportunity to get together with other working LP/VNs. You discover similarities in challenges and satisfactions. Ideas are shared on how to deal with difficult situations in the work setting. It is a good idea to keep a running record of all inservice programs, seminars, and workshops taken, including dates, CEUs, and topics, for future reference. Ask for these records to be included in your file at your place of employment as well as copies for yourself. Many states now require CEUs for relicensure.

Certification Opportunities

We encourage LP/VNs to take advantage of the knowledge available from certification seminars or self-study courses. The knowledge is the basis for improved nursing skills and safety in client care. In many states/agencies, certification is also the basis for salary increases and advancement.

Certification in Managed Care (CMCN)

An intensive two-day seminar prepares the LP/VN to take the examination. Upon successful completion of the examination, the nurse is certified and may use the extension title of CMCN. A recertification plan is currently being planned. To inquire about the managed care certification, contact:

American Association of Managed Care Nurses
Contact Person: Sloan Reed or Susan Wermus
4435 Waterfront Drive, Suite 101
Glen Allen, Virginia 23060
Phone: 804-747-9698
http://www.aamcn.org

Certification in Pharmacology

The National Association of Practical Nurse Education and Services (NAPNES) pharmacology certification requirements vary according to the individual nurse and/or sponsoring agency. If desired, the LP/VN may take the challenge examination without benefit of a course. Courses are available, and a sponsoring agency may designate the course as an initial step. Recertification is required every five years, and continuing education requirements vary from 48 to 120 CEUs. For information, contact:

NAPNES Recertification Office
ATTN: Helen Larsen
1400 Spring Street, Suite 330
Silver Spring, MD 20910
Phone: 301-588-2494

Critical Thinking Exercise

Imagine that your state does not recognize certification in long-term care. List the pros and cons of becoming certified.

Certification in Long-Term Care (CLTC)

This home study certification program was developed by NAPNES and the National Council of State Boards of Nursing (NCSBN). It covers pharmacology, aging, pediatrics, and key topics that enhance your competence. Once you successfully complete the certification examination, you will receive a certificate and pin and may use the extended title CLTC. To be eligible for certification, you must hold an LP/VN license in the United States or its territories and have practiced long-term care for 2000 hours within the last three years.

Harcourt Health Sciences offers a home study guide for long-term care, titled *Long-Term Care Certification* (1996). To obtain the book, call 800-426-4545 and ask for book number 08151 31704. Or you may use the Web at www .HarcourtHealthSciences.com.

Recertification is required every five years. For additional information about the certification and testing, contact:

Nancy Chornick
NCSBN
Phone: 800-240-2376

Certification in Addiction (CALPN)

The National Nursing Society on Addiction is developing a certification program for LP/VNs. Upon successful completion it will include the extension title CALPN. For information, contact:

Dottie Chemler, MS, CARN, CADC
President, Illinois Nurses Society on Addiction
2221 64th Street
Woodridge, IL 60517
Phone: 630-968-6477

Moving Up

If you are an LP/VN who says "I want to be an LP/VN. I have no desire to be an RN," good for you. You have obviously given careful consideration to your personal goals. Satisfaction in nursing both for you and the clients you care for is closely related to clear-cut goals. If you decided that you want to be an LP/VN, chances are that you will be satisfied with your choice and will provide satisfactory care to your clients. If, however, someone else decided that you should be a nurse, chances are that you will never be entirely satisfied with the choice. This lack of satisfaction will be mirrored in the care you give to clients. The same process is true in regard to making a decision to become an RN. If you do not want to become an RN, avoid letting anyone push you into it. Only when a goal is truly your own will you be motivated to do your best both in the educational process and in the care of clients.

If, however, you want to enter an RN program, it is important to know what is available educationally. A major problem in developing upward mobility programs for LP/VNs is the belief held by some educators that a practical nursing course is terminal in nature; that state boards of nursing will not permit such programs, nor will credit be given by professional nursing programs. Although the same reasoning continues to be held in some parts of the country, other directors of nursing have successfully negotiated with state boards of nursing to develop progressive LP/VN-to-RN programs. Contact your state board of nursing for a list of available professional nursing programs within your state.

Educational Mobility for Nurses

Critical Thinking Exercise

Your sister, who is an RN, insists that you, too, become an RN. How will you decide what to do?

In *Career Ladder,* the author states, "I believe that historically the Helene Fuld School of Nursing at the Hospital of Joint Diseases and Medical Center (New York City) is the first program to demonstrate the belief that practical/vocational nursing is indeed a part of the nursing profession, and that a curriculum can be constructed that effectively articulates with one that prepares for registered nurse licensure with minimal repetition" (Ahl, 1975, p. 143). The program, initially a 15-month course trimmed down to 47 weeks, was initiated in 1964. Justine Hannan, hospital Director of Nursing, worked with the Board of Nursing within New York State's Education Department, and by 1968 the department granted full registration to the program. By 1970, it was accredited by the NLN. "The school has had an impact on the quality of nursing in its home hospital, and has sent graduates into dozens of other health care facilities throughout New York and fifteen other states. It has willingly shared its experience with educators who have made inquiries about its work, and has demonstrated that career ladder education is both valid and appropriate for a large number of persons who have the aptitude and commitment to such a goal" (Ahl, 1975, p. 150).

Career-ladder programs are carefully planned to avoid duplication of content. "The curriculum is not a Practical Nursing curriculum for the first year and an Associate Degree Nursing curriculum for the second. It is a totally new curriculum designed in terms of essential learnings for beginning nursing competencies. It allows the student to be a competent Practical Nurse practitioner at the end of one year of study and a competent Registered Nurse practitioner at the end of an additional year" (Story, 1974, p. 2).

A unique program approved by the Minnesota Board of Nursing is available through seven northern Minnesota technical, community, and four-year colleges involved in the Itasca Nursing Education Consortium (INEC). It was developed in 1982 to help the student move through the upper levels of nursing education. Students may enter the practical nursing program at four of the schools and participate as a full- or part-time student. On completion of the program the graduate practical nurse becomes eligible to apply to take the NCLEX-PN.

The second year is available at two community colleges. INEC LPNs who are admitted to the second year are granted 23 credits. Students take a three-credit nursing transition course. Students must receive a C or higher in all nursing courses and must maintain a 2.00 cumulative grade point average. A total of 64 nursing credits is required to receive an associate degree. The graduate becomes eligible to apply to take the NCLEX-RN.

The nursing associate degree (ADN) RN may choose to continue her education to receive a baccalaureate in nursing. This degree is available through two four-year colleges that are members of the Consortium. For information contact:

Mary Vnuk
Associate Degree Nursing Program
Lake Superior College
2101 Trinity Road
Duluth, MN 55811
Phone: 218-725-7713 or 1-800-432-2884
FAX: 218-733-5937
e-mail: mvnuk@lsc.mnscu.ed
online: http://www.lsc.mnscu.edu/

Career ladder programs exist in many areas of the country. Your state board of nursing is an excellent resource of information about programs in your area. See Appendix A for state board listings.

ADN Advanced Standing for LP/VNs

An innovative "progression to the nursing associate degree" program has evolved at the Northeast Wisconsin Technical College in Green Bay, Wisconsin. The **progression program** is available for Wisconsin LPNs who have graduated from an accredited program. The person must hold a current Wisconsin license as an LPN. For those in the 0 to 5 years after graduation category, no proficiency testing or work experience is required. For those LPNs applying six or more years after graduation, no proficiency testing is required if during the last three years the LPN has (1) work experience of 1000 hours in a licensed health care facility/agency, or (2) completed an approved refresher course. Students who do not meet these requirements must test (NLN Mobility and LPN Gap Test).

Advanced standing credit is granted for all students upon successful completion of Introduction to

Associate Degree (AD) Nursing, ten credits of Nursing Process (three courses), and Applied Nursing Pharmacology. Non-nursing credits may be transferred from colleges or vocational programs (subject to college policies). LP/VNs licensed in other states who wish to apply without a Wisconsin license may request individual approval. Graduation from an approved practical/vocational nursing program is required. A total of 57 credits of nursing and non-nursing courses is required to complete the associate degree nursing curriculum. For additional information, contact:

Carol Rafferty, Associate Dean of Health and Community Services,
or Jim Clark, Counselor
Phone: 1-800-422-NWTC

Regents College of Albany, New York, has the first long distance learning nursing program in the United States. More than 22,000 individuals from around the world have earned associate and baccalaureate degrees in nursing from Regents College. It is accredited by the Middle States Association of Colleges and Schools, Commission on Higher Education. Its nursing programs have been accredited by the National League for Nursing (NLN) Accreditation Commission since 1977. Regents College examinations are recognized by the American Council on Education, Commission on Educational Credit and Credentials for the award of college level credit. The college is founded on the premise that what you know is more important then where you learned it. Previous credits, military training, continuing education programs, Internet-based programs, and so on are all evaluated by college faculty when you apply. Generous learner support is made available to students. Students are able to study and prepare at their own pace while maintaining their jobs. Performance evaluation is available regionally and theoretical evaluation is available at Sylvan Testing Centers located throughout the country. For information contact:

William M. Stewart,
Director of Public Relations
Phone: 1-518-464-8775 or 1-888-647-2388
e-mail: pr@regents.edu
website: www.regents.edu

No-Credit RN Programs

Turf issues continue to exist in nursing at all levels: nursing assistant to LP/VN to ADN to BSN to MSN. Plan to be a part of the solution, not the problem, when you are in a position to make a difference.

There continue to be RN programs that do not recognize the worth of a practical/vocational education. These programs insist that LP/VNs start from the beginning and repeat all previously covered theory and skills courses, including basic nursing skills. The bottom line is that a number of programs are available throughout the country that can be used by the LP/VN to become an RN—if that is what is right for that nurse.

There are two resources for locating approved nursing programs. First, there are the state boards of nursing (see listing in Appendix A). Request a list of board-approved professional nursing programs preparing for registered nurse licensure. Second, a list of all nursing programs in the United States is available from the NLN in the publication called *State-Approved Schools of Nursing,* which lists addresses, telephone numbers, and types of programs available. It is available in some libraries, or call (212) 989-9393, extension 138, to order.

Summary

- ☐ A majority of LP/VNs work in long-term care facilities or hospital-based medical units.
- ☐ Employment of LP/VNs is expected to increase faster than the average for all occupations through the year 2006.
- ☐ During 1988–1999, salaries ranged from $11.25 to $13.24/hour for the largest number of LP/VNs.
- ☐ Licensed practical nursing is considered a fairly large occupation in British Columbia, Canada.
- ☐ Nursing characteristics vary according to the work involved. Overall, nurses must be emotionally *stable, physically healthy, caring* and *empathetic.*
- ☐ Postgraduate certification courses are available for LP/VNs. They increase knowledge and skill, and in many states, the salary and position. They also help you keep up-to-date.
- ☐ LP/VN to RN programs are available throughout the country. Contact your state board of nursing or NLN for listings.
- ☐ Regents College of Albany, New York, developed the first long-distance learning nursing program in the United States.
- ☐ Turf issues continue at all levels of nursing: nursing assistant to LP/VN to ADN to BSN to MSN. Plan to be a part of the solution, not the problem, when you are in a position to make a difference.

Review Questions

1. What is the primary area for LP/VN jobs in the United States and Canada?
   A. Doctors' offices and clinics
   B. Temporary help agencies
   C. Long-term care facilities
   D. Hospital-based medical units

2. Why become certified in areas after becoming an LP/VN?
   A. The certifications are designed to increase your nursing knowledge and skill
   B. You will be able gradually to assume the work of an RN without becoming an RN.

C. Use of the extended title(s) will improve your status among other employees and peers.

D. Unless your state board of nursing acknowledges the certification, it serves no purpose.

3. Which type of program will allow you to become an LP/VN after one year and an ADN after one more year?

A. A career ladder program

B. A progression program

C. No-credit RN program

D. An accelerated/advanced standing ADN program

4. What aspects of being an LP/VN would you stress when competing for a job (such as OR) with an unlicensed applicant?

A. Personal characteristics such as reliability

B. Lack of competent instructors for unlicensed personnel

C. Agency responsibility to hire licensed staff

D. Nursing process skills such as data collection (assessing)

5. Which program will give you credit for nursing courses taken in the practical/vocational nursing program, and, once you meet general education requirements for the first year of the ADN program, make it possible to become an associate degree nurse in one year?

A. A career ladder program

B. A progression program

C. No-credit RN program

D. An accelerated/advanced standing ADN program

References

Ahl ME. In Lemburg C (ed). *Open Learning and Career Mobility in Nursing.* St. Louis: C. V. Mosby, 1975.

Bright job future. Practical Nursing Today 1:11–18, 1999.

Bureau of Labor Statistics. *Occupational Employment Statistics 1997; National Occupational Employment and Wage Estimates.* December, 1998. Homepage: oes-info@bls.gov.

Bureau of Labor Statistics. *1998–1999 Occupational Outlook Handbook: Licensed Practical Nurses.* February, 1999. Homepage: OOHinfo@bls.gov.

Gilmore J. Shoulder to shoulder. Practical Nursing Today 1(1):9–12, 1998.

National Council of State Boards of Nursing. *1997 Job Analysis of Newly Licensed Practical/Vocational Nurses.* Vol. 18(4). Chicago, 1998.

Story D. *Career Mobility.* St. Louis: C. V. Mosby, 1974.

Bibliography

Constantly changing. Practical Nursing Today 2(1):14–17, 1999.

Do you carry the NAPNES pharmacy certification card? AJPN, June 1997, p. 32.

Licensed Practical Nurse Certification. AJPN 4(4):11, 1997.

Long-term care certification for LP/VNs is here. AJPN 4(4):16, 1997.

Nurses can get managed care certification through AAMCM. AJPN 4(4):11, 1997.

Regents College receives grant for developing high-tech health care curriculum. AJPN 5(2):37, 1998.

Some LPNs are better trained for RN candidacy than RN students. AJPN 4(6):57, 1998.

U.S. Bureau of Labor Statistics. Salary levels vary, depending upon area and responsibilities. Practical Nursing Today 2(1), 1997.

Ventura M. Nurses go underground. Practical Nursing Today 2(1):42–43, 1999.

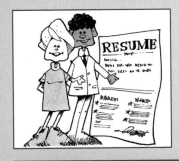

PART **SIX**

How to Get There

Chapter 18

Nursing Ethics and the Law

Outline

Values, Morals, Ethics, and Law
Critical Thinking and Ethical Decisions
Importance of General Legal Aspects
Legal Aspects of Nursing and the Legal System
Types of Legal Action
Specific Legal Terms and Concepts
    Nurse Practice Act

Principles of Ethics
    Autonomy (Free to Choose)
    Beneficence (Doing Good)
    Nonmaleficence (Do No Harm)
    Fidelity (Be True)
    Justice (Fair to All)

Practical Application of Ethics and the
    Law in Difficult Situations
    Accountability in Nursing
    Situations and Documentation
    Telephone Logs

Key Terms

abandonment
advance directives
assault
autonomy
battery
beneficence
breach of duty
civil action
common law
confidentiality
criminal action
depositions
durable power of attorney
ethics

fidelity
futility
general consent
informed consent
intentional torts
justice
law
liability
libel
living will
malpractice
mandatory licensure
morals
negligence

nonmaleficence
nurse practice act
paternalism
permissive licensure
preponderance
privacy
proximate cause
slander
standard of care
statutory laws
unintentional torts
veracity

Objectives

Upon completing this chapter you will be able to:

1. Explain the relationship between nursing ethics and the law.
2. Discuss five principles of ethics.
3. Describe the differences among ethics, morals, and values.
4. List seven steps needed for critical thinking and ethical decision making.
5. Discuss legal and clinical competency.
6. Discuss what is meant by the patient's bill of rights.
7. Differentiate between civil action and criminal action.
8. Using the correct terms, list the five steps of the legal process.
9. Explain the purpose of the nurse practice act, an example of statutory law.
10. Define terms commonly used in nurse practice acts:
    a. Basic nursing care
    b. Basic nursing situation
    c. Complex nursing situation
    d. Delegated medical act
    e. Delegated nursing act
    f. Direct supervision
    g. General supervision
11. Differentiate between mandatory and permissive licensure.
12. Describe how the nursing standard of care has come into being.
13. Review the four elements necessary to prove negligence.
14. Explain liability as it applies to the student nurse and instructor.
15. Describe three intentional torts.
16. List six common causes of recurring liability for nurses.
17. Discuss how to document client information in a legally correct way.
18. Differentiate between a living will and a durable power of attorney.
19. Explain how nursing standards, ethics, and the law influence the decisions you make in difficult clinical situations.

Values, Morals, Ethics, and Law

Personal values and morals are the building blocks of ethics. *Value* means the worth you assign to an idea or an action. **Morals** refer to the customs of society or the ethical habits of a person. **Ethics** refers to our system or code of behavior. Personal values are freely chosen and are affected by age, experience, and maturity. A child usually embraces family values during childhood. The teen years are a time of trying out the family values and either incorporating them or rejecting and replacing them with new values. Values may continue to be modified throughout one's lifetime, with input from new knowledge and experience. Based on changes in values, morals can be shifted, as can one's personal code of behavior (ethics). Your personal ethics are the basis of your nursing ethics. "Law is the minimum ethic, written down and enforced; behavior that is not merely desired but mandated" (Hall, 1996, p. 49).

Ethics in nursing deals with rules of conduct—what is right and what you ought to do in a particular situation. "In general, 'good' nursing lends to good nursing ethics, and those ethical values in turn are the basis of nursing law" (Hall, 1996, p. 6). Almost 75% of Americans surveyed in a November, 1997, Gallup Poll rated nurses high or very high in honesty and ethics. This rating placed them higher than any other profession, including health care professionals (High public esteem, 2000, p. 21). The **law** (legal aspects in nursing) has to do with rules and regulations that control the practice of nursing. The state nurse practice act is your legal guideline in nursing.

Sometimes ethics and the law are in conflict. For example, you may be ethically opposed to abortion; however, abortion in the United States is legally permitted under certain conditions. You may ethically refuse to assist with the abortion procedure, but you cannot refuse to give nursing care to the woman involved. "You may not abandon your patient," in the words of Sr. M. Antonette, a former Director of Nursing at Sacred Heart Hospital, Allentown, Pennsylvania. See Table 18–1.

TABLE 18-1: Nursing Ethics Versus Personal Values		
NFLPN Code for Licensed Practical/Vocational Nurses	**A Statement of My Personal Value System**	**Adjustment Needed**
Know the scope of maximum utilization of the LP/VN as specified by the nursing practice act and function within this scope		
Safeguard the confidential information acquired from any source about the patient		
Provide health care to all patients regardless of race, creed, cultural background, disease, or life style		
Refuse to give endorsement to the sale and promotion of commercial products or services		
Uphold the highest standards in personal appearance, language, dress, and demeanor		
Stay informed about issues affecting the practice of nursing and delivery of health care and, where appropriate, participate in government and policy decisions		
Accept the responsibility for safe nursing practice by keeping oneself mentally and physically fit and educationally prepared to practice		
Accept the responsibility for membership in NFLPN and participate in its efforts to maintain the established standards of nursing practice and employment policies that lead to quality patient care		

From *Nursing Practice Standards Booklet*. Raleigh, NC: National Federation of Licensed Practical Nurses (NFLPN), 1991.

Critical Thinking and Ethical Decisions

Critical thinking plays a major role in sorting out ethical choices and legal responsibilities in regard to the client. As a student nurse and as an LP/VN, know the steps for moral and ethical reasoning as presented by Alfaro-Lefevre (1999). See Box 18–1.

Fortunately, you have excellent resources to assist you in the ethical decision-making process (Box 18–2). The client's knowledge of choices regarding care also affects ethical decision-making. Be sure as a student nurse and as an LP/VN to confirm your final ethical decisions with the RN supervisor *before* acting.

Importance of General Legal Aspects

As practical/vocational nursing responsibility increases for involvement in the nursing process and accountability for providing high-quality nursing care, it becomes even more important for you to understand the basic concepts of the laws that gov-

Box 18–1. Steps for Moral and Ethical Nursing

1. Clearly identify the issue based on the perspective of the *players* involved.
2. Recognize your personal values and how they may influence your ability to participate in health care decision-making.
3. Identify the alternatives.
4. Determine the outcomes of the alternatives.
5. List the alternatives and rate them, on a scale from Best, Better, Good, Bad, Worse, to Worst, according to which would produce the least harm or the greatest good, based on the *client's* values.
6. Develop a plan of action that will facilitate the best choices.
7. Put the plan into action and monitor the response closely.

Adapted from Alfaro-LeFevre R. Steps for Moral and Ethical Reasoning. In *Critical Thinking in Nursing; A Practical Approach,* 2nd ed. Philadelphia: W. B. Saunders, 1999, pp. 105–106.

sets the precedent for a ruling on a case with similar facts in the future.

Laws developed by the legislative branch of the state and the federal government are called **statutory laws.** The **nurse practice act,** which governs the practice of nursing, is an example of a statutory law. Each state has its own nurse practice act. States can make these laws as long as the items in their laws do not conflict with any federal statutes. States involved in multistate licensure will have similar laws in their nurse practice acts.

Types of Legal Action

The two classifications of legal action are civil action and criminal action. A **civil action** is related to individual rights. It involves the relationship between individuals and the violation of those rights. For example, if you cause harm by administering an incorrect medication, the client can bring a civil action suit against you. Guilt on the part of the nurse can be established by a **preponderance** (majority) of the evidence. If the nurse is found

ern your nursing performance. This knowledge base will be valuable to you in making decisions. Such knowledge also will help you protect yourself against acts and decisions that could involve you in lawsuits and criminal prosecution.

Legal Aspects of Nursing and the Legal System

To understand the connection between legal aspects of nursing and the legal system in the United States and Canada, a brief review of the legal system is in order. The legal system in both countries originates from English common law. Because it originates in the courts, **common law** is called judge-made law. Common law is one way of establishing standards of legal conduct. It is useful in settling disputes. Once the judge has made a decision, this decision

Box 18–2. Resources for Making Ethical Decisions

1. Your instructors
2. Clinical nurses and physicians
3. The NFLPN Code for Licensed Practical/Vocational Nurses (Table 18–1)
4. The NFLPN Nursing Practice Standards (Appendix C)
5. The NFLPN Specialized Nursing Practice Standards (Appendix C)
6. The NAPNES Code of Ethics
7. The NAPNES Standards of Practice for Practical/Vocational Nurses (Appendix B)
8. The philosophy, mission, and policies of your health agency
9. Your job description
10. The health agency staff
11. The agency ethics committee

guilty, monetary compensation is a typical punishment.

A **criminal action** involves persons and society as a whole. It involves relationships between individuals and the government. If a nurse takes it upon herself to remove a life-sustaining device and the client dies, this is considered murder. A criminal action suit would be filed against the nurse. Guilt on the part of the nurse needs to be established by the production of proof beyond a reasonable doubt. Punishment can be death, imprisonment, fines, or restriction of personal liberties. When a criminal case is completed, it is possible to be sued in a civil court.

Specific Legal Terms and Concepts

Nurse Practice Act

The duties and functions that nurses can perform are defined on the state level by the *nurse practice act*. The nurse practice act of each state defines what nursing is, what it is not, and under what circumstances it can be practiced for compensation. The nurse practice act provides the administrative rules and regulations under which a nurse functions as an LP/VN.

It is necessary for practical/vocational nurses to understand that they must limit their work to the area of nursing defined in their state's nurse practice act. This defines your scope of practice. Practical/vocational nurses must realize that *no physician, registered professional nurse, or agency can give them the right to do more than what their license says they can do.*

In 1981, the National Association of Practical Nurse Education and Service (NAPNES) issued a statement of responsibilities required for practice as a practical/vocational nurse (Box 18–3). Statements from official nursing organizations do not carry the weight of law. They are useful as a guide for behavior and may be used in a court of law as a point of reference. *The nurse practice act of your state is your final authority.*

Box 18–3. NAPNES Statement of Responsibility for LP/VNs

1. Recognizes the LPN's or LVN's role in the health care delivery system and articulates that role with those of other health care team members.
2. Maintains accountability for one's own nursing practice within the ethical and legal framework.
3. Serves as a client advocate.
4. Accepts a role in maintaining developing standards of practice in providing health care.
5. Seeks further growth through educational opportunities.

From NAPNES, 1981.

Terms Used in Nurse Practice Acts

Terminology remains standard in many states. As you study the scope of practice for licensed or trained practical/vocational nurses in your state, knowledge of the following terms may be helpful.

BASIC NURSING CARE. Nursing care that can be performed safely by the LPN or LVN, based on knowledge and skills gained during the educational program. Modifications of care are unnecessary, and client response is predictable.

BASIC CLIENT SITUATION. Client's clinical condition is predictable. Medical and nursing orders are not changing continuously. They do not contain complex modifications. The client's clinical condition requires only basic nursing care. The professional nurse assesses whether the situation is a basic care situation.

COMPLEX NURSING SITUATION. Client's clinical condition is not predictable. Medical or nursing orders are likely to involve continuous changes or complex modifications. Nursing care expectations are beyond that learned by the LPN or

LVN during the educational program. The professional nurse assesses whether the situation is a complex nursing situation.

DELEGATED MEDICAL ACT. Physician's orders given to an RN, LPN, or LVN by a physician, dentist, or podiatrist.

DELEGATED NURSING ACT. Nursing orders given to an RN, LPN, or LVN by an RN.

DIRECT SUPERVISION. Supervisor is continuously present to coordinate, direct, or inspect nursing care. Supervisor is in the building.

GENERAL SUPERVISION. Supervisor regularly coordinates, directs, or inspects nursing care and is within reach either in the building or by telephone.

Principles of Ethics

Five ethical principles assist in determining a right course of action: **autonomy, beneficence, non-maleficence, fidelity,** and **justice.** Each of these principles will be discussed separately. Related issues are reviewed to assist in understanding how the principle applies in nursing.

Autonomy (Free to Choose)

Autonomy allows the competent client to maintain control over health care decisions. Clients make informed choices based on knowledge of their condition and treatment options. For example, a young woman is diagnosed with breast cancer. She has decided not to receive treatment and requests discharge as soon as possible. You will support the decision and continue to provide your finest care whether or not the client's ethics regarding treatment agree with your ethics.

The following issues related to autonomy are discussed: privacy, access to medical records, general consent, informed consent, authorized consent, advance directives, no-code orders, removal of life support systems, euthanasia, and organ donation.

Privacy

Autonomy includes client **privacy.** This is why your instructor asks the client directly for permission to allow students to observe a particular treatment or procedure. It is also the reason why the client is not exposed needlessly in the course of routine care.

Access to Medical Records

The medical record belongs to the hospital. The client has the right to see the record. The practical/vocational nurse, however, does not have the authority to give the record to the client. Refer client requests to view the medical record to your supervisor and the physician.

General (Implied) Consent

General consent for treatment is obtained upon admission. It may be obtained by the LP/VN or by an admission clerk during a routine admission. The fact that a person has voluntarily sought admission to a health care agency and willingly signs a general admission form is an example of general consent. A client may revoke this permission verbally.

Informed Consent

Informed consent must be obtained for invasive procedures ordered for therapeutic or diagnostic purposes (for example, surgery). Informed consent means that the client is told in nontechnical language

- What the treatment is
- What the risks are
- What the alternative treatments are
- Who will perform the treatment
- Whether the treatment is really necessary

The client must indicate that he *understands* this information. Remember that the client's understanding of the information must be documented.

In most states, informed consent is the responsibility of the physician because he or she must explain the implications and complications of the procedure to the client before written permission is obtained. The client may revoke this permission verbally.

"Being asked to witness a patient's signature on a consent form is no small responsibility. Your signature attests to three things: that the patient gave his consent voluntarily, that his signature is authentic, and that he appears to be competent to give consent" (Sullivan, 1998, p. 59).

Authorized Consent

Parents cannot give informed consent for the treatment of their children, but they can *authorize treatment* for their children up to a certain age. Courts of law recognize that parents generally authorize what is appropriate for their children. In most states, "minor" is defined as under age 18 years. Some states allow minors to give their own consent for substance abuse treatment, mental health problems, pregnancy, and sexually transmitted diseases (STDs). Emancipated minors are defined as those living on their own and managing their own finances or who are married and have children. They are competent to give their consent.

Advance Directives

Two types of written directives are available to clients as a way of stating their personal wishes regarding future health care. These directives are the **living will** and the **durable power of attorney.** Both are written by the client while he or she is mentally competent.

LIVING WILL. This document is filled out by the individual and witnessed by a person who will not benefit by the death of that individual. Living wills are recognized as legal documents in 38 states in the United States and the District of Columbia. They are not recognized as legal documents in Canada. The individual generally is advised to give a witnessed copy to the health care provider and a trusted friend or relation and to keep one copy for

self in a location that is easily accessible. If a person is moving to or spending time in another state, he or she is advised to determine whether the living will is considered legal in that state. Otherwise, he may discover too late that the written directive will not be honored.

DURABLE POWER OF ATTORNEY (DPOA). This document, sometimes known as the *durable medical power of attorney,* is a legal document throughout the United States. As an LP/VN, it is necessary for you to understand the scope and execution of the DPOA in your state or province. Choice in Dying (CID) is a national nonprofit organization dedicated to serving the needs of dying clients and their families. This organization has pioneered in making advance directives for over 25 years. CID advocates the right of clients to participate fully in making decisions about their medical treatment at the end of file. For information, contact:

> Toll Free-Hot Line 1-800-989-WILL, or
> www.choices.org, or write or Fax
> Choices in Dying National Office
> 1035 30th Street NW
> Washington, DC 20007
> 1-202-338-9790
> Fax 202-338-0242

The DPOA has three major provisions:

1. It identifies who will make decisions for the person in a medical situation if he or she is unable to speak for self.
2. It identifies the extent of treatment desired by the person if the person is in a coma or a persistent vegetative state.
3. It lists the medical treatments that the person would never want performed.

The role of the next of kin in making decisions about care for the client differs from state to state. "The biggest challenge: no advance directive and family opposition." Only about 15% of clients have advance directives in the form of a living will or health care proxy [DPOA]" (Haynor, 1998, pp. 27–28). Sometimes providers ignore client advance directives. The instructions provided by the client may be vague, the physician might assume that the client did not know about an available treatment or simply defers to the wishes of family members. Sometimes clients have not discussed advance directives with their physician, or a facility has a policy that a written physician's order of Do Not Resuscitate (DNR) must be in the chart in order to comply with the client's wish. For your legal protection, know what your state and facility policies are and whether the client has a written advance directive that the physician is aware of (Wolfe, 1998, pp. 51–56). "Do Not Hospitalize (DNH) orders may be more effective than DNR orders in limiting treatment and preventing unnecessary or unwanted patient transfer from a long-term care to an acute care facility" (Legal side when long-term residents require emergent care. 1998, p. 56).

No-Code Orders

No-code orders are legal orders not to resuscitate a client, written by the physician, and they do not have to be updated unless the client changes her or his mind. If a written no-code order does not exist and the nurse does not code the client, the nurse is in effect making a medical decision. The nurse is practicing medicine without a license and may be subject to a lawsuit. There is no such thing as a partial or slow code. All care givers must know when a written no-code order exists. Check your state and agency policy regarding no-code orders. Some policies include specific modified codes that must be followed.

Removal of Life Support Systems

The physician must pronounce the client dead and document this status *before* the nurse turns off the ventilator.

Euthanasia

The term itself means a good or happy or painless death. As used today, euthanasia refers to assisting with a killing *actively* or permitting the death of a person who has a painful or a prolonged illness (example: removing life support). Euthanasia is not the same as a no-code order written by a physician based on a decision made by the physician and the client or the family. A no-code order is a *passive* action, with the goal of avoiding prolonging life unnecessarily, not actively ending it. "The ANA, as well as the AMA and the National Hospice Association, has issued position statements expressly declaring opposition to nurse or physician participation in assisted suicide" (Daly et al, 1997, p. 209).

Nurses must know the legal and moral aspects of assisted suicide. Laws vary from state to state. Nurses, as primary care givers, may be involved in caring for the client involved. Abandonment of the client is not an option.

Legislation passed in Oregon in 1994 permits physicians to provide "aid in dying to qualified citizens requesting such assistance." In 1998, eight men and seven women—all of whom were terminally ill and whose average age was 69 years—used Oregon's Death with Dignity Act (Report tracks impact, 1999, p. 16). The United States House of Representatives has passed a bill by which any physician who prescribes drugs for the purpose of causing death faces a 20-year prison sentence. As of November 29, 1999, it has not passed in the Senate. The same bill allows physicians to order controlled substances in doses necessary to relieve pain.

With the permission of the instructor, divide into groups. Choose a viewpoint you do not usually hold. Be prepared to present reasons for the viewpoint. Choose a spokesperson to summarize the group views.

- Group 1: Terminally ill clients have the right to choose death by physician-assisted suicide.
- Group 2: Terminally ill clients must wait to die of natural causes.
- Group 3: The nurse's personal ethic conflicts with the decision of groups 1 and 2. Discuss the nurse's rights, roles, and responsibilities to the client.

Refer again to the critical thinking steps on page 298 to assist you in making your decision.

Organ Donation

Organ donations are voluntary. At this time organs cannot be bought or sold. Although many clients and families give permission for organ donation after death, the demand for organs far exceeds supply. You may have been asked to agree to personal organ donation at the time you got your driver's license. Many states participate in this effort. It has been suggested that money be given for organs to cover funeral expenses and so on to increase the number of donors.

Body tissues that can be donated include skin, cornea, bone, heart valves, and blood. One example of a successful body tissue transplant was the transplantation of umbilical cord blood for a rare genetic bone disease at the University of Minnesota in 1995. Approximately one cup of blood taken from a newborn's discarded umbilical cord and placenta was donated. Donated body organs include the heart, liver, kidneys, lungs, and pancreas.

Organ donation has raised both ethical and legal questions in some instances—for example, having a baby so select organs or body tissues can be used to save a sibling.

 Critical Thinking Exercise

What ethical and legal issues do you see in the issue of organ donation?

Beneficence (Doing Good)

Beneficence involves *doing good* with your nursing actions. It may also involve preventing harm and removing harm. It does not conflict with the principle of autonomy. You provide care according to nursing care standards. For example, if you give the wrong medication, you report it as soon as you recognize your error. Your ethical concern is to prevent harm to the client. Beneficence is a greater good than concern for yourself in regard to the error.

Paternalism is a form of beneficence that does intrude on autonomy. If you deceive, threaten, or manipulate a client into performing a therapeutic activity, the activity itself may be beneficial, but you have taken away the client's right to make the final decision (autonomy). To avoid paternalism, the following method was presented by a lactation counselor at a public health nursing seminar: "I wish all women would breast-feed their babies. The value to the mother and the child is a scientific fact. I present the facts and respond to their questions, but the final decision belongs to the mother. I respectfully support their decision."

The following issues related to beneficence are discussed: rights of clients, unintentional torts, liability of student nurses and instructors, common causes of nursing liability, charting, incident reports, malpractice insurance for nurses, limits of employer liability, steps in bringing a legal action, and giving testimony.

Rights of Clients

It is recognized that a personal relationship between the physician and the client is essential for the provision of medical care. The traditional physician-client relationship takes on a new dimension when care is rendered within an organizational structure. Legal precedent has established that the institution itself also has a responsibility to the client. It is in recognition of these factors that the rights of clients are affirmed.

Clients have become increasingly concerned and vocal about the level of care they expect to receive. Many agencies now issue "client's rights" statements upon admission. Some require that the client or a family member acknowledge receiving the statement by signing a form. Table 18–2 provides examples of issues addressed in a state's "Patient's

TABLE 18–2: Patient's Bill of Rights
1. Information about rights
2. Courteous treatment
3. Appropriate health care
4. Physician's identity
5. Relationship with other health services
6. Information about treatment
7. Participation in planning treatment
8. Continuity of care
9. Right to refuse care
10. Experimental research
11. Freedom from maltreatment
12. Treatment privacy
13. Confidentiality of records
14. Disclosure of services available
15. Responsive service
16. Personal privacy
17. Grievances
18. Communication privacy
19. Personal property
20. Services for the facility
21. Protection and advocacy services
22. Right to communication disclosure and right to associate. (Additional rights in residential programs for chemically dependent or mentally ill minors or 24-hour services for emotionally disturbed minors.)
23. Isolation and restraints
24. Treatment plan

Summary of issues addressed in Minnesota Statute 144.651, Patients' Bill of Rights. Published by Minnesota Hospital and Healthcare Partnership, 2550 West University Ave, Suite 350S, St. Paul, MN 55114. Aug. 1995, revised Aug. 1998.

Bill of Rights." Review your own state's Patient's Bill of Rights.

Unintentional Torts

A tort is a wrong or injury done to someone that violates his or her rights. Tort law is based on the premise that in the course of relationships with each other there is a general duty to avoid injuring each other.

Negligence and **malpractice** are examples of **unintentional torts.** "Negligence is the unintentional tort of *acting* or *failing to act* as an ordinary, reasonable, prudent person with resulting harm to the person to whom the duty of care is owed" (Bolander, 1995, p. 52). Malpractice means negligence by a professional. In nursing, it relates to an action or lack of action, not to what you intended to do. Good intentions do not enter in. As a nurse you are held responsible for your conduct. *Student practical/vocational nurses are held to a level of a licensed practical/vocational nurse's performance.* The LP/VN's conduct, not his or her intention, is the issue.

ELEMENTS NECESSARY FOR NEGLIGENCE. (1) Duty, (2) breach of duty, (3) damages, and (4) proximate cause are the four elements that must be present to cause an action for negligence against the nurse. Each of the four elements must be proved by the client to receive compensation. *Duty* refers to the nurse's responsibility to provide care in an acceptable way. The nurse has a duty based on education as well as the expectations and standards of his or her place of employment. **Breach of duty** means that the nurse did not adhere to the nursing standard of care. What was expected of the nurse was not done (omission) or was not done correctly (commission). *Damages* means that the client must be able to show that the nurse's negligent act injured him or her in some way. The client must prove actual damage. **Proximate cause** means that a reasonable cause-and-effect relationship can be shown between the omission or commission of the nursing act and the harm to the client. Did the nurse's negligent act cause the injury in question?

Liability of Student Nurses and Instructors

Student nurses are held accountable for the nursing care they give. They are held to the standards of a licensed practical/vocational nurse. This emphasizes the necessity of:

1. *Preparation for working in the clinical area.* The instructor is held responsible for making sure that the student assigned to a client has the necessary knowledge base and skill to give safe nursing care. The instructor is also expected to provide reasonable supervision for the care given by a student.
2. Requesting additional help or supervision if needed.
3. Complying with agency and school of nursing policies.

Common Causes of Nursing Liability

Many of the errors leading to common nursing liabilities can be avoided by following the guidelines you learned in nursing school.

Learning Exercise: Major Areas of Clinical Evaluation

In what major areas are you evaluated during each clinical rotation?

The major areas of **liability** can be categorized as lack of safety, knowledge, skill, observation and reporting, documentation, and acceptance of responsibility for nursing actions—all of which are part of the usual clinical evaluation. The most common errors are drug errors, most of which can be avoided if you follow the guidelines you learn in basic nursing and practice in the clinical areas. See

Box 18–4 for other recurring areas of liability. One of the best defenses against malpractice is development of rapport with the client. The very best defense is not to err in the first place. Always function within the standard of care.

Charting

Documentation is part of your job. It is not busy work. Legal documentation is basic nursing in all institutions. The forms may be different, but the basics remain the same. The chart is a legal document and can be used in court. Be sure to review the charting procedure for your specific institution and adhere to it. Legal charting is also an opportunity for you to show that you have a legitimate knowledge base. It gives credibility to practical/vocational nursing as a vocation. Charting gives you the opportunity to show that you functioned within the standard of care.

General Guidelines for Legal Documentation

Traditional methods of charting include (1) source-oriented (narrative charting), and (2) problem-oriented (*S*ubjective *O*bjective *A*ssessment *P*lan

---

Box 18–4. Recurring Areas of Liability

1. Client falls.
2. Failure to follow physician orders or established protocols.
3. Improper use of equipment.
4. Failure to remove foreign objects (as in the OR, or during other invasive procedures).
5. Failure to provide sufficient monitoring (physician's orders or agency policy).
6. Failure to communicate (between nurse and client and other health professionals).

From Eskreis TR. Recurring areas of liability. In Seven common legal pitfalls in nursing. Am J Nurs 98: 34–38, 1998.

[SOAP], *S*ubjective *O*bjective *A*ssessment *P*lan *I*ntervention *E*valuation [SOAPIE], *S*ubjective *O*bjective *A*ssessment *P*lan *I*ntervention *E*valuation *R*evision [SOAPIER], and *S*ubjective *O*bjective *P*lan [SOP] charting). These traditional methods are being replaced by (1) focus charting (use of focus to label nurse's notes, categories of data, action and response, and flowsheets), and (2) charting by exception (nurse/physician order flowsheets used to document assessments and intervention). All formats are adapted to the computer.

Regardless of which method of charting is used by an institution, the following guidelines apply:

1. Date and time should accompany each entry.
2. Each entry should be accurate, factual, specific, and objective. Nurses must constantly remind themselves to avoid subjective comments when charting. Subjective comments are judgments made by you. Avoid them. Eliminate the word "appears" except when the client is sleeping.
3. Each entry must be legible, spelled correctly, and grammatically correct. A lawyer can question your ability to give competent nursing care if you do not have command of the English language. Print, if this is an agency policy or if your handwriting is hard to read. Use correct punctuation, because the meaning of a sentence can change based on punctuation. Sloppy charting may be interpreted as sloppy or unsafe nursing care. It communicates that you did not take the time to write, and a lawyer could accuse you of not taking the time to care.
4. Place entries on the chart as soon as possible after the events occur. Charting entries are always entered in chronologic order. This indicates when the event happened in the time column. If someone else charts before you are able to record an entry or if you have forgotten to record an entry, a late entry may be used. Put the actual charting time in the time column for the late entry and include the actual date and time of the events in the nurses' notes.

5. For written entries, use permanent ink (no erasable pens) in the color identified in the institution's procedure manual. The trend is toward use of black ink and military time. Avoid using highlighters on any chart form. Many do not show up on photocopies or Fax copies.
6. Do not leave blank lines. If an item on a flowsheet does not apply, write in N/A (not applicable). If other staff persons need to make an entry, do not save lines. They can make a late entry. Write your signature and title on the right. Use a line to fill in any empty space before your signature.
7. Ditto marks are never used.
8. *Use only approved abbreviations as found in the institution's policy and procedure manual.* This assists in communication and reduces errors.
9. Document medical and nursing treatments performed and the client's response to these treatments. If the client refuses these treatments, document the reason for refusal.
10. When seeking help in difficult situations, document communication with supervisors by name and content of conversation.
11. As an LP/VN, do not co-sign for nursing students. If you must sign off a client chart that is not for one of your clients, write, "I'm signing this to complete the record; I have no knowledge of the client."
12. Do not add any notes once charting is complete unless you use a *late entry format.*
13. Do not delete notes or correct errors with "white out" ink on written notes. When an error is made in charting, draw a single line through the error, write in the date and time, and sign. Do not write "error" above the entry; instead, write "mistaken entry." A court may interpret the term "error" as incorrect care.
14. Record all abnormal observations, including changes in the client's condition and to whom these observations were reported.
15. Record care actually given, not care that will be given in the future.

16. Each dated and timed entry must be signed using your full, legal title as determined by your state.
17. If you did not chart it, you did not do it, and a lawyer will surmise that you did not care!
18. Avoid treating flowsheets casually. If you place a symbol indicating normal findings, be sure you have reviewed the institution's parameters for normal findings. These can usually be found on the flowsheet.
19. For computer charting, consider your sign-on code as equivalent to your signature. Use only your code and do not let anyone else use yours. *Protect the client's right to confidentiality by not leaving personal information available for viewing during charting or when you have completed your charting.*
20. "Document every intervention or patient instruction" (Murphy, 1997, p. 147).

Incident Reports

Incident reports are intended to provide in-house improvements in care. They are administration records required by federal law so that agencies can see patterns and correct them. Incident reports are written as soon as possible after the occurrences by the health providers who witnessed the incident. They are objective. Let others draw conclusions. They should be written with the thought that they may be viewed by attorneys on the "other side." The client's description of what happened should be included. The report should be legible, factual, and objective; it should be in permanent ink, and it should not be worded to accept or place blame, e.g., if someone is found on the floor, the report should state "found on floor," not "fell." Although the incident itself is also recorded on the client's chart, avoid writing "incident report filed" on the chart.

Malpractice Insurance for Nurses

More nurses are being named in lawsuits. Nurses are responsible for their own acts. Although the employing agency may assume responsibility for the nurse during a lawsuit, it can then turn around and sue the nurse. Did you know that you can also be held responsible for the "neighborhood advice" you give—for example, telling a neighbor how to care for her sick child?

Each nurse must carefully consider whether it is necessary to purchase a malpractice insurance policy. Although incidents of suing for malpractice continue, as an LP/VN your chances of being sued are statistically small. Look carefully at the circumstances that are a part of the agency of which you are an employee. See Table 18–3.

TABLE 18–3: Malpractice

Reasons for Your Own Malpractice Insurance Coverage

1. The jury's award could exceed the limits of your agency's coverage.
2. Your employing agency could pay out an award to a plaintiff and then countersue you.
3. You acted outside the scope of employment and the agency argues it is not liable.
4. Your employer's policy covers you only on the job.
5. An agency might carry a policy that covers you only while you are employed by that institution. A suit may come up years after you have stopped working for the employer. It is suggested that nurses purchase occurrence coverage and not claims coverage. For this reason, occurrence coverage protects the nurse for each incident regardless of present employer.
6. Agency may decide to settle out of court. Plaintiff could pursue a case against the nurse.
7. Has your employer paid the insurance premium?
8. After a settlement, insurers could turn around and sue the nurse.
9. With your own coverage, you will have your own lawyers, not the lawyers also defending the agency.

Limits of Employer Liability

The employer may be held responsible for acts performed by the nurse within the scope of employment. However, the employer may sue the nurse to recover fees and other monies involved while defending him or her.

Steps in Bringing a Legal Action

Legal actions follow an orderly process. See Box 18–5 for steps in bringing a legal action.

Box 18–5. Steps for Bringing a Legal Action

1. The client believes that his or her legal rights have been violated by the nurse.
2. The client seeks the advice of an attorney.
3. The attorney has a *nurse expert* review the client's chart to see whether the nurse has *violated the nursing standard of care.* If it is determined that a standard of care has been violated, a *lawsuit* is begun. This is not based on floor routine if it violates the standard of care.
4. The client (the plaintiff) files a *complaint* that documents the *grievance* (violation of rules). This is served to the defendant (the nurse).
5. The defendant responds *in writing.*
6. The *discovery* period (pretrial activity) begins. Statements are taken from the defendant nurse, witnesses, nurse expert, client (plaintiff), and other care givers. Policies and procedures of the health care facilities are reviewed.
7. During the *trial,* important information is presented to the judge or jury. A *verdict* (decision) is reached. The plaintiff (the client) has the burden of proof (evidence of wrongdoing) during the trial.
8. An *appeal* (request for another trial) can be made if the verdict is not considered acceptable by either the plaintiff or the defendant.

Giving Testimony

Your attorney will review types of questions you can expect. He or she will also prepare you for types of questions that may slant your testimony. Your attorney will not tell you what to say, but will suggest appropriate ways to respond. Dempski (2000, p. 59) provides the following tips:

1. *Take your time.* Think about what is being asked and how you will answer it. The pause also gives your attorney a chance to object if needed. Your attorney will signal you if you should answer the question.
2. *Be specific.* Answer "yes" or "no" whenever possible, without adding details. The attorney will ask a follow-up question if he or she wants to learn more.
3. *Resist the urge to say more.* There is a temptation to fill silence. Don't.
4. *Stick to the facts.* **Veracity** (telling the truth) is important. Avoid trying to be clever and do not guess. If you do not remember, say so. Say "I do not remember" rather than "I do not know."
5. *Refer to the client record/documents* as needed.
6. *Correct mistakes and misconceptions*—do not assume you understand. Ask that a question be rephrased as needed. Correct any statements you may have stated incorrectly.

Depositions usually take place in an attorney's office. You may be able to request that it be in your attorney's office. Anyone involved with the lawsuit may attend. A court reporter or stenographer will record your testimony. A few weeks after the deposition, you and your attorney may be able to review the testimony and make corrections. You may be asked about the corrections in the trial.

Once the deposition is scheduled, provide information on where and how you can be reached. Look professional (as you would for a job interview). Do your utmost to be calm and polite no matter how rude others, including the opposing attorney, are toward you.

You may ask for a break as needed. This is a

good idea, especially if you are tired and/or not thinking clearly (Dempski, 2000, p. 60).

Nonmaleficence (Do No Harm)

Hippocrates said, "At the least, do no harm." *Nonmaleficence* means *primum non nocere:* first do no harm. Nonmaleficence is the basis for many of the "rules" promoted by your instructors. Examples include the "rule of 5" in dispensing medications, checking the temperature of bathwater, checking the temperature of formula, lowering the bed to its lowest position after completing a treatment or preparing to leave the room, and not abandoning your clients when their ethical principles conflict with yours.

Included in this segment to assist you in understanding nonmaleficence is licensure, unlicensed assistive personnel, standards of care, intentional torts, functioning beyond the scope of practice and experience, physical and emotional abuse, and Good Samaritan acts.

Licensure

The practice of licensing was instituted by nurses themselves. Nurses were concerned about the nursing care that they delivered and the safety of their clients.

Upon completion of a state-approved LP/VN nursing education program, a graduate is eligible to apply to take a national licensing examination in practical/vocational nursing. See Chapter 19 (NCLEX-PN). Each state has established its own criteria for passing the examination. States also have made arrangements for interstate *endorsements* for nurses who choose to work in other states. This means that it is possible to work in another state without repeating the NCLEX-PN if you have met that state's criteria for passing. Multistate licensure is now the law in select states. Check Appendix A for the location of your state licensing board. All nurse practice acts address nursing licensure. Depending on the state in which you work, licensure will be mandatory or permissive.

Mandatory licensure protects, by law, the role of the nurse (that is, what nurses do). This means that anyone who practices nursing must be licensed. **Permissive licensure** protects the title of the nurse but not what nurses do. This means that the practical/vocational nurse may practice nursing without a license but cannot use the title LPN or LVN. Because of permissive licensure, unlicensed persons may perform nursing skills performed by the practical/vocational nurse.

 Learning Exercise: Nursing Licensure

Which kind of license is required in your state?

Some boards of nursing are instituting on-line verification of nursing licensure. The Minnesota Board of Nursing reported in 1995 that it has contracted with the Minnesota Department of Administration to provide on-line verification of information about licensed practical nurses (Minnesota Board of Nursing, 1995, p. 4). The Board provides public information about nurses who have current registration. The verification system enables callers to obtain a nurse's license number, registration expiration date, and whether any Board action has taken place. The service is available 24 hours a day, every day. Employers will be able to use this option to comply with requirements for written verification of a nurse's registration by the Joint Commission on Accreditation of Healthcare Organizations.

All states and provinces have examining councils that provide nursing examinations for licensure and review complaints that can lead to revocation of a license. Because of the sheer numbers of complaints received and the small number of board members, it is difficult to review all complaints. (Some states employ a compliance officer, who investigates cases of suspected drug or alcohol abuse.) Revocation (removal or elimination) of a license is a serious matter. Some boards of nursing are taking a rehabilitative rather than a punitive stance to drug abuse. All boards of nursing may limit, suspend, revoke, or deny renewal of a license because of violations of the nurse practice act.

Critical Thinking Exercise

What happens to the LP/VN whose license is revoked because of drug abuse and who remains untreated?

Unlicensed Assistive Personnel

The use of unlicensed assistive personnel (UAP) to provide client care has grown dramatically in recent years. It is expected that the trend will continue. These unlicensed persons are trained to perform a variety of nursing tasks. Supervision of UAPs by the RN to ensure safety of client care is a major concern. The responsibility for the act delegated can never be given away. There is concern that because of the lack of licensed nurses in an agency, duties will be delegated inappropriately to UAPs. It is the RNs and LP/VNs who stand to lose their jobs and licenses if the care provided by UAPs does not meet the standards of safety and effectiveness. The training program for UAPs does not provide the same depth in education and experience that programs for licensed nurses provide. Licensed nurses are also accountable to both their employers and their state nursing boards.

Standards of Care

A phrase used in nursing has important legal implications: You are held to the nursing **standard of care.** The standard of care is based on what an ordinary, prudent nurse with similar education and experience would do or not do in similar circumstances. Resources for the nursing standard of care are found in Box 18–6.

Box 18–6. Resources for the Nursing Standard of Care

1. Nurse practice act: Identifies the minimum level of competence necessary for you to function as an LPN or LVN in your state.
2. Nursing licensure examination (NCLEX-PN): Tests for *minimum* competence.
3. Practical/vocational nursing programs: Based on guidelines provided by the board of nursing, these programs guarantee a minimum knowledge base and clinical practice necessary to provide safe nursing care. Curricula, textbooks, and instructors are resources for information about the standard of care.
4. Written policies and procedures: The agency for which you work provides a standard of nursing care for you to follow. This is the reason why it is important for you to read the policies of the agency to find out whether verbal directions are supported by written policies. If a question about care ever comes up in court, a lawyer will use the agency policy and procedure manual as one guide to expected behavior. Remember that policies and procedures *do not* overrule your state's nurse practice act and educational preparation. However, institutional policies may be stricter than state law.
5. Custom: An unwritten, usually acceptable way of giving nursing care. Expert witnesses would be called to testify to "the acceptable way," not your coworkers.
6. Law: Decisions that have been arrived at in similar cases brought up before a court (judge-made law).
7. Statements from the NFLPN and NAPNES. See appendixes B and C.
8. Nursing texts and journals.
9. Administrative rules of your board of nursing.

Intentional Torts

Intentional torts require a specific state of mind, that is, that the nurse involved intended to do the wrongful act. Significantly, not all insurance companies cover intentional torts in their malpractice insurance policies. Check your policy. Examples of intentional torts follow.

■ **Assault and battery: Assault** is an unjustified attempt or threat to touch someone. **Battery** is actual physical harm to someone. Remember this when a client refuses a treatment or medication. The client gives implied consent (permission) for certain routine treatments by entering the institution. Clients retain the right to refuse verbally any treatment and may leave the institution when they choose unless they are there for court-ordered treatment. Nurses can protect themselves from assaultive clients but can use only as much force as is considered reasonable to protect themselves.

According to the Emergency Nurse Legal Bulletin (1982, p. 2.), "Treating a client without consent is a battery whether or not the treatment is medically beneficial." For example, a physician may attempt to get a court order to allow a blood transfusion for someone opposed on religious grounds. However, "when the client is fully competent, is not pregnant, and has no children, a court is unlikely to compel a life-saving blood transfusion over the client's refusal." When faced with a similar situation, the practical/vocational nurse respects the client's belief system and notifies the supervisor for further advice or interpretation.

■ **False imprisonment and use of restraints:** *False imprisonment* is keeping someone detained against his or her will. It can include use of restraints or seclusion in a room without cause and without a physician's order. Restraint by verbal threats of physical harm is also included in this category.

■ **Defamation:** *Defamation* means damage to someone's reputation through false communi-

Critical Thinking Exercise

How does the Patient's Bill of Rights relate to the care of an elderly confused client?

cation or communication without their permission. **Libel** is defamation through written communication or pictures. **Slander** is defamation by verbalizing untrue or private information (gossip) to a third party. Clients have the right to expect that you will share information about them only with health care providers who are actively involved in promoting their health. This is called **confidentiality.** The client has the right to expect you to speak the truth. Additional unnecessary conversation with coworkers and those outside the agency can result in a charge of defamation. The same is true of all documented information or of invasion of privacy by taking unwanted photographs or showing the client affliction to others, students included, without permission. The client's privacy is protected by law. Remember: Loose lips may sink your ship.

You and other health care providers have the same right to privacy. You often are privy to information about the personal lives of nurses, physicians, and other coworkers. Although the desire to repeat the information you hear may be tempting, it is best left unsaid.

Beyond the Scope of Practice and Experience

As an LP/VN, you might be asked by an RN or physician to perform nursing duties beyond your scope of practice or experience. It is up to you to speak up. For example:

I am not comfortable doing something beyond the LP/VN nurse practice act.

I have never done this before.

I will be glad to learn if you teach me, watch me demonstrate in return, and write a memo for my file that this has been done.

I was taught to do this while in school but did not have a chance to _____ a real person. Please demonstrate and then watch me do it before I do it on my own.

My orientation here did not include how to do _____. I need to be shown (or told if safe just to follow directions). Will you do that or assign someone else to show me? I learn quickly so it will be time well spent.

You have provided a detailed orientation, but I do not feel ready (or qualified) to assume a charge nurse position. I think I need more _____, so I can function effectively and within my nurse practice act.

Also, be sure that when you are seeking employment you check out the philosophy, mission statement, and policies of your potential place of employment. Ask what is included in your job, the period of orientation you will receive, what the information will cover, and who will do the orientation. If you discover during your inquiry that your work will cover more than you have learned or is beyond the scope of practice, say so. Listen also to your affective response: what is your intuition saying? Getting a job just to get a job may result in being fired and/or losing your license as quickly for what may not be your fault. The ideal of ethics is that all share your ethics and are fair. The reality of ethics is sometimes quite different.

Physical and Emotional Abuse

In the course of your career in practical/vocational nursing, you will probably suspect or actually see the results of some type of abuse. As a practical/vocational nurse, you have a legal responsibility to report your suspicions or observations of abuse by following your facility's abuse policy. Note that a "suspicion" is a nagging doubt. Refer to your state's abuse laws for specific rules that govern your responsibility for reporting abuse. It is important to be empathetic (as opposed to sympathetic)

so that your observations or reporting will be as objective as possible. Becoming a part of the client's emotions may lead you to jump to conclusions or accept a particularly convincing but untrue explanation. Whether the client is a child, woman, man, or elder, reputations are at stake. Once an accusation has been made, it is difficult to be truly free from it, even when it has been proved groundless.

Follow your facility's policy for reporting abuse. The social services department can be helpful in helping you report abuse. Offer concrete, specific observations. Quote statements made and avoid offering a personal interpretation. Let the facts speak for themselves.

Good Samaritan Acts

Good Samaritan acts stipulate that a person who renders emergency care in good faith at the scene of an accident is immune from civil liability for his or her action while providing the care. All 50 states and the District of Columbia have enacted Good Samaritan laws (Brown, 1999, p. 65.) The state statutes are of special concern to nurses and physicians who provide emergency care outside of the agency that employs them. The statutes vary, so check with your state board of nursing or agency risk manager for information on your state Good Samaritan laws. You could also check the National EMS Information Exchanges data base on Good Samaritan laws to see whether your state's law is posted at https//naemt.ort/nemsie/immunity.htm.

Fidelity (Be True)

The fourth ethical principle of fidelity encompasses the entire scope of nursing practice. It challenges each nurse to be faithful to the charge of acting in the client's best interest when the capacity to make free choice is no longer available. This does not include rescuing behaviors and becoming paternalistic in making decisions for vulnerable clients. This ultimately includes knowing the difference between the personal feelings of the nurse and the client's wishes (Turner et al., 1998, p. 7). To assist in understanding fidelity, the topics of client competency, confidentiality, casual transmission, and information that must be revealed are included.

Client Competency

You can expect to hear increased use of the term competency in both a legal and clinical sense. The following details provide a brief framework to help you use this term correctly.

Client competency has both a *legal* meaning and a *clinical* meaning. Some client rights issues are based on proof of competency or incompetency within the court system.

Legal competency refers to a client who is:

■ Eighteen years old or older.
■ Pregnant or a married woman.
■ A self-supporting minor (referred to as a legally emancipated minor).
■ Competent in the eyes of the law (incompetency is determined by the court).

Clinical competency refers to a client who is able to:

■ Identify the problem.
■ Understand the options for care and the possible consequences.
■ Make a decision.
■ Provide sound reasons for the option he or she chooses.

Confidentiality

Confidentiality is involved in the principle of fidelity. The client has the right to have information shared only with his or her immediate health care providers. For example, your neighbor is admitted. You are not assigned to his care. However, you want to know about his condition. Based on confidentiality, you are violating his confidentiality by reading his chart.

What is the difference between privacy and confidentiality? "*Privacy* refers to the right to be left alone and free from intrusion, including the right to choose care based on personal beliefs, feelings, or attitudes; the right to govern bodily integrity (accepting or rejecting treatment or exposure of the body); and the right to control when and how sensitive information is shared. *Confidentiality* refers to the nondisclosure of information regarding patients" (Badzek and Gross, 1999, p. 52). These days breaches in privacy and confidentiality occur more readily. Computer charting has already been noted on page 307. Fax transmission of sensitive data is common, information is e-mailed to other facilities, documents are copied.

Where is the Fax located in the clinical area?
Is it possible for visitors, etc. to see what has been Faxed?
Who on the unit is responsible for checking in Fax transmissions?
Is there a facility policy that helps limit who has access to incoming and outgoing Fax transmissions?

Casual Transmission

Sometimes confidentiality is breached by discussing a client in a public area like the cafeteria.

 Critical Thinking Exercise

Suppose you overhear a couple of LP/VNs speaking disrespectfully about an obese client and complaining how difficult it is to move him. What would you do?

Often it is not necessary to mention a client's name for others to know who is being discussed. Confidentiality has been breached, as has dignity. "Dignity is the condition or quality of being esteemed, honored, or regarded as worthy of respect. Such esteem comes not only from a sense of self-worth but from how others perceive us" (Haddad, 1998, p. 21).

Information That Must Be Revealed

There are laws that require reporting of certain client information without their consent. The purpose is to protect the public. For information that many states require be reported, see Box 18–7.

Justice (Fair to All)

Justice, a fifth ethical principle, means that you must give clients their due and treat them fairly. This implies that patients with the same diagnosis should receive the same level of care (Challey and Loriz, 1998, p. 17). Consider the current topic of **futility.** Health care is expensive, but medicine often can extend a life past the point of natural death.

Box 18–7. Information That Must Be Revealed

1. *Communicable disease* to the local health department or the Centers for Disease Control. This includes AIDS, but the nature of the disclosure varies.
2. *Vaccine-related adverse reactions* to the Department of Health and Human Services. (Reporting of some reactions are mandatory; others voluntary. Call 800-822-7967 for the FDA's reportable events table.)
3. *Criminal acts.* All states mandate reporting of rape cases. Some mandate reporting of injuries by gunshot or sharp instruments. Some states require reporting of blood alcohol levels (BAL) beyond the legal limit.
4. *Equipment-related injuries.* When use of a medical device results in injury or death, it is reported.
5. *When there is a clear and present danger.* Most common are laws mandating reporting of client mistreatment or professional misconduct.
6. *Abuse and neglect of a client or elderly person,* usually to police or social services.
7. *Incompetence or unprofessional acts* as defined by state law. Facilities have policies for how to report (Ventura, 1999, pp. 61–64).

At what point is treatment considered futile and the client allowed to die? Consider the following questions presented by a medical ethicist from your own point of view.

   Critical Thinking Exercise

Health care is expensive. So is insurance. At what point do we limit what treatments insurance companies and government pay for?

_____

_____

Should all treatments be available to all people? Who pays?

_____

_____

_____

_____

"In a democracy, being fair (being just) does not mean giving all people the same things; it does mean treating all the same, at least within the legal process" (Hall, 1996, p. 300). As a nurse you make daily decisions in order to give clients "their due." For example, the clients on your floor represent different levels of wealth, social status, culture, religion, and moral and value systems. All are acutely ill. The newest client has Kaposi's sarcoma, a defining component of acquired immune deficiency syndrome (AIDS). Do you classify AIDS as a life-threatening illness or as a retribution for behaviors you consider unethical? If your ethics interfere with the care you give, you may find yourself (1) giving this client more time than needed and doing less than needed for other acutely ill clients, or (2) providing minimal care for him and lavishing attention on those who "deserve the care."

There are many daily care issues relating to justice. Listen to your inner talk: "He's so young—so much living left to do; she's had a full life already; she's an alcoholic—never took care of her kids"—and so on.

Critical Thinking Exercise

At the end of your next clinical day, take time to reflect on your reaction to clients and how it affected your client care. Did the word "deserve" enter in your thoughts, or did you provide justice for all?

Practical Application of Ethics and the Law in Difficult Situations

You have learned that nursing demands that you be responsible. This means being reliable and trustworthy. At no time can you expect a peer, supervisor, or client to say to you, "It's OK that you didn't come to work today because your car isn't functioning properly," or "It's OK if we talk about your interests and problems today" (rather than those of the clients), or "It's OK that you didn't do the work you were assigned because you're having a bad day." Nursing says, "I'm sorry that you have problems to cope with that are heavy, but it's up to you to deal with them because your priority, in this vocation, is the client."

Accountability in Nursing

The word accountability means that you are answerable. As a nursing student, you are answerable to yourself, to your assigned client, to the team leader, to the physician, and to your instructor, who constantly evaluates your work. As an LP/VN, accountability to the instructor is replaced by accountability to the employing agency. You are held accountable for all the nursing actions that you perform or are assigned to perform. The measures of accountability are the nursing standards of practice.

Situations and Documentation

If you are asking "How can I apply what I have just learned? It seems so remote from real nursing," we want to assist you in jump-starting your critical thinking process. "Situations and documentation" is offered as a method of practical application of ethics and the law. Use the information now as needed and again as reference when you graduate. We begin with three suggestions:

1. Know your state nurse practice act. It is the final authority legally as an LP/VN.
2. Be familiar with your agency policy. Remember that agency policy cannot give you permission to function beyond your state nurse practice act.
3. Be familiar with the NAPNES standards of practice, the NFLPN nursing standards, and the NFLPN code for practical/vocational nursing. They recommend minimal acceptable standards of nursing behavior.

SITUATION. LATE ENTRY: When you get home after the shift you realize you forgot to chart or forgot to chart something important. There is no law against making entries out of order.

Documentation. If the information is very important, such as giving a medication, call the nursing unit immediately. Speak to the nurse assigned to your client and ask him or her to chart the information for you. As soon as possible, usually the next day, countersign the charting.

SITUATION. DOCUMENTING UAP CARE: Know the agency policy. Many agencies have UAP checklists for routine care. The LP/VN follows up on the data as necessary. If you are documenting nonroutine care, you want to be sure that you have either witnessed or verified that the care was given.

Documentation. Write in the name, followed with UAP. For example, "Signe Hill, UAP, reported that _____." Follow with what you observed to verify that actual care was given.

SITUATION. DOCUMENTING SOMEONE ELSE'S CARE: If a nurse on the unit asks you to document care given by him or her that you did not witness and you do it, you could be at risk legally.

Documentation. This is quite different from having a staff member call in after he or she is off duty to ask you to make an entry. When the nurse is right there, refuse to do it. Offer, instead, to assist in completing his or her work so that he or she will be able to chart.

SITUATION. ILLEGAL ALTERATION OF A CLIENT'S RECORD: Tampering with client records includes (1) adding to someone else's notes, (2) destroying all or part of the record, (3) rewriting all or part of the record, (4) omitting important facts, (5) purposely writing inaccurate information, or (6) falsifying a date or time or adding a late entry without identifying it as a late entry (*Surefire Documentation,* 1999, pp. 260–261). Alteration can result in a person being charged with fraud. The usual reason someone tampers with a record is to cover up improper or ineffective care.

Documentation. When you discover a tampered entry, immediately contact your nursing administrator or risk manager. It is not a good idea to try to correct the documentation. The administrator will probably copy both your notes and the tampered entries. Continue to document honestly. You may be asked to write an incident report.

SITUATION. PERSONAL CRITICISM OF YOU IN CLIENT'S RECORD: This form of criticizing your client care goes against accepted nursing standards.

Documentation. Once in the record, you may not alter the charting or add an entry to defend yourself. Notify your administrator and speak to the nurse who made the entry. Perhaps he or she will be willing to complete a truthful incident report, noting only what he or she saw without blaming you or anyone else. If this problem is noteworthy, the administrator may choose to have an inservice program on proper use of nursing notes.

SITUATION. ILLEGIBLE PHYSICIAN'S OR-DER: It happens! Ask for clarification. If you cannot reach the physician, contact your supervisor and he or she will follow a chain of command to obtain clarification. Also, don't forget that there may be another nurse on the unit who has no problem reading the physician's writing. If you find that you have problems reading certain physician's orders, get used to checking the order with him or her before the person leaves the unit.

Documentation. Document your attempts to reach the physician and the method used. A telephone log book works well for this. When you finally have clear orders, write an entry on the physician's order sheet. For example, date, time, clarification of orders for date, time (of original entry), t.o. (telephone order), Dr. _____, your name and title.

SITUATION. TELEPHONE ORDERS: When used, physician orders conveyed by telephone should be given directly to the nurse, who repeats the order back to the physician. Spelling of medications or treatments is checked if necessary. So many medications sound alike, and doses can be confusing. If it is a sensitive order, meaning one that carries special risk, two people should listen to the order. (This is suggested for all telephone orders.)

Be sure to check the policy of your employer about the legality of an LPN accepting phone orders.

Documentation. The order is entered on the physician's order sheet as quickly as possible. Note the date and time of the order and that it was a telephone order (t.o.). Write your full name and credentials. If another nurse listened to the conversation with you, have him or her sign after your name. The order is then carried out the usual way. If the physician called the order in response to your data collection (assessment), write your reason in the nurse's notes for calling the physician as well as the data you collected on the client prior to the call. Once the order is carried out, collect data (assess) regarding the client's response to the intervention ordered.

SITUATION. VERBAL ORDERS: Verbal orders should not be accepted except in emergency situations. Written orders by the physician protect the physician, the client, and the nurse. It is difficult to explain to a court why the physician, who has access to the chart, did not write the order. *Verbal orders should be repeated for accuracy* using the physician's exact words. Ask for names of medications to be spelled if any confusion exists.

Documentation. Record the order on the physician's order sheet as soon as possible. Note the date, time, and that it was a v.o. (verbal order). Write your name and credentials. Example: Ellen A. Zaic, LVN, charge nurse for Frederick Jones, MD. (Many agency's policies require that the physician co-sign the order within 24 hours.) Transcribe the order the usual way. Document data collection (assessment) you have done before and after following the order.

SITUATION. QUESTIONABLE ORDER: A physician's written or verbal order is a legal order that the nurse must carry out. However, the nurse has the responsibility to recognize whether an order may harm the client and refuse to carry it out. Deal directly with the physician first. If this is unsuccessful, use the nursing chain of command, beginning with your immediate supervisor. If the problem is not resolved through the nursing channels, it must reach the physician chain of command quickly to avoid harm to the client.

Documentation. Never change the order on your own. The physician will usually rewrite the order or give a new telephone order. If not resolved at this point, document your refusal, data collection as rationale, discussion with the physician (include name), and whom you contacted.

For additional help, record their responses. Remember to note carefully the times of contact. A follow-up letter to the nursing administrator may be needed for the record. Be as objective as possible in discussing the event. Some agencies have special forms and procedures for documentation.

SITUATION. GIVING ADVICE: It has probably happened already that someone sought your advice for a remedy or the name of a competent physician. It probably even felt flattering. Be careful: you may have crossed the line into practicing medicine by suggesting something as simple as an over-the-counter medication. Giving the name of a specific physician may open you up to slander or libel. Give a list of physicians, if you must, rather than naming one (advice to your neighbors puts you in the same legal bind).

Documentation. In an agency setting, share the client's questions with the head nurse or physician. Document the dates, times, and persons with whom you discussed the client's concerns.

SITUATION. UNDERSTAFFED UNIT: "Floating" is working in an area that is not your usual work area. In 1991, the Joint Commission on Accreditation of Healthcare Organizations (JCAHO) revised its nursing care standards that are used as a basis for making accreditation decisions. One of the standards states that nursing staff should be competent to fulfill their assigned responsibilities. Directives from the Joint Commission include the need for timely and adequate orientation and cross-training. Practical/vocational nurses need to receive adequate orientation, cross-training, and education for float duty. You are responsible for informing supervisors if you do not feel competent to work in any assigned area.

Some agencies will fire you for not "floating." Instead of refusing the assignment, negotiate with the nurse in charge regarding priorities of care. "Nice to do" tasks may have to be left undone. If you do not know how to do something, ask for instruction.

Notify your supervisor if you are short-staffed. There is a legal concern regarding **abandonment.** You may not leave your place of employment until you can transfer the care of clients to your replacement.

Documentation. Follow this with a memo because a memo is more effective than verbal notification alone. Keep a copy for yourself.

SITUATION. SIGNING A WILL: Nurses may witness the signing of a will if they do not stand to gain personally from the will. Check your agency policy before doing so. As a student, check with your instructor before you agree to witness the signing of a will.

Documentation. Document in the client's record that you witnessed the signing of a will.

SITUATION. POSSIBLE NEGLIGENCE: Be sure you have all the facts before acting on your suspicions. Collect data from the client, anyone who witnessed the behavior, client's chart, etc. Report possible negligence to the nursing supervisor.

Documentation. Fill out an incident report with facts only. Record events and client and witness statements. Include names and titles of persons to whom you have made a report with dates/times. In the nursing notes, describe any intervention you have taken to prevent further harm to the client.

SITUATION. STANDING ORDERS: Some states do not allow standing orders except in intensive and coronary care units. Because standing orders call for making judgments, the practical/vocational nurse must always check first with the RN before carrying them out. If you are a charge nurse, request that standing orders be reviewed by the physician on a regular basis.

Documentation. Document data collection (assessment) that has caused you to be concerned about particular standing orders. Document to whom you have expressed your concern—date and time.

SITUATION. DISCHARGE INSTRUCTIONS AND CLIENT EDUCATION: The professional nurse, physician, podiatrist, or dentist initiates health teaching for clients. The practical/vocational nurse reinforces this teaching. Teaching is the domain of the professional nurse, and LP/VNs play a supportive role in it, once the instruction or education has been started by the RN. Discharge instructions are given verbally and in writing, with the client signing a form indicating that he or she understands the information. Preprinted information forms are valuable and are available in many agencies. The practical/vocational nurse initiates client teaching in the area of basic health care. See Box 18–8 for suggestions.

Documentation. All interventions, including client teaching, whether reinforced or initiated, must be documented in the client's chart. Be descriptive. Saying that discharge instructions or client education was provided is not enough if there is a legal question after discharge.

Telephone Logs

Telephone logs can be used routinely to document the time, problem, and advice received or given. Also, attempted calls to physicians or supervisors should be logged in.

Excellent additional information is available in Mosby's *Surefire Documentation* (1999) on documentation during client care, in challenging client situations, and for difficult professional problems.

Box 18–8. Basic Health Care Teaching for the LP/VN

- How to avoid constipation
- Pyramid diet
- Cleanliness
- How to avoid colds
- Babysitting hints
- Parenting techniques

Summary

☐ Personal ethics are the building blocks of your nursing ethics. They are made up of what you believe in, value, and practice in your personal life. Your personal and professional ethics modify as you continue your personal and professional growth. Critical thinking provides the steps that allow sound ethical decisions to be made.

☐ Sometimes your ethical views differ from legal realities. In nursing, your state's nurse practice act provides the basis for the legal parameters governing your nursing practice. *Know it well.* When ethical questions arise, the legal system becomes involved in determining what can and cannot be done.

☐ Nursing ethics are based on the principles of autonomy, beneficence, nonmaleficence, fidelity, and justice. Autonomy says, "The client has the right to decide." Beneficence says, "Do good." Nonmaleficence says, "Do no harm." Fidelity says, "Be true." Justice says, "Give all clients their due." These are basic principles to keep in mind as new ethical questions arise.

☐ Tort law is based on doing no harm in relationships. In nursing it refers to the professional relationship between the client and the nurse. Torts are either unintentional or intentional. Negligence and malpractice are examples of unintentional torts—"performance less than the standard of practice." Assault and battery, false imprisonment (including use of restraints without orders), and defamation of character are all examples of intentional torts.

☐ Check out the philosophy, mission statement, and policies of your potential place of employment *before* you accept the job. You cannot abandon your client in the middle of a legal procedure because your ethics differ from those of the client.

☐ The living will and the durable power of attorney are two ways in which an individual can express his or her wishes in regard to medical interventions in a major medical event. The living will is legal in most but not all states in the United States. It is not legal in Canada. The durable power of attorney provides for a legal decision maker if the client is unable to make decisions. It is legal in all states, but each state form may differ.

☐ You have the responsibility of knowing the law—the nurse practice act of your state. It is a major resource for the nursing standards of care. Nurses are held accountable for their nursing actions, and ignorance of the law is not accepted as an excuse for illegal or unethical practices.

☐ Common areas of nursing liability most often can be avoided by following the guidelines learned in basic nursing. Medication errors are number one on the list of recurring liabilities. To avoid liability, function within the standard of care. Keep current. Take classes. Read journals. The worst questions an LP/VN can hear from a lawyer are, "You haven't taken *any* classes since you graduated?", "You do not subscribe to a nursing journal?", and "You do not belong to your professional organization?"

☐ Pay attention to the ethical guidelines put forth by your professional organization. Join your professional organization and take advantage of current updates. Have a voice in what becomes the law.

☐ Guidelines for nursing ethics have been developed by the International Council of Nurses (ICN), the National Federation of Licensed Practical Nurses (NFLPN), and the National Association of Practical Nurse Education and Service (NAPNES) for practical and vocational nurses.

☐ Evaluate your personal values and compare them with the accepted codes of nursing ethics. Difficult decisions about topics such as AIDS, abortion, organ transplantation, confidentiality, maintenance of life through life-support systems, and refusal of treatment due to religious convictions are some of the many ethical and legal issues facing nurses today.

Review Questions

1. What dictates the legal duties and functions of a practical/vocational nurse?
   A. The employer
   B. The U.S. Constitution
   C. The state nurse practice act
   D. The professional nursing organization
2. To what level of performance is a student practical nurse held?
   A. Student nurse
   B. Graduate practical nurse
   C. Licensed practical nurse
   D. Registered nurse
3. What is meant by being sued for breach of duty?
   A. The nurse was behind in her 8 PM meds.
   B. The nurse was hired to give meds and do treatments, not toilet residents.
   C. The nurse was guilty of poor time management techniques.
   D. The nurse did not perform her duties according to the standard of care.

4. How can the LP/VN explain the difference between the living will and the durable power of attorney to a relative?
   A. "There is essentially no difference between the two documents."
   B. "The living will is the superior of the two documents."
   C. "The living will states everything you want and do not want to have done for you under all circumstances."
   D. "The durable power of attorney names a proxy who will decide what medical treatment you will receive when you are unable to specify for yourself."
5. What can the LP/VN be sued for, for discussing details about the supervisor's sex life that is damaging to his/her reputation?
   A. Libel
   B. Battery
   C. Slander
   D. Assault

References

Alfaro-LeFevre R. *Critical Thinking in Nursing: A Practical Approach,* 2nd ed. Philadelphia: W. B. Saunders Company, 1999, Chapter 4.

Badzek L, Gross L. Confidentiality and privacy. Am J Nurs 99(6):52–54, 1999.

Bolander VB. *Sorensen and Luckmann's Basic Nursing,* 3rd ed. Philadelphia: W. B. Saunders Company, 1994.

Brown SM. Good Samaritan laws: Protection and limits. RN 62(11):65–68, 1999.

Challey PS, Loriz L. Ethics in the trenches: Decision making in practice. Am J Nurs 98(6):17–20, 1998.

Daly BJ, Berry D, Fitzpatrick JJ, Drew B, Montgomery K. Assisted suicide: Implications for nurses and nursing. Nursing Outlook 45:209–214, 1997.

Dempski K. If you have to give a deposition. RN 63(1):59–60, 2000.

Emergency Nurse Legal Bulletin. Westville, NJ: Med/Law Publishers, 1982, p. 2.

Haddad A. What Would You Do? RN 61(7):21–24, 1998.

Hall JK. *Nursing Ethics and Law.* Philadelphia: W.B. Saunders, 1996.

Haynor PM. Meeting the challenge of advanced directives. Am J Nurs 98(3): 27–32, 1998.

High Public Esteem for Nurses. Am J Nurs 100(1):21, 2000.

Legal side when long-term residents require emergent care. Am J Nurs 98(9):56, 1998.

Minnesota Board of Nursing. Board implements on-line verification. For Your Information 2(3):4, 1995.

Murphy RN. Legal and practical impact of clinical practice guidelines on nursing and medical practice. Nurse Practitioner 22(3):138–148, 1997.

National Association of Practical Nurse Education and Service. NAPNES Standards of Practice for Licensed Practical/Vocational Nurses. 1976, 1981, 1993.

NFLPN. Nursing Practice Standards Booklet. Raleigh, NC: NFLPN, 1991.

Patient's Bill of Rights. St. Paul, MN: MHHP. 8/1/95 (revised 8/1/98)

Report tracks impact of Oregon's assisted suicide law. RN 62(5):16, 1999.

Sullivan GH. Getting informed consent. RN 61(4):59–62, 1998.

Surefire Documentation. St. Louis: C. V. Mosby, 1999.

Turner SL, Bechtel GA, Davidhizer R. Ethical principles in enhancement of patient care. Am J Practical Nurs 48(1):6–9, 1998.

Ventura MJ. When information must be revealed. RN 62(2):61–64, 1999.

Wolfe S. When is it time to die? RN 61(11):50–56, 1998.

Bibliography

Anderson G. Medicine vs. religion: The case of Jehovah's Witnesses. Health Soc Work, 1983.

Haddad A. Ethics in action. RN 62(1):23–25, 1997.

Haddad A. Ethics in action. RN 62(9):25–28, 1997.

Hustad GL, Hustad JH. *Ethical Decision Making.* St. Louis: C. V. Mosby, 1995.

Mason DJ. On human perfection. Am J Nurs 99(3):7, 1999.

Ventura MJ. Are these nurses criminals? RN, December 1997, pp. 26–29.

Ventura MJ. Where nurses stand on abortion. RN 62(3):44–47, 1999.

Wolfe S. When care givers endanger patients. RN 61(12):28–32, 1998.

The Final Is NCLEX-PN

Outline

Key Terms

boards
CAT
cursor

enter key
mock examinations
multistate licensure

NCLEX-PN
space bar

Objectives

Upon completing this chapter you will be able to:
1. Explain what is meant by NCLEX-PN.
2. Explain what is meant by computerized adaptive testing (CAT).
3. Discuss the requirements of your state board of nursing for eligibility to take the licensing examination.
4. Explain how multistate licensure works.
5. Differentiate between a temporary work permit and licensure.
6. Discuss minimum competency.
7. Practice exercises to reduce test-taking anxiety.
8. Discuss review books and mock examinations.

Almost without exception, when student nurses are asked about their goal for the year, they respond by saying, "I want to pass the **boards**," meaning, pass the licensure examination.

Does the thought of having to take a test leave you feeling numb? Welcome to the club. Some anxiety about test taking is normal. It can work to your benefit. Without it you would probably watch television instead of studying. Once again the research results are on your side. Some learners blame fear and anxiety in test-taking situations for their poor test performance. Research has indicated that if you do not do well on tests, odds are that one or more

of the following reasons apply to you: (1) you are less intelligent than the average student, (2) you have poor study habits, or (3) you have weak test-taking skills. The first reason does not apply in your situation because you would not have been admitted to the practical nursing program if it were true. Chapter 6 deals with overcoming poor study habits and with test-taking skills.

In our experience, lack of preparation of the subject matter and poor test-taking skills are the most common reasons for low test scores. Occasionally a learner has such great fear and anxiety about test taking that it interferes with what was studied. This situation requires a knowledge of relaxation techniques, or even drugs, but this is the exception, not the rule.

What Is the NCLEX-PN?

The **NCLEX-PN** is the National Council Licensing Examination for Practical Nurses. "To ensure public protection, each jurisdiction requires a candidate for licensure to pass an examination that measures the competencies needed to practice safely and effectively as a newly licensed, entry-level practical/vocational nurse" (NCLEX-PN Test Plan 1998). The NCLEX results provide the basis for licenses granted to practical/vocational nurses by boards of nursing. The boards of nursing are the only agencies that can release the test results to candidates.

The same examination—the NCLEX-PN—is given in the United States, American Samoa, the District of Columbia, Guam, the northern Mariana Islands, Puerto Rico, and the Virgin Islands. This makes it possible to provide licensure by endorsement from one board of nursing to another. Endorsement means that an LPN or LVN may apply for licensure without retesting when moving within this jurisdiction. Your state or territory may already be involved in **multistate licensure** endorsement for nursing regulation.

An easy way to understand this model is to think about your driver's license. Once you have a valid license in your state, you can drive in any state provided you follow the driving regulations of that state. The same principle applies in multistate licensure. If you are licensed in a state with multistate licensure, you will be able to practice in other states that have passed multistate licensure legislation. You will have to adhere to any differences in licensure within each state.

Utah is the first state to enact multistate licensure, followed by Arkansas, Maryland, North Carolina, Texas, Iowa, Nebraska, South Dakota, Wisconsin, and Mississippi. Maine, Delaware, and Idaho anticipate adoption soon. The effective date for the multistate licensure legislation was January 1, 2000,

to match completion of NURSYS, a system for tracking nursing licensure and discipline (Ventura, 1999, p. 58).

 Learning Exercise: Multistate Licensure

Contact your Board of Nursing (address in Appendix A):

1. Has your state or territory adopted multistate licensure since the publication of this text?
2. How does the mutual recognition model of nursing licensure differ from the current licensure model?

Content of the NCLEX-PN

The National Council of State Boards of Nursing developed the NCLEX-PN. A document entitled Test Plan for the National Council Licensure Examination for Practical Nurses is available from the National Council of State Boards of Nursing, 676 St. Clair Street, Suite 550, Chicago, IL 60611-2921. Phone: (312) 787-6555. Website: http://www.ncsbn.org. The 1999 NCLEX-PN examination reflects the outcome of Yocom's (1997) *Job Analysis Study for Licensed Practical/Vocational Nurses,* the National Council's Examination Committee, and 1997 Job Analysis Panel of Experts. Over 10,000 LP/VNs were involved in the job analysis. The NCLEX-PN is a secure examination, so no actual test questions are included in the Test Plan. However, the document is helpful in explaining the general content areas of the test. It is worthwhile to send for and read the entire document.

The test plan consists of concepts, principles, and nursing process integrated throughout a one-content dimension: Client needs. The four major categories of client needs are

- Safe, effective care environment
- Health promotion and maintenance
- Psychosocial integrity and
- Physiologic integrity

All content categories reflect client needs across the life span in a variety of settings.

Computerized Adaptive Testing (CAT)

Since April, 1994, practical/vocational nursing graduates (candidates) have taken the NCLEX-PN by computer. This method is called computerized adaptive testing **(CAT).** Testing centers are located across the United States and its territories.

Major Benefits of CAT

The computer selects the items you will answer while you are taking the examination. This gives you the best chance to demonstrate your competence.

As you answer an item on the examination, the computer adapts the examination to your answer. This is possible because the computer has a large number of test items stored in its memory. As you answer the standardized multiple-choice items, the computer chooses next the best item to measure your competence. The computer goes down a "pathway" or "branch." Questions are based on the candidate's previous answer. Testing stops when the minimum number of questions is answered if it can be determined with certainty that the candidate passed or failed. Otherwise the testing continues until a clear pass/fail decision can be made, the maximum number of questions is reached, or time runs out. Practical/vocational nurses answer a minimum of 85 questions. The maximum number of questions during the five-hour maximum testing period is 205 (National Council Completes 1997 job analysis. Issues, 1997, p. 1).

The computer indicates that you have completed the test. Your state board of nursing is informed of the results and notifies you in approximately two to three weeks. Test results are not available over the phone. Candidates who do not pass receive a NCLEX-PN Diagnostic Profile. It identifies areas for improvement as well as areas of strength. An "X" near the "higher performance" on the right does not mean that the candidate necessarily performed well in that area. It just means that the performance was higher than in other "X" areas. Truly high areas are not reported for failing candidates. The bottom of the profile shows the relative performance in the content areas. An "X" far to the left indicates weakness and a need to restudy content. If the "X" is equally located to the left, spend most of the time restudying the area with the most content area in the test. Remember, however, that the examination is scored on the overall performance on the whole test, not the sections.

Additional Benefits of Computer Testing

Because of the computer method, *year-round testing* is available in centers scattered throughout the United States. Your nursing instructor can identify the specific areas available in your state. Your state board of nursing gives you permission to take the licensure examination after you graduate and apply for licensure. They authorize you to make an appointment at a testing center. The testing center will schedule you within 30 days after you call to make your appointment unless you specify a later date. Call for an appointment soon, even if you do not want to take the test immediately. Waiting to schedule can limit the available dates. If you wait until the authorization to test is near to expiring, you may not get in to test before expiration. The dates of authorization to test cannot be extended regardless of the reason. This will require reregistering and repaying to test (National Council of State Boards of Nursing, 1997, p. 4).

Practical/vocational nursing candidates will find the computer method *less stressful,* even if they lack previous computer experience. Each testing room is limited to no more than 15 candidates. The test-taking area is quiet and relaxed. There is enough time to answer each question. Just pace yourself. There are two breaks; one is mandatory. The computer lets you know how much time you have spent on the test. The testing time is shorter with the computer, and notification is quick.

A newly licensed practical nurse called her former instructor to say she passed the NCLEX-PN. "All I needed was one finger to operate the computer. The directions were easy and the sample items before the exam eased my mind."

NCLEX-PN Test-Taking Tips

Types of Items

Items in the NCLEX-PN are all multiple choice at the cognitive levels of knowledge, comprehension, application, and analysis (NCLEX-PN Test Plan, 1999, p. 3). There are two types of items: (1) case scenario, and (2) stand-alone items (i.e., miscellaneous items that do not pertain to an ongoing scenario). Read the scenario or stand-alone item carefully. Remember that some of the items presented may be for validation. Validation items are being tried out for use in future NCLEX-PN tests. You will not be penalized for answering them incorrectly. The only problem is, NCLEX-PN will not identify these items as validation items.

(Hint: Stay calm when you read a situation or item that you think you have never heard of. It could be a validation item. Or it could be a situation in which you could apply information from another area you know well.)

Answering the Items

Items appear one at a time on the computer screen. You can review the item as long as you like. However, once you have recorded your answer you can-

not go back and change it. You may not leave an item without answering it. Answer each item even if you must guess at the answer. This permits the computer to continue and to choose the next item for you.

Recording Answers

No prior computer experience is necessary or beneficial for taking the NCLEX-PN computer test. Prior to taking the NCLEX-PN, all candidates receive instructions about how to record their answers and a practice session. Three sample questions provide actual practice. "Sample" is printed on each sample question on the screen. Once the word "sample" is no longer there, the actual test has begun (National Council of State Boards of Nursing, 1997, p. 5). The information you need to know about the computer to take your licensing examination is limited to two computer keys and an item called a cursor. A description of these three items follows. All other computer keys are locked off so that nothing will happen if you accidentally push them.

- The **cursor:** A blinking light that the candidate moves to each of the four choices that are provided for each item.

  The **space bar:** A long bar located at the bottom of the keyboard. The space bar moves the cursor among the answer choices when pushed.

  The **enter key:** A key on the computer marked *enter*. After the cursor is moved to the choice the candidate thinks is the right answer, the answer is recorded when this key is struck TWICE. You will not be able to go on to the next item until the answer is entered. The computer needs the entered answer to select the next item. ■

Keeping Track of Time

Bring a watch. There are no clocks in the room. Avoid spending long periods of time on any one item. This will allow you to pace yourself.

Test-Taking Etiquette

The National Council of the Boards of Nursing have selected National Computer Systems, Inc. (NCS) as the new test service for the NCLEX examination beginning October 1, 2002. There will be no interruption in testing for nurse candidates. The NCLEX Examination Program will continue to be administered by the current test vendor, the Chauncey Group International, until the new contract begins (Minnesota Board of Nursing, 1999, p. 5). The testing takes place at existing testing centers to ensure test security. Until October 1, 2002:

1. Call to arrange for an appointment.
2. Arrive one-half hour early. If you arrive late you may be seated if there is space. Otherwise you will have to reschedule the test and pay a new fee.
3. Present your Authorization to Test letter, which is mailed to you after your application has been processed by the board of nursing.
4. Sign in on a log, entering the time you check in and the type of test you are taking. (The person in the carrel next to you may be someone other than a nurse candidate.)
5. Along with your Authorization to Test letter, present a picture ID and another form of identification.
6. Look to one monitor and view your demographic data (from your application) to verify data.
7. You are fingerprinted (right thumb).
8. Belongings, including the contents of your pockets, are placed in a locker; you keep the key. You may bring a snack to keep in your locker to eat at break. Candy, chewing gum, food, drinks, purses, wallets, pens, pencils, beepers, cell phones, post-it notes, study materials or aids, and calculators are not allowed in the testing room (National Council of State Board of Nursing, 1997, p. 1.)
9. Sit on a chair.
10. A small camera will record your facial image. You can see this on the monitor. The image is frozen and accompanies your test results and thumb prints for scoring (security

purposes). If the monitor does not work, three Polaroid snapshots will be taken.
11. Enter the testing room.
12. Take your seat and adjust the height.
13. Adjust the monitor (lighter or darker).
14. Bright pink scrap paper (six sheets counted) are given to each candidate. Raise your hand if you need more. They are counted and returned at the end of the test.
15. Pencils are provided.
16. Do the practice exercise and begin the test.
17. A video and audio recording is made of the examination period. An attempt to cheat will result in expulsion from the testing area. You lose.

If you are testing after October 1, 2002, ask your instructor for any changes in directions.

Preparing for the NCLEX-PN

Requirements

To help erase some of the mystique that often surrounds the licensure examination, it is worth remembering that the examination tests *minimum competence*. This means that if you have met the requirements for attending a state-board–approved school of practical/vocational nursing and have successfully completed all theory and clinical requirements, chances are excellent that you will pass the NCLEX-PN.

A detailed NCLEX-PN instruction booklet will be provided, in addition to licensing information from your board of nursing. Your instructor will assist you in applying for the licensure examination. The general rules are:

1. Submit proof of graduation.
2. Apply for licensure from the state board of nursing and submit the required fee. Some jurisdictions have additional fees.
3. Complete application for NCLEX-PN and submit fee to the testing service.
4. When you receive your Authorization to Test letter in the mail after your board of nursing

has made you eligible, register with the testing center. You cannot make an appointment to take the examination until your board of nursing declares you eligible and you receive the Authorization to Test letter in the mail. Information regarding scheduling will be included with your Authorization to Test letter.

5. Schedule a date and time to take the examination (within 30 days of your phone call unless you request a later date).
6. Take the NCLEX-PN.

Your instructor will also assist you with an application for a temporary permit so you will be able to work as a graduate practical or vocational nurse (GPN or GVN). Once the result of the NCLEX-PN examination is in, this permit is automatically revoked. Passing the NCLEX-PN means that you will work as a fully licensed practical or vocational nurse (LPN or LVN). If you fail the NCLEX-PN, you will have to surrender your temporary permit and will work as a nursing assistant.

Reducing Anxiety Prior to Testing

Normal anxiety is your friend. It is this "cause-and-effect" type of anxiety that actually makes you sharper and more alert during a test. Only when anxiety overwhelms you does it become your enemy. Accept the energy resulting from normal anxiety as your partner. Total personal comfort is not the key. Normal anxiety leaves you somewhere between too much relaxation and too much tension: perfect for testing.

Make your daydreams and positive thinking work for you. Think about what you think about. Are you in the habit of seeing yourself failing or just squeaking by? Because everyone daydreams and sets the stage for their reality, daydreaming is a natural way to practice being confident and successful. Practice the following exercises on successive days. Find a time when you can visualize without interruption.

Continue to repeat the parts of the exercise in sequence until you find yourself less threatened by the idea of testing—any testing.

 Learning Exercise: Visualizing the NCLEX:PN

Part 1

Close your eyes. See yourself arriving at the testing center one-half hour before testing begins. See yourself entering a waiting room in an office-like environment, welcoming and pleasant. Registration and sign-in go as planned. Everything, including the picture-taking and fingerprinting, goes smoothly. Candidates are coming in and going out continuously. You are asked to enter the testing area. As you enter you note that the room has beautiful soft-color carpeting. The carrel you are seated in reminds you of a large library carrel. Your instructor has already told you that there are 15 carrels in a room. The test room is glassed-in on two sides. Each carrel has an IBM computer with a mouse (which you do not use), a banker's lamp, and a chair with arm rests. You see yourself sitting down, adjusting the height of the chair and the monitor. You are confident and ready to begin.

Part 2

Close your eyes and imagine yourself in the same setting. Remember to include the detail. This time, the examination seems really hard for you. Rather than giving up, you do your best on every item, focusing on the item rather than on the outcome of the test. Take all the time permitted. When you get up to leave, remind yourself that you have done your best.

Remember: Your whole life does not depend on one test.

Spend the evening before the licensing examination relaxing. Little will be accomplished by worrying or by last-minute cramming. Read something light and entertaining, watch television, or do what you already know will relax you.

Get a good night's sleep by going to bed at your usual time (whatever meets your sleep requirements). Going to bed extra early and not falling asleep may result in a new worry for you to contend with.

Follow through with your usual morning habits. Do not force your system to adjust to a new demand.

Casual attire is appropriate. Think of comfort for sitting and writing. Wear layers of clothing that can be adjusted to your needs.

A Word About Review Books and Mock Examinations

New review books based on the NCLEX-PN format have been developed by the major nursing publishing companies. Each review book basically includes an outline of practical/vocational nursing content, items with explanations, and references for the answers. Items are intended to simulate the NCLEX-PN format. Please realize that the test items of the NCLEX-PN itself are highly guarded and confidential. Actual NCLEX-PN test items are not included in any review book. Some review books contain computer disks with test items. These disks do not simulate CAT testing, but they do provide computer experience.

Review of content and test items are developed by instructors who teach specific areas of practical/vocational nursing programs. The best preparation is to study faithfully from the beginning of the program to its conclusion and also on a regular basis until you take the examination. Do not put all your eggs in one basket. Merely reading a review book without studying the content will rarely help you pass boards.

Mock examinations are available for a fee. They offer practical/vocational nursing students an opportunity to assess their level of readiness for NCLEX-PN. After taking mock examinations, a student receives a readout of his or her test performance.

This includes:

- A percentile score for each category of client needs.
- The items the student got wrong.
- A book listing the correct answers, rationale, and explanations for correct answers and distractors for each item.

If students have an idea of their strong and weak areas, they can better focus their study efforts. Be sure to check publishers' offerings of mock examinations. Choose the one that most closely resembles the actual format of the NCLEX-PN. As a practical/vocational nursing student you can benefit from tests during the year that encourage problem solving and the application of knowledge. Some of these systems provide adaptive testing as used by NCLEX-PN. Use these experiences as additional means of preparing for your nursing licensure examination.

Good luck! Keep a positive mental attitude.

Summary

- ☐ Lack of preparation of subject matter and poor test-taking skills are the most common reasons for low test scores. Occasionally fear and high anxiety are involved, but these are exceptional cases.
- ☐ The NCLEX-PN is the National Council Licensing Examination taken by graduate practical/vocational nurses to become licensed. This examination is administered by computer, using computerized adaptive testing (CAT).
- ☐ Prior to scheduling the NCLEX-PN, all practical or vocational nursing course work must be completed.
- ☐ Each candidate takes a different track during the CAT method of testing. The track is based on your answers to previous items and provides a way for you to demonstrate

your competency in practical/vocational nursing. Results are available in about two to three weeks.

☐ Remember to continue your positive mental attitude. If it needs polishing, stop and do it now!

Review Questions

1. If you were going to explain what the NCLEX-PN tests for, what might you say?
   A. Just in case I have to assume RN responsibilities during the night shift, for example, I must know what she or he does.
   B. This test covers everything that I have learned and practiced on the clinical unit during the year.
   C. The NCLEX-PN tests for the minimum amount of knowledge and skills that I must have to be safe and competent at a beginning level.
   D. As you know, nurses assume the work of other medical professions on the evening and night shift, so it tests multidisciplinary knowledge.
2. How is nursing process related to the NCLEX-PN?
   A. It is one of the major content dimensions of the examination.
   B. Nursing process is integrated throughout the catagories of the examination.
   C. Each step (phase) of the nursing process is weighed by a percentage.
   D. Nursing process is no longer considered a valuable part of modern nursing.
3. How does the computer select questions for you during the NCLEX-PN?

A. Using the answer to your previous question.
B. By your overall gradepoint during your schooling.
C. You may be selected randomly to answer all the questions.
D. Test bank questions are individualized.
4. What happens to your temporary work permit after you receive the results of the NCLEX-PN?
   A. You may continue to work using the permit until you successfully complete the NCLEX-PN.
   B. Nothing, because the use of the temporary permit is limited anyway.
   C. You keep the permit so that you will be able to work as an aide as needed.
   D. The permit is rescinded if you do not complete the NCLEX-PN successfully.
5. How does anxiety relate to test taking?
   A. A moderate amount of anxiety is desirable.
   B. A high level of anxiety provides the drive.
   C. A low level of anxiety motivates you best.
   D. It is immaterial since it is your will power that counts.

References

Minnesota Board of Nursing. For Your Information 15(3): Fall, 1999.
National Council completes 1997 job analysis of newly licensed practical/vocational nurses. Issues, 1997. Homepage: Http://www.ncsbn.org.
National Council of State Boards of Nursing. Questions

about taking the NCLEX examination are answered. Issues, 1997. Homepage: http://www.ncsbn.org.
*NCLEX-PN Test Plan for the National Council Licensure
Examination*. Chicago: National Council of State Boards
of Nursing, 1998.

Ventura MJ. The great multistate licensure debate. RN
62(5):58, 1999.
Yocom C. *1996 Job Analysis Study for Licensed Practical/
Vocational Nurses*. Chicago: National Council of State
Boards of Nursing, 1997.

Bibliography

Examination Committee Contemplating Changing NCLEX-
PN Test Plan. Issues 18(4), 1997. Chicago: National
Council of State Boards of Nursing Homepage, 1997.
http:www//ncsbn.org.
Heaman D. The quieting response (QR): A modality for
reduction of psychophysiologic stress in nursing stu-
dents. J Nurs Educ 34(1):5–10, 1995.
Minarik PA, Price LC. Multistate licensure for advanced
practical nurses? Nursing Outlook, March/April, 1999.
Multistate Regulation Taskforce. Communique. Chicago:
National Council of State Boards of Nursing, April, 1998,
and July, 1988.
National Council of State Boards of Nursing. Constructing
an activity list for use in job analysis studies. National
Council Homepage, 1997. http://www.ncsbn.org.
National Council of State Boards of Nursing. Mutual recognition model for nursing regulation: Frequently asked
questions. National Council Homepage, March 1998.
http://www.ncsbn.org.

National Council of State Boards of Nursing. National Coun-
cil concludes 1999 annual meeting. New NCLEX exami-
nation test service selected by delegates. Chicago: Na-
tional Council Publications, August 2, 1999.
National Council of State Boards of Nursing. Utah enacts
nursing regulation—Interstate Compact Bill. National
Council Homepage, March 1998. http://www.ncsbn.org.
Newswatch Professional Update. Utah makes it easier for
RNs to practice across state lines. RN, June, 1998.
Nursing Data Source 1997. Volume: *Focus on Practical/
Vocational Nursing*. New York; NLN Division of Re-
search, 1997.
"Testing." Issues 18(4), 1997. Chicago: National Council of
State Boards of Nursing.
Wendt A, Brown P. 1999 NCLEX-PN Test Plan: Responding
to changing nursing practice. Journal of Practical Nurs-
ing 48(4):December, 1998.
Wendt A, Clark S. *National Council Detailed Test Plan for
NCLEX-PN Examination*. Chicago: NCSBN, 1998.

Chapter 20

Finding a Job

Michael S. Hill, MS. CRC, ABDA

Outline

Key Terms

artful vagueness
conditional job offer
follow-up illusion
hidden job market

illegal questions
informational interviews
interpersonal styles
networking

reference hierarchy
resignation courtesy
résumé
working the room

Objectives

Upon completing this chapter you will be able to:

1. List employment opportunities available to practical/vocational nurses.
2. Determine interpersonal styles and how to use them to achieve interpersonal rapport.
3. Describe and use individuals within your job search network.
4. Effectively participate in an informational interview.
5. Discuss how and where best to target job leads.
6. Role play employer telephone contacts and respond positively to hard interview questions.
7. Develop résumés that will get an employer's attention.
8. Convey positive nonverbal messages at the interview.
9. Have an insight into the cultural and age differences of the interviewer.
10. Discuss the importance of employer follow up both at the time of application and after the interview.
11. Anticipate a successful pre-employment physical examination and drug screening.
12. Write an effective resignation letter with style.

Graduation: Closer Than You Think

If you are reading this chapter, you are near to graduation or about to graduate, with the expectation that employers will be beating down your door. You may also be concerned about your career opportunities after investing so much money in your education.

You are to be congratulated for having become a member of one of the fastest growing employment areas: health services. In *America's Top Medical and Human Services Jobs* (Farr, 1994), Farr states that the job outlook for nursing has a growth rate that is faster than average through the year 2005. This is a response to the long-term care needs of a rapidly growing elderly population and the need for general health care.

Job growth and opportunities vary from region to region at different times. Employment opportunities vary according to each individual's tenacity, geographic location, and sometimes just luck. Your job search will be more successful if you consider looking into the areas such as those listed in Chapter 17.

Critical Thinking Exercise

1. What type of environment do I want to work in? Direct health care, state/federal government, private duty, insurance-related, sales, industry . . . or other?

_____

2. What population, type of client, do I find most rewarding to work with?

_____

_____

_____

3. What kinds of nursing skills do I find most challenging and rewarding? Additionally, what new areas would I like to be involved in?

_____

_____

Now What Do I Want To Do?

Many job ads in newspapers, the Internet, and professional publications require the candidate to have had prior experience. By completing your program, you have gained practical experience. Now it is a matter of convincing the employer that it is to his or her benefit to hire you. Think about what your education has provided you.

It is a distinct advantage if your educational program has included clinical (hands-on) nursing experience in the areas you are most interested in. These nursing experiences include clinical rotations, special projects, computer, or work with a temporary permit prior to taking the NCLEX-PN.

Your practical work experiences will lead to clarification of your school lessons, help you hone your skills, and provide valuable work references. Think about it: By taking advantage of the clinical rotations and work experiences available to you, a significant step in the job search has already been taken while you were finishing your education. You have had an opportunity to learn about and develop skills that are valued in the major areas of nursing employment.

Using Interpersonal Styles to Your Benefit

What are **interpersonal styles,** and which style fits you? Think for a moment about the contacts you have made in the classroom, in the clinical areas, and among your school friends. You have the unique opportunity of making contacts with nurses at all levels who can be instrumental in helping you obtain a job.

First, however, you must ask yourself: (1) Who am I? (2) How am I seen? The first question enables you to look at yourself in relation to your values and interests and determine what motivates you. The answer to this question will provide you with information about which work environments to consider for employment.

Through the second question, you can learn how others see you and whether what they see is congruent with the messages you think you are sending (Kuntz, 1995). A positive impression will go a long way to develop networks and work references.

Mercer (1994) suggests that to master an interpersonal style, it is necessary to foster a spirit of cooperation and to meet others on their own terms. He indicated that to achieve rapport, people use four major interpersonal styles: results-focused, detail-focused, friendly-focused, and party-focused.

Results-Focused

Individuals with a results-focused style prefer to get information quickly and act upon it immediately. Signs of this style include "a tendency to talk fast, finish other's sentences, and act irritated when others don't get right to the point."

You may want to respond to these individuals by "making your points brief, describing what you have done and plan to do next. Speak rapidly and avoid getting sidetracked."

Detail-Focused

These individuals are interested in every detail about a subject, no matter how large or how small. They are perfectionists who would rather have a task performed correctly than quickly. Signs of this type include "speaking slowly and deliberately to absorb all information, often asking for additional details."

In responding to these individuals in an employment situation, you will want to bring a portfolio of information that covers seminars, classes, volunteer work, and so on. "Carefully explain each element of what you have done to date and plan to do. Make sure that the individual is comfortable with every aspect of your work."

Friendly-Focused

These individuals expect to have an easy-going conversation initially. Signs of this style include "talking about themselves or conversations about your personal life along with discussing weekend plans, hobbies, and nonwork activities." When the small talk is completed, they tend to shift to either a results-focused or detail-focused style.

To respond to these individuals, you may want to "chat with them for two to five minutes about nonwork activities." Following this you will want to "state that you will need to return to school/work and then discuss the business at hand." Then watch for clues to whether the person switches to the results- or detail-focused style.

Party-Focused

"These people love to laugh, tell jokes, and have a good time before getting down to business." Once this is done they, like the friendly-focused person, will shift to the results- or detail-focused style.

The best way to respond is to laugh along with them or, if you are good at it, tell a few jokes of your own.

To make a good impression on people, it is important to (1) listen to what they have to say; and (2) if you disagree with someone with whom you want to maintain rapport, use "artful vagueness." **Artful vagueness** is responding to another's comments without implying that either of you are wrong. An example would be to respond to a statement with "You've got a point there" or "You may be right."

Networking Your Way to Success

1. What are the best methods of networking?
2. What is the worst networking mistake?
3. What is the best way to "**work a room**"?

Smart **networking,** influential people in your school and clinical work experiences can lead to finding new jobs, better pay, faster promotions, and greater job satisfaction. Consider, for example:

- Instructors who are willing to write a positive recommendation if your work warrants it. *Be sure to ask for permission prior to bringing in a form or giving out his or her name.* Do not assume that an instructor will give you a positive reference. Specifically ask, "May I list your name for a positive reference?"
- Unit managers, supervisors, team leaders, staff RNs, and LP/VNs are sources of information about job openings in their areas and can be approached for recommendations. Some students think that they are "invisible" in the eyes of regular facility staff. Not so! Frequently staff offer feedback to instructors and nurse managers about future employees.
- School placement people are a source of information when you register with the school's career service center and can inform you about Job Service Centers and so on.

Listen carefully when feedback is passed on to you. You often have to work directly with the primary nurses or team leaders. Identify the nurses whose work you admire and ask for their evaluation and suggestions about your work.

Before you complete a clinical rotation, *ask se-lect nurses* whether they would be willing to write a positive reference letter for you. If the answer is "yes," write down the nurse's name (spelled correctly), title, work address, and work phone number. I strongly encourage you to ask what he or she will say about you. When discussing your references during an interview, it is to your advantage to allude to what they say about you. If you don't ask what the person will say about you, you are risking the possibility that he or she will also discuss all your flaws.

A brief courtesy letter about your need for a positive reference letter should be sent at the time you begin your job search; follow-up telephone contacts to reference persons four to five days after sending the letter will remind them of you and their promise. Your telephone contact might sound something like this:

> "Hello, Ms. Anderson, this is Katelyn Bieser. I'm calling to follow up on the letter I sent you last week, to see whether you have had an opportunity to write the letter of recommendation we discussed at the end of the last rotation."
>
> If the answer is no: "I know that you've been pretty busy lately. Would it be possible to follow up with you next week when you have had more time? Great, I will call back then. Have a good day!"

Offer to write a letter yourself for their review and signature. A letter to the reference writer and a letter of recommendation might look like those in Box 20–1 and Box 20–2.

Additionally, when networking, use other contacts that you have made, or be willing to meet new people who can help you, such as:

- Family and friends with nursing contacts. Let them know that you are looking for work. Ask for job leads and names of contacts. Follow up with these people every two weeks until you get the job you want. Remember to thank these people for all their help once you get the job. You never know, you may need their help again in the future. Job opportunities are often

Box 20–1. Sample Letter to Reference Writer

*May 8, 200_*

Ms. Jennifer Abbinante, Nursing Administrator
Veterans Hospital
1000 Veterans Lane
Minneapolis, MN 55402

Dear Ms. Abbinante,

Thank you again for agreeing to be a work reference for me. My experiences on the medical-surgical unit were both challenging and rewarding. I am pleased that I now have the opportunity to use the skills you taught me.

I am actively seeking employment in medical-surgical units at hospitals within the metro area. A letter of reference from you is definitely an asset to my job search.

Knowing your busy schedule, I have enclosed a possible letter of reference for your review and signature. However, if you prefer to write your own letter you may wish to mention my ability to work under pressure, ability to administer medication on time, communication skills with staff and patients, computer proficiency, and my willingness to take on new assignments.

Your assistance in helping me secure employment is greatly appreciated. I plan to give you a call next week to let you know how my job search is going and answer any questions you may have regarding the reference letter. I look forward to talking with you soon. My phone number is (612) 555-2728.

Cordially,

Katelyn Bieser
2001 Putt Drive
Cottage Grove, MN 55016

Encl.: Reference Letter

located not by what you know as much as by whom you know.

- Former health care employers. If you are interested in a nursing position, contact the employer.

- Newspapers, nursing journals, the school alumni office, telephone yellow pages, the school's career placement office, state Job Service, and local county agencies.

- If you browse on the Internet, there are some

Box 20–2. Sample Letter for Reference to Complete and Place on Letterhead

May 15, 200__

Dear Employer:

Please accept this as a letter of recommendation for Ms. Katelyn Bieser, whom I supervised during her medical-surgical rotation. Katelyn was enjoyable to work with and displayed a high degree of skill as a student practical nurse.

Specifically, she learned new tasks quickly, attended to client vital signs, was proficient on the computer, provided nutritional care, and administered medication promptly. Katelyn was able to follow both physician and RN orders and had the keen sense to know when to ask for help.

I believe that Katelyn will make a positive contribution to any hospital/company she chooses to work for. Should you have further questions about Katelyn's skills and abilities as a nursing professional, please feel free to contact me.

Cordially,

Jennifer Abbinante, RN,
Surgical Care Charge Nurse

Box 20–3. Internet Sites for Careers

Messmer Carier Site Suggestions

www.ajb.dni.us; www.careerbuilder.com; www.careermag.com; wwwcareermosaic.com; www.careerpath.com; www.careers.org; careers.wsj.com; www.cweb.com; www.coolworks.com; www.headhunter.net; www.hotjobs.com; www.jobbankusa.com; www.jobtrak.com; www.monster.com; www.nationjob.com; aol.com:career center; and careers.yahoo.com.

From Messmer M. Career Search Sites: Job Hunting for Dummies, 2nd ed. New York: IDG Books Worldwide, 1999.

Michael Hill Career Site Suggestions

http://altavista.digital.com; http://www.excite.com; www.dejnews.com; http://hotbot.com; http://www.lycos.com; http://webcrawler.com; www.nursejobz.com; www.springnet.com; www.afreserve.com; www.wwnurse.com; www.medhunters.com; www.nurse-recruiter.com; www.careershop.com; and kforce.com.

general career search sites that can be used/ explored to find job opportunities. Box 20–3 lists several Internet sites for careers that will prove useful.

Locally, also consider checking to see whether the facilities that you wish to work for have web pages of their own. This provides you an opportunity to learn about job openings and what the facility is about. This can be done by searching the Internet and/or contacting the receptionist at those facilities and asking for their Internet address. Hint: When using the Internet, it will take time to locate job and career opportunity areas. After entering the career/job area, try using the search box and type in "licensed practical (or vocational) nurse" or "nurse" as a possible shortcut. The beauty of the Internet is that you can search locally, by state, and in different countries.

- Attend professional conferences or training sessions and then begin **"working the room."** Meissner (1995) has recommended the following steps: (1) arriving early to obtain your name badge and to see who else is attending; (2) not bringing your spouse with you; (3) avoiding sitting at tables with other students; sit instead with people already working in the field; (4) identifying the people who hire by their more professional appearance and avoidance of eye contact with others; (5) sitting down at the table and introducing yourself to the people next to you; (6) requesting business cards; and (7) not leaving these events early or immediately after the event ends. Contacts can often be made by opening a conversation with a remark such as, "I found Ms. Smith's comment about the _____ interesting. Have you heard about that before?"
- Call a prospective employer and ask, "Are you hiring?" If the answer is no, ask "Do you know of anyone else who is hiring?" If yes, ask for the contact person's name, if known.

Critical Thinking Exercise

Who can you think of that is a part of your job network? List the individuals in the spaces below.

Name	Phone

Networking should be a never-ending process even after you have found your dream job. You never know when that dream job might come to an abrupt end owing to reorganization and downsizing. Additionally, remember that networking is a means to job satisfaction and advancement.

Not networking while you are in school or working is the worst mistake you can make.

As a rule, whether you are happily employed or looking for another job, the successful person is the one who makes a point of meeting someone new each day either by telephone or in person. This includes (1) displaying a positive affect with clients, (2) seeking your supervisor's input on how to build your career, (3) working on building relationships with key people in the facilities in which you work, (4) building positive peer relationships by being willing to lend a hand, and (5) treating everyone as you would like to be treated. This will lead to access to other networks.

Information Interviews to Create Future Expectations

Critical Thinking Exercise

1. How might informational interviews help your career?
2. Whom do you trust to tell you how your voice sounds? Who will help you understand how it needs to sound?
3. With whom can you practice the informational interview telephone request?

List three names: _____

Chances are that at some time during your educational program you will be asked to visit community health facilities. Your instructor will provide objectives and questions to help make the experience worthwhile. Objectives or questions may focus on the following areas:

- Purpose
- Staffing patterns
- Hours or shifts
- Facility specialty

Viewing this assignment as an **informational interview** will create an additional personal focus for you. The informational interview will allow you to find out how the facility works first-hand, assist you in determining whether you would want to work there, and allow you to meet the employer before you actually seek a job.

To obtain an informational interview with an employer, it is important to practice with another individual prior to making the telephone contact. It may be tempting to make the phone call and read the example without practicing in advance. But if you do this, remember that is exactly how it will sound—as though you are reading!

This is the time to concentrate on how your voice sounds to the employer with respect to pitch and intonation. Franklin (1995) reported that several studies of spoken English have shown that "low-pitched, clear voices were judged to be more mature, truthful, and competent than high-pitched ones."

Also, "nasal voices signaled low status, were uninviting, and grated on the listener." Monotones, such as occur when reading aloud, were boring to the listener. Loud, fast talkers were viewed as dynamic but shifty. Finally, individuals with whiney voices were a definite turn-off.

The key is to find someone who will give you an honest opinion about how you sound. When you approach that person, explain the reason you are asking for his or her opinion. Explain that you view it as another learning experience toward achieving your goals.

The following is an example of a telephone informational interview request:

1. Hello, my name is _____.
2. Can you give me the name of the person in charge of hiring? (Emphasis is on first learn-

ing the name of the right person. Don't begin by asking, "May I speak to the person in charge of hiring?")

Box 20–4. Follow-Up Letter After Informational Interview

January 17, 200__

Ms. LeAnn Lemberger, Director of Nursing
St. Joseph Hospital
1000 Writers Lane
Minneapolis, MN 55402

RE: Informational Interview

Dear Ms. Lemberger:

Thank you so much for meeting with me on Wednesday, January 16, 200__. The information that you provided was both valuable and interesting. Your suggestions about what employers are looking for and which areas to focus my schooling on were very much appreciated.

I found that the variety of programs offered was progressive and individualized to meet the needs of the client. The tour that followed supported your comments about the positive interactions between staff and clients.

I can only hope to be fortunate enough to work at such a Center following my graduation this June. Thank you again.

Sincerely yours,

Katelyn Bieser
2001 Putt Drive
Cottage Grove, MN 55016
(612) 555-2728 or kbieser@spacestar.com

3. May I speak with Mr./Ms. _____?
4. Hello, Mr./Ms. _____. My name is _____.
5. I am a student practical nurse at _____ (school's name).
6. As a part of my learning experience, I would like to visit your facility for an informational interview.
7. Would it be possible to set up an informational interview on _____ (day) at 9:00 AM or 2:00 PM, or another time?
   A. If yes: Great! I'll see you at _____. Thank you!
   B. If no: Is there someone else whom you recommend that I contact?

There is usually no problem with speaking directly to top nursing management during an informational interview. Management likes to "get the word out" about what their facility really is like. However, do not make the mistake of turning this into a job interview. No one likes to be tricked, and management tends to have a long memory.

Look sharp during the informational interview. These are not "T-shirt, shorts or jeans and sandals" side trips. Consider them as future career opportunities. In a safe place, keep a copy of the information you obtained with name, address, and phone number, for the time your job search begins. Follow up the informational interview with a thank you letter. See Box 20–4.

How to Look for Employment Openings

Critical Thinking Exercise

1. Is it true that it is pointless to look for work during the holidays?
2. Where is the most effective job search performed?
3. Why is waiting for the employer to contact you a lost cause?

It is important to begin to apply for employment approximately two months prior to graduation if you expect to work shortly after graduation. Obtain a telephone answering machine or use a telephone "voice mailbox" service so that you do not miss any employer calls. If your graduation is in December, do not fret. It is a myth that the November–December holiday season is the worst time to hunt for a job. The holiday season is among the best times to look for a job as employers are already looking at staffing patterns for the new year.

You need to do some homework in preparation for seeking employment. Find out all you can about the facility at which you wish to work. Facilities often provide free pamphlets as part of their advertising. Obtain the "mission statement" of the facility if it is not in a pamphlet. Also remember the information you have acquired and stashed away during your education.

Your nursing program director will also have policy manuals for affiliated facilities. Ask to see those manuals. It is very important to try to find out the name of the person who does the hiring or influences hiring. This is the person whom you will want to contact. You may be referred to another department, but there is a good chance that your name will be remembered later.

According to *The Job Hunting Handbook: Job Outlook to 2005* (Dahlstrom & Company, 1995), 75% of jobs available are not advertised. Do not wait for an ad to appear to apply to an employer. Through their research, Dahlstrom & Company discovered that people use the following methods to get jobs and to tap into the **hidden job market.**

Assistance from family and friends
Direct application to employer
Response to newspaper advertisement
State Job Service or Work Force Centers
Private employment agencies
Civil service examinations
School placement offices
Union hall hiring

Assistance from family and friends has the highest rate of success in getting a job. One area often overlooked in the past was job fairs.

Another means of applying directly to employers is sending a letter to a prospective employer. Make a follow-up telephone contact to arrange an interview or at least to use as a networking opportunity for additional job leads.

Often a brief, to-the-point letter accompanied by a résumé addressed to the director of nursing at the facility to which you are applying is helpful. Your cover letter might appear as in Box 20–5.

Avoid including a personal reference list or a photograph of yourself with the cover letter. Retain the reference list for your interview and provide it only on request. *Do* follow through by calling for an interview on the day stated in your letter.

The timing of employer contacts has not changed since the 1990s. It is best to use Sundays and Mondays to research job opportunities and then contact employers from Tuesday forward. The best time to call employers has traditionally been from 9:00 AM on for interview scheduling and follow-up contacts.

As a rule, employers no longer have the luxury of contacting every prospective candidate owing to time constraints and the demands of their own jobs. Those candidates who wait to be contacted should prepare to be disappointed when contacts do not occur.

If your resource for a job opening is the newspaper, call for an interview (unless the ad specifically says to write). The reason for this is that others are looking at the same ad, and in such cases, "The candidate who hesitates is lost." Ask to speak to the person in charge of hiring. Your conversation will tend to reflect the following example:

1. Hello, my name is _____.
2. Who is in charge of hiring?
3. May I speak with Ms. _____?
4. Hello, Ms. _____. My name is _____.
5. I will be graduating from the (school name) practical/vocational nursing program in (city name) on (date).
6. Do you have any practical/vocational nursing staff positions open?
   6A. If yes: Would it be possible to set up an interview on (date) at 9:00 AM or perhaps 2:00 PM? If no: What would be a

---

Box 20–5. Sample Cover Letter for Employment

*April 10, 200_*

Ms. Debra Palmsteen, Director of Nursing
Chicago Lakes Hospital
2031 Lakeside Drive
Chisago, MN 55890

Re: LPN Staff Nurse Position

Dear Ms. Palmsteen:

I will graduate from the Fairview Hospital practical nursing program this June. While doing a medical nursing rotation at your hospital, I was impressed by the quality of client care, staff professionalism, and learning opportunities.

In addition to this rotation, my work experiences have included client care planning, plan review, direct client care, passing medications, computer entry, and team participation.

I am interested in obtaining employment at your hospital and being able to work with your staff again. I will contact you on Tuesday, April 17, 200_, to see whether you have received my résumé and to determine when we might arrange an interview. Should you wish to contact me prior to this time I can be reached after 3:30 PM. I look forward to speaking with you.

Cordially,

Katelyn Bieser
2001 Putt Drive
Cottage Grove, MN 55016
(612) 555-2728 or kbieser@spacestar.com

better time and date? . . . Great! I will see you then.

6B. If the answer is no, we are under a hiring freeze, catch your breath and don't be put off. The *Job Hunting Handbook* recommends the following response:

6B (1) Oh, I understand. A lot of institutions have hiring freezes at this time of year. But those hiring freezes can't last forever. I'd like to be the first on your list when you lift your hiring freeze. Would you take a few minutes to meet with me and see where I might fit in once your hiring freeze is lifted? If yes, see 6A. If no: Do you know of anyone who might be hiring? (2) If yes: Would you also know the contact person and/or have the telephone number?

_____ _____ _____
(facility) (contact) (telephone)

(3) If no: I appreciate your time. Thank you. (or)

(4) If no: Thank you for trying. Would it be possible for me to come in for an informational interview?
If yes: See 6A.
If no: Well, thank you again. Goodbye.

Deflect the employer's questions until the interview because you do not want to be "washed out" by a phone conversation. If the employer begins to ask you questions about your background, education, or work experience, you might respond, "I have completed an accredited practical/vocational nursing program and have the required work experience. I would like the opportunity to discuss my qualifications during our interview." As in point 6A, earlier, say, "Would it be possible to set up an interview with you on Wednesday? . . . (etc.)".

The tone of your voice makes a significant difference on the telephone. If you smile while talking, you will project a positive tone. Practice the preceding format in advance with a friend. Write notes for yourself if necessary.

Even if you are not ideally qualified for a job opening, apply if it appeals to you. Advertisements often describe the ideal candidate for the job, and the ideal is usually not available. If you do lack some skills that are required and are able to obtain an interview, an employer will be impressed if you ask whether facility in-service programs, orientation, and continuing education courses are offered by the employer to enhance your job skills.

References: A Timeless Treasure

 Critical Thinking Exercise

List the persons in your reference hierarchy.

Prospective employers will be more interested in some work references than in others. There is a **reference hierarchy** of individuals who act as references. Ranging from most to least important are:

1. Current or former nursing instructors, staff from clinical sites where you worked rotations, and supervisors from past work and volunteer experiences.
2. Personal references or friends. (Note: Employers generally don't bother to contact personal references and put little value in their opinions.)

On reference sheets, include the person's name, job title, address, and work phone number. Three is the usual number of references requested. Pick and choose from your list of resources for maximum impression.

The statement "References on Request" can be placed at the end of your résumé. It is a matter of personal choice. References should be listed on the reference list and given to the interviewer if he or she requests them. References, however, are "treasures." Avoid giving them out if you are not interested in the position.

Résumés: The Contributions You Will Make

Critical Thinking Exercise

1. What items should not be included in a résumé?
2. Why are job duties written in sentence form not used?

Development of a paper scannable/personal and a plain text electronic **résumé** is a must! It focuses on your work skills, experiences, and qualifications. Résumés are not used as a confession or "tell-all" script. They should not include such items as reasons for leaving past jobs, salary requirements, personal photographs, and personal data including marital status, race, religion, height, weight, or number or age of children.

Ethridge (1995) also recommends omitting an "Objective" statement, often located at the top of the résumé. Additionally, it has been noted that employers don't care about your "personal goals" and that statements like "excellent health" are a waste — who would report that their health was bad?

Unfortunately, many résumés are never read because they are too cluttered or wordy or contain the areas noted earlier that have turned the interviewer off. Use only short bulleted sentences no more than two to four words in length.

Résumés may be varied according to the job you are seeking. Remember, you want to let the employer know that you can fill the job.

Essentially, all résumés have a format of personal data, education, work experience, licenses/professional memberships, and possible military experi-ence. It is recommended that you stop and think about what specific classes or job tasks you have performed and record them in your résumé. Don't assume that the employer knows what you mean when saying "performed nursing duties."

For work/military experiences, it is recommended that years of experience be listed rather than specific dates. Additionally, for older workers, do not dredge up your entire work history but stop after ten years. Also avoid listing experience/training on outdated technology.

Remember that it is important that your résumé be truthful. Employers may look for inconsistencies, work experiences that are too good to be true, or a résumé that appears purposely vague. Keep your résumé consistent and well balanced.

The initial impression made by the résumé is significant. Basic factors to consider for scannable/ personal and electronic plain text résumés are listed in Box 20-6.

Three sample résumés, two typed (Boxes 20-7A and B) and one electronic (Box 20-8), were found to be very successful.

Cover Letters: Tailored to Fit the Job You Want

Critical Thinking Exercise

Why do cover letters need to be sent in with résumés?

It is essential to include a cover letter with each résumé. The cover letter may be submitted by mail or dropped off with an application for the employer. Cover letters directly answer newspaper and Internet ad requirements and qualifications or follow up the unsolicited phone calls you made inquiring about job openings. Neatness, correct spelling, and proper grammar are mandatory. Each letter should be one

Box 20–6. Basic Résumé Factors Scannable/Personal Résumé Factors to Consider

- Length. Two pages are the maximum. One page is preferred.
- Paper. Quality bond. Stay with colors such as white, cream, beige, or gray. Use matching paper for the cover letter and envelope.
- Typing. Absolutely no spelling or grammatical errors or extra marks. Type your résumé on a computer and use a laser printer. The computer allows for painless corrections. Updating is performed quickly. It is worth going to a quick print shop to make résumé copies. Standard copy machines provide poor-quality copies.
- Faxing. Copy your résumé onto white paper. By sending the Fax on white paper, the transmission will be faster and the Faxed copy will be clearer and easier to read.
- Balance and space: An uncluttered, balanced design is desirable so that the résumé is easy to read. Because most managers don't have time to read, a "bulleted" style is recommended when listing job skills and past duties.
- Emphasis: Depends on whether you have a strong or a limited work history.

Electronic Plain Text Factors to Consider

Dixon (1998) has suggested that plain-text electronic (ASCII) résumés are the number one choice among employers. Development of this type of résumé includes an absence of "italics, underlining, bold, hollow bullets, or any type of pretty formatting."

By eliminating these frills, employers with standard personal and Macintosh computers are able to read the ASCII résumé. It is recommended that your résumé be no longer than one and one half pages in length, with one page preferred. One acceptable way to do this is to taper the job duties toward the end of the résumé.

After completion of the résumé, you are encouraged to forward it to yourself to download and print. This is a great way to check that what you are sending is received as intended.

page long, an original (never photocopied) with no "white-out" ink applied, and in a block letter format.

If an employer asks for specific experience, be sure to list this in your cover letter even if your experiences are not listed on the résumé.

Note: You may use the same cover letters that you send out by post for your electronic mail. It is recommended that you "paste" your résumé to the end of the electronic cover letter and send this out as a whole unit rather than as attachments to the e-mail message. Depending upon the computer that the employer has, she or he may be unable to open your attachment.

See the sample cover letters to an employer contacted through an unsolicited telephone call (Box 20–9A) and through a newspaper ad (Box 20–9B).

Proactive Follow Up Today

Learning Exercise: Follow Up

1. What is the percentage of people who do not follow up with employers after submitting résumés or participating in interviews?
2. When is the best time to make a follow-up call?
3. How might you get past the secretary to find out whether you have been hired?

Follow up after a job interview is essential. It is a constant source of amazement to employers that 90% of the people who interview never follow up to see whether they will get the job. Recent graduates and even nurses who have been working in the field for some time are under the **follow-up illusion** that it is the employer's responsibility to contact them. She or he who hesitates will be disappointed!

Text continued on page 348

Box 20–7A. Sample Typed Résumé Starting with Work Experience

KATELYN BIESER

2001 Putt Drive, Cottage Grove, MN 55301
kbieser@spacestar.com (612) 555-2728

WORK EXPERIENCE

KESA Temp. Health Care Agency Plymouth, Minnesota	Contracted Services	**Licensed Practical Nurse** 1998 to Present
• Personal Care Services • Assisted Medical Staff • Medical Equipment Operation	• Administered Medications • Flexible Shift Scheduling • Charted Observations	• Responded to Patient Calls • Quality Assurance • Computer/Dictaphone Use
Forest View Nursing Home Hastings, Minnesota	Part Time to Attend School	**Certified Nursing Assistant** Two Years
• Assisted Physicians/Staff • Health Care Intervention	• Direct Patient Care • Injury Prevention	• Obtain/Chart Vital Signs • Promote Daily Living Skills
The Small Town Cafe Bloomington, Minnesota		**Waitress** 2½ Years
• Direct Customer Service • Assisted w/Food Preparation	• Time Management • Cleaned Tables/Dishes	• Cashiering • Maintained Work Area

EDUCATION

Fairview School of Nursing Minneapolis, Minnesota	Practical Nursing	Diploma 1997
Cottage Grove High School Cottage Grove, Minnesota	General Education	Diploma 1992

LICENSES/MEMBERSHIPS

State of Minnesota Board of Nursing St. Paul, Minnesota	License 1997 to Present
National Federation of Licensed Practical Nurses Garner, North Carolina	Membership 1997 to Present

REFERENCES

Available on request.

Box 20-7B. Sample Typed Résumé Starting with Education Experience

KATELYN BIESER

2001 Putt Drive, Cottage Grove, MN 55301
kbieser@spacestar.com (612) 555-2728

EDUCATION

Fairview School of Nursing Minneapolis, Minnesota	Practical Nursing	Diploma 1997

• Nursing Care Principles • Clinical Nursing • Maternal/Child Nursing	• Medication Administration • Professional Communications • Psychosocial Development	• Med-Surgical Principles • Health Care Delivery • Nutritional Care

Cottage Grove High School Cottage Grove, Minnesota		Diploma 1992

WORK EXPERIENCE

Forest View Nursing Home Hastings, Minnesota	Certified	Nursing Assistant Two Years

• Assisted Physicians/Staff • Health Care Intervention	• Direct Patient Care • Injury Prevention	• Obtain/Chart Vital Signs • Promote Daily Living Skills

Bieser & Associates Cottage Grove, Minnesota		Domestic Manager 1993 to present

• Budgeting/Inventory Control • Coord. Daily Living Activities	• Health Care Management • Mediation/Planning	• Quality Control • Crisis Intervention

LICENSES/MEMBERSHIPS

State of Minnesota Board of Nursing St. Paul, Minnesota	License (In Progress)

National Federation of Licensed Practical Nurses Garner, North Carolina	Membership 1997 to Present

REFERENCES

Available upon request.

Box 20–8. Sample Electronic Plain-Text Résumé

KATELYN BIESER

2001 Putt Drive, Cottage Grove, MN 55301
(612) 555-2728 (or) *kbieser@spacestar.com*

SUMMARY OF QUALIFICATIONS

Direct patient care, medication administration, computer operation, time management, obtaining/charting vital signs, professional communication, and willingness to take on new tasks.

EDUCATION

2003 Practical Nursing Diploma	Fairview School of Nursing	Minneapolis, MN
Nursing Care Principles	Medication Administration	Medical-Surgical Nursing
Clinical Nursing	Professional Communication	Health Care Delivery
Maternal/Child Nursing	Psychosocial Development	Nutritional Care Services
General Education Diploma	Cottage Grove School System	Cottage Grove, MN

Emphasis on educational skills enhancement, including mathematics, English, reading, spelling, and academic learning skills.

WORK EXPERIENCE

2½ Years Waitress	The Small Town Café	Bloomington, MN
Direct Customer Service	Time Management	Sales & Product Marketing
Assisted w/Food Preparation	Cashiering/Food Discounts	Maintained Work Area
2 Years Child Care	Bieser Babysitting, Inc.	Cottage Grove, MN
Personal Care Services	Flexible Scheduling	Nutritional Feeding/Care
Recreational Development	Cooking/Cleaning	Safety Intervention

LICENSES/MEMBERSHIPS

(In Progress) License	State of MN Board of Nursing	St. Paul, MN
2001 to present Membership	NFLPN	Garner, North Carolina

REFERENCES

Available upon request.

Box 20–9A. Sample Cover Letter: Unsolicited Phone Call

August 14, 200__

Ms. Taru Molander, RN, Director of Nursing
St. Helen General Hospital
8354 177th Lane
St. Paul, Minnesota 55000

RE: LPN Staff Nurse Position

Dear Ms. Molander:

Thank you for taking the time to speak with me about the Practical Nurse staff position. As we discussed, I believe that my clinical work experiences and skills are a good match for the job.

In addition to two plus years of experience as a Nursing Assistant, my job skills and abilities include:

- *Direct patient care*
- *Charting observations*
- *Communication*
- *Graduate of accredited program*
- *Safety orientation*
- *Medical staff assistance*
- *Personal health intervention*
- *NCLEX-PN license (in progress)*

I will contact you on Tuesday, August 19, 200__, to see whether you have had an opportunity to review my résumé and determine when an interview may be arranged. I look forward to speaking with you soon.

Cordially,

Katelyn Bieser
2001 Putt Drive
Cottage Grove, MN 55301
(612) 555-2728 or kbiesers@pacestar,com

Encl: Résumé

Box 20–9B. Cover Letter: Newspaper Ad Response

*August 13, 200_*

Ms. Christine Johnson, RN, Director of Nursing
St. Helen General Hospital
8354 177th Lane
St. Paul, Minnesota 55000

Re: LPN Staff Nurse Position

Dear Ms. Johnson:

Please accept my résumé as application for the Licensed Practical Nurse position advertised in the Minneapolis Star & Tribune newspaper. I believe that my work experiences through the Fairview Nursing Program and at the nursing home are a good match for the position.

As a recent graduate of the Fairview Nursing Program, I will be taking my NCLEX-PN on September 20, 200_. My clinical work experiences include client care planning, plan review, direct client care, administering medications, and team participation. Additionally, I have worked as a Certified Nursing Assistant for two years at the Forest View Nursing Home in Hastings, Minnesota, performing the above duties, plus more.

I will contact you on Tuesday, August 21, 200_, to see whether you have had an opportunity to review my résumé and determine when an interview may be arranged. I look forward to speaking with you soon.

Cordially,

Katelyn Bieser
2001 Putt Drive
Cottage Grove, MN 55301
(612) 555-2728 or kbieser@spacestar.com

Encl: Résumé

While the information is fresh in your mind, write a thank you letter to the interviewer the same day you interviewed. Write before you become distracted by other projects. Remember, the more often the employer sees or hears your name, the better your chances of being hired rather than being the person waiting for the phone call. A thank you letter may be as simple as that in Box 20–10.

Box 20–10. Thank You Letter for an Interview

August 28, 200__

Ms. Cheryl Sundquist, Director of Nursing
St. Helen General Hospital
8354 177th Lane
St. Paul, Minnesota 55000

RE: LPN Staff Nurse Position

Dear Ms. Sundquist:

Thank you for meeting with me today to discuss the LPN staff position. Following our conversation about the job duties and the tour of the hospital floor, I feel that my work experiences and education are a good match.

Specifically, I look forward to the opportunity to work on the pediatric floor, as this is a special interest of mine. Through our work together the clients will receive timely, quality care.

I remain very interested in the position. I will contact you on Wednesday, September 4, 200__, to see whether you have made a decision or whether a second interview should be arranged. I look forward to speaking with you soon.

Cordially,

Katelyn Bieser
2001 Putt Drive
Cottage Grove, MN 55301
(612) 555-2728 or kbieser@spacestar.com

Remember to follow up with the employer! Call the employer on the date stated in your letter. Make it a practice not to make follow-up contacts on Mondays. These days are traditionally reserved for staff meetings and other duties and are just plain full. The best times to make your follow-up calls are after 9:00 AM. The key to a successful follow-up call is to be courteous but firm with the secretary. Ask to speak with the person in charge of hiring.

The following is a sample follow-up contact to an employer:

> *Secretary:* Good morning. Ms. George's office.
>
> *You:* This is Katelyn Bieser calling. May I speak with Ms. George, please?
>
> *Secretary:* I'm sorry, she's away from her desk/on another line/in a meeting. May I take a message?
>
> *You:* Ms. George and I met last week about the LPN staff position and she said that I should follow up.
>
> *Secretary:* One minute, please.

Although the employer might be away from the office, or on another line, the secretary will probably check to see whether your call should be taken. If the employer is not available, ask the secretary to tell you the best time to reach him or her.

Answers to Application Questions

 ### Learning Exercise: Application Questions

1. What are reasonable responses to employment gaps on applications?
2. What are employers doing to check on application falsification?
3. What are illegal questions?

You will be asked to fill out an application either before or after the interview. It is important that you answer the questions truthfully. If you have had three or more jobs in the past three years, an employer will be concerned about this and will expect you to supply good reasons for leaving. Reasons for leaving might include work interfered with schooling, lay-off, relocation, career exploration, and job stagnation. Gaps in employment between jobs might be explained by responses such as laid off, job hunting, returned to school, travel, and family responsibilities (Dahlstrom & Company, 1995, p. 35).

If there are questions you wish to defer until the face-to-face interview, write in "N/A" (for not applicable), or "Will explain," or leave the space blank. One such area might include expected wage and wages with former employers. For the current wage expected, write "Open;" don't specify a dollar amount. With wages in former employment, leave the spaces blank if you know that you were underpaid or tell the truth if the wage was fair.

Be aware that you do not have to answer questions about age, religion, marital status, children, physical data (unless these are specific requirements for the job), and criminal record (unless it relates to security clearance, housing, or perhaps employment in schools, child facilities, and nursing homes).

An employer's eyes will naturally gravitate toward any blank spaces. Therefore, answer every question you can even if it does not apply to you (e.g., for military service, write N/A in the space if you didn't serve).

Critical Thinking Exercise

If the questions asked are illegal, will you decide to answer the questions or leave the spaces blank?

Some employers view blanks or "Will explain" as an automatic screen for someone they do not want to employ. Should you choose to answer **ille-**

Box 20–11. Sample Answers to Illegal Questions

Have you been hospitalized within the past five years?

Answer: I do not have any health problems that would interfere with fulfilling the advertised position.

Have you ever been on workers' compensation?

Answer: N/A (not applicable)
or
I had a (type of injury) in (year), from which I recovered. It taught me better body mechanics and that if I have any concerns about job tasks to ask for help.

Do you have a criminal record?

Answer: I made a mistake that resulted in a _____. I have paid for that error in judgment and am now wise enough not to repeat it.

gal questions, the examples in Box 20–11 might be helpful.

Do not attempt to falsify information because this will provide grounds for dismissal after hiring. Personnel departments will contact your references, schools, former employers, and others to verify the information on your job application and résumé. The *Job Hunting Handbook* (1995) further emphasized this point when it noted that personnel departments often check your credit records to see whether you are a responsible consumer. This is especially true if the job pays more than $20,000 per year.

Preparing for the Interview

During an interview, *you* are also interviewing the potential employer. If you have prepared adequately, you will be able to evaluate whether your job skills or physical abilities match the objectives

Critical Thinking Exercise

1. What will the employer try to determine during the interview?
2. What is the best way to work with an employer when the person is different from yourself?

of the facility. Remember to bring along a copy of your résumé, LPN license (if you have passed NCLEX-PN), CPR card, and medical records documenting tuberculosis skin tests, hepatitis B, and tetanus vaccinations in case they should be requested (Anderson, 1997).

Interviews are stressful not only for you but also for employers. The employers have to fit interviews into their regular work duties, justify why one candidate should be hired rather than another, and be on constant guard not to discriminate in matters of age, sex, race, and so on. Knowing that there are concerns on both sides—yours and the interviewer's—will help you be less defensive. It will also help you understand the meaning of the questions asked and help you answer them in an honest and reassuring way.

Part of your responsibility is to help the interviewer become comfortable with who you are and why you should be selected for the job. Yeager and Hough (1990) have suggested example responses to deal with age and cultural differences encountered in an interview. See Box 20–12.

Interview Questions and Answers: A Challenging Opportunity

Often the first interview question, "Tell me a little bit about yourself," is an ice breaker designed to make you comfortable and to determine what is important to you. Take advantage of the question to put both you and the interviewer on even ground.

Box 20–12. Tips for Handling Differences Between You and the Interviewer

- If the interviewer is younger than you, statements such as "I bring a lot of experience to this position" will have a more positive effect than "I know I am older than the typical candidate, but . . . ." If the interviewer is older than you, statements such as "I have always worked very hard and feel that learning is a lifelong process" will help establish your maturity.
- With respect to cultural background, when there are differences between you and the interviewer you need to remember that different groups have different norms concerning eye contact, personal distance, body language, and other subtle aspects of communication.
- To work through the differences, it is recommended that you follow the interviewer's lead in the course of communication. Don't mimic the interviewer's specific style but allow her or him to establish some norms concerning how to communicate.

Additionally, avoid giving answers to unanswered illegal questions. For example, don't volunteer that you are married, have children, were brought up in a dysfunctional family, and so on.

Practice the sample responses given in Box 20–13 to typical interview questions as part of your preparation for the interview. Do this as role play-

Learning Exercise: Interview Preparation

1. What is the best way to prepare for an interview?
2. Why is silence from an interviewer something to watch out for?

Box 20–13. Sample Interview Questions and Answers

Tell me about yourself.

Answer: Would you like to know about my work history or my personal life?

For the work history, provide a brief description of your recent schooling and past jobs. If your personal life: I recently graduated from school after living in this area for the past several months. I have a family, consider this my home, and plan to be here for some time. (This demonstrates stability and responsibility.)

Have you ever done this type of work before?

Answer: Yes, in fact some of my experiences include direct care of clients during clinical rotations, volunteer work as a Candy Striper and . . . .

Why do you want to work here?

Answer: The (facility's name) has an excellent reputation in the community and job opportunities for which I am trained. Additionally, your mission statement of _____ reflects my views on _____.

Why did you leave your last job?

Answer: As you know, I am a recent graduate and am looking for employment in my field of study.

Note: If you have worked as a LP/VN: I am looking for a new position to expand my work skills, keep the job interesting, and provide better advancement opportunities.

Tell me about your last employer.

Answer: I really enjoyed my work at _____, which has an excellent reputation for _____. But, now it is time to move on to new opportunities.

What have you done to keep your clinical skills current?

Answer: Well, in addition to participating in several clinical rotations during school, I recently joined (professional organization) to keep abreast of new developments in nursing.

What kind of salary or wage do you expect?

Answer: I know that you will pay me what you feel I am worth and I can't ask for more than that.

Note: If an employer insists that you give a wage quote, give a wage range using your bottom dollar and a realistic top salary. A possible salary resource at your public library is the book by Wischnitzer and Wischnitzer—see References.

Additionally, if you are considering relocation to another city/state, you are encouraged to use www.homefair.com to determine how much salary you would need to maintain your current standard of living. For instance, during the year 2000, an individual earning $22,000 per year in Duluth, Minnesota, needed to earn $28,845 in Arlington Heights, Illinois.

Answer: I would think that we could agree on a salary between $00,000 and $00,000 (Seitzer, 1995).

How do you compare your verbal skills with your writing skills?

Answer: Organizations are more dependent than ever on their employees communicating well both verbally and in writing. I am constantly taking advantage of opportunities to develop both areas by asking for feedback and utilizing the feedback I receive.

Box 20-13. Sample Interview Questions and Answers continued

Why should we hire you instead of someone else?

Answer: I think that my references can best answer that question. I am sure that when you contact them they will agree that I am hard working, dependable, and get the job done right.

When are you available for work?

Answer: Right away. Or: I would need two weeks to resign from my current job because I owe this to my employer. This will provide time for me to tie up any loose ends and allow my employer to find a replacement.

Note: If the prospective employer insists that you terminate your position immediately, you are witnessing a power play. You need to ask yourself whether you really want to work for this individual. This could be the tip of the iceberg for future power plays.

How is your health? Are there any parts of the job that you won't be able to perform?

Answer: I have always been very healthy. I see myself as being able to perform all parts of the job. I think that the best approach to any job is using common sense. If I need help, I am not afraid to ask for it.

What are your greatest strengths?

Answer: I would have to say that my strengths include (1) _____, (2) _____, (3) _____, (4) _____, and (5) _____.

Note: Your responses should be consistent with what your references say about you.

What are your weaknesses?

Answer: If I make a mistake I find that no one can be harder on me than me. I want the job done right.

What was your last employer's opinion of you?

Answer: Great! My employer always appreciated the fact that I was willing to take on new responsibilities and got the work done correctly.

Note: If you were "fired" by your last employer or if you left on bad terms: My last employer will tell you that my work was excellent. We did not work well together. Rather than have the situation continue, the decision was made to leave. It has worked out for the best.

What are your long-term goals?

Answer: Eventually, I would like to work as a charge nurse here at this facility. While my aim is not to replace the current charge nurse, it is my goal to learn all I can. Then I will be a contributing member of the team, and you will feel confident that the work is being taken care of.

Can you work under pressure?

Answer: Yes, I have experienced working under pressure for many years. This has meant meeting deadlines, dealing with difficult people, and having my employers know that their jobs would be done right.

Note: Be prepared to give an example, because many employers will ask for one.

continued

Box 20–13. Sample Interview Questions and Answers continued

Will child care be an issue?

Answer: No. I have found a good day care setting for my children. If they can't go to day care, I have worked out a system of alternating days with another provider or relative to take care of them so that my work is minimally affected.

Note: Although some individuals believe that this is an illegal question, I believe that the employer has a right to know. A stable staffing pattern is needed to maintain quality client care.

Do you have any questions?

Answer: Yes, I would like to know if it would be possible to take a tour and to find out when I can start.

Note: Unless offered the job now, this is not the time to ask about wages. Wait until the job is offered to you, which will allow you some negotiating room. If offered the job at the time of the interview (or afterward), ask about (1) pay rate, (2) benefits, (3) vacation, and (4) starting date.

If you need a higher wage, now is the time to negotiate it because the employer has expressed a desire to hire you. One strategy to use if the starting wage is lower than you desire is to review your new job duties with the employer.

Ask the employer to agree to meet two or three times during the year to review your work performance and wage. Should you choose this strategy, ask the employer to put it into writing. Your work performance and increased wages are a goal you are both working toward.

Would you be willing to work overtime?

Answer: Yes, if it will help the unit.

May we contact your current employer?

Answer: Yes, but after a firm job offer has been made. I would appreciate, however, that before you contact my employer you allow me to talk with my supervisor first as a courtesy.

Is your spouse employed? Will there be a conflict?

Answer: Yes, my spouse has a job. No, I don't see that there would be a conflict. We are both looking forward to my working for you.

Note: Although some individuals may believe that this is an illegal question, I believe that the employer has a right to know the answer. A stable staffing pattern is needed to maintain high-quality client care.

Aren't you overqualified for this job?

Answer: I may be more qualified than other individuals you are considering, but this simply means that I will be able to hit the ground running, and make an immediate contribution. After learning your system, I hope to be eligible for advancement opportunities within the organization.

---

ing, with another person in the role of the interviewer. Ask the person to mix up the order of the questions to prepare you better. You may also want the mock interview to include so-called illegal questions. This will prepare you to handle these questions effectively if they are asked. Successive practice sessions will make you appear to be confident when the time comes for the actual interview.

Also, by being prepared you will not fall victim to the interviewer's most powerful interview tool: silence. Candidates will usually try to fill the void of silence by providing more information—often revealing details beyond their prepared answers to standard interview questions.

Here is an example of "too much information." *Question:* Why did you leave your last job? *Answer:* As you know, I am a recent graduate and am looking for employment in my field of study and I've never done anything before but work as a babysitter".

Making a Lasting Impression

Learning Exercise: Interview Preparation

1. What are the best clothes and make-up to wear for an interview?
2. What is the value of a good handshake?

The kind of person you are is an additional concern to the interviewer. The impression you make includes everything that has been discussed previously plus your appearance and habits during the interview. Suggestions for all nurses are included in the following.

Personal Hygiene

Bathe. Hair should be clean and arranged in a moderate style. Men's hair and beard should be neatly trimmed. Nails should be clean and nicely manicured (avoid polish). If you are a smoker, yellow finger stains may be removed with bleach and water. Use a nonperfumed deodorant.

Recent mouth care may be needed to remove bad breath (remember not to indulge in food or drink with a heavy unpleasant odor near the time of the interview). Floss and brush your teeth, tongue, palate, and inner cheeks with a soft toothbrush. Use a breath freshener. Go easy on the aftershave or perfume, and don't sprinkle any on your clothing. Limit yourself to light perfume (a "clean" look goes a long way).

Clothing

Dress conservatively. When choosing clothing, both men and women should try on many different suits or blazers to determine which fits best and hangs right. A poorly fitting suit looks bad and wears out faster. When buying clothing, the reality is that students may not always be able to afford the ideal. You can always look your best in clothes that are clean and ironed and shoes that are polished. Check out thrift stores and consignment shops, because they are resources waiting to be discovered. Additionally, you might check out community organizations, such as Clothes Closets, that will loan clothing (e.g., the YMCA or YWCA). When looking for clothing, consider the following points:

MEN. Wear a long-sleeved white dress shirt, a solid or pin-stripe navy blue or gray suit, and a medallion patterned red or navy tie that is 3 inches wide. Dark shoes, long dark socks, and a belt that matches the shoes are also a must.

WOMEN. Choose solid or pin-stripe navy or blue dresses, jacket dresses, or suits. Look for simple straight or pleated skirts that reach at least knee level and are comfortable to sit in. Remember that a skirt that is too short may be viewed as being "too sexy." Wear dark, low-heeled shoes with closed toes.

Women with larger hips may want to avoid wearing short jackets. Short jackets flatter women who are petite. Additionally, women who wear gray jackets will want to keep the gray away from their faces by wearing a crisp white blouse or a soft beige sweater. Gray clothes near your face may "drain your complexion."

Make-Up

Conservative make-up is always appropriate. Make-up should be kept to a minimum; wearing too much is the most common mistake. Remember that it is the confidence you display in the interview that makes you attractive to the employer.

Accessories

Wear simple jewelry or none at all. Simple necklaces such as pearls and colored beads work well. Avoid hanging earrings and bracelets that clank, and rhinestones and fake rubies. Plan ahead what purse or briefcase you will carry. You will want to limit yourself to one or the other and have it small enough to avoid getting in your way, yet big enough to hold any papers. If you have a coat or umbrella, ask politely where you can hang or lay them. The main point is to avoid holding items or balancing them on your lap. The fewest distractions will help keep you calm and focused on the interview.

Posture

Walk tall and sit erect but not entirely at the back of your chair. Both feet should rest on the floor, and your head should be upright. Arms and hands should be in an open position and not crossed (remember, you have nothing to hide). Keep your hands inactive. If you must fidget, consider bringing a paper clip to the interview to hold in your hands.

Manner

Your manner should be assured. Do not interrupt the interviewer. Pause to think as needed, then answer without hesitating. Ask for an explanation or repetition of any questions you do not understand.

Eye contact is essential, especially when answering questions. If you are uncomfortable with making eye contact, two techniques can be used to correct this: looking at the employer's nose or looking at the space between the eyebrows. Both give the illusion of eye contact. Remember to look away periodically. Avoid making negative statements or comments about school, former jobs, or personal problems.

Courtesy

When meeting the employer, smile and extend your hand for a firm handshake. Do not use a "bone-crusher" grip or a limp, "dead fish" handshake. Find someone to practice with prior to the interview to get your handshake right. Additionally, if your palms tend to sweat, rub your hand along the top of your thigh when standing up. It will remove the moisture while appearing very natural.

After the handshake, say, "Mr. (Ms.) Smith, my name is _____." Similarly, when the interview is over, stand up, look the person in the eyes, and offer your hand for a firm handshake. Address the employer by surname: "Mr. (Ms.) Smith, thank you for the opportunity to interview with you. Based on what I have learned here today, I know that I can do the job. I would like to call you in four days to see if you have made a decision. Would that be all right?" If you want the job, give the employer a list of your work references or letters of recommendation.

Habits

Do not chew gum or smoke while in the waiting room or during the interview. Also, don't smoke outside the building and then come in for the interview. Although the nicotine may make you feel calm, you will be bringing in the fresh smell of smoke, which is often offensive to nonsmokers. Politely refuse an offer for coffee or tea or cigarettes. In addition, do not read any materials on the employer's desk.

Anticipate Pre-Employment Physical Examinations and Drug Screenings

Learning Exercise: Pre-Employment Issues

1. Does a conditional job offer mean that you got the job?
2. If you fail a drug test, does it mean that you have a chemical abuse problem?

More and more employers are requiring pre-employment physical examinations as a part of conditional job offers. A **conditional job offer** states that you have been offered the job contingent upon your passing a physical examination or drug screening. If you fail, the job offer is withdrawn.

For a physical examination: You will be required to meet with a doctor specified by the employer, who will perform an examination and can legally ask you about your past medical history. Think about any past surgeries, workers' compensation injuries, allergies, and family history, including cancer and heart trouble. Be prepared to provide the dates of these occurrences and the names of the physicians who provided treatment. If you have any personal concerns about the answers your physician might provide, call your doctor prior to the pre-employment physical examination to discuss the job and obtain his or her opinion.

For a drug-screening examination: If you are taking medications, be sure to notify your employer prior to the screening. You will want to reaffirm in the employer's mind that you are taking a medical prescription that will not interfere with your work.

Be aware that although drug-screening accuracy is improving, it is not 100% accurate. Many legal drugs and common foods, such as a poppy seed bagel, could trigger a positive result. Holtorf (2000) reported that there were many "common foods, vi-tamins, and medications that will cause false positives, including ibuprofen (Advil, Nuprin), vitamin B_2, and over-the-counter remedies such as Nyquil, Contac, Sudafed, and Dimetapp."

According to Sakson (1995), any positive test should be followed by a second and more rigorous test, as many drug screening tests have between a 5% to 25% error rate. Discuss with the employer that you are aware of the reliability problems with initial drug screening tests. State that you would like to take a more rigorous test, and that the employer can name the time and place of the screening. The key is sincerity; if you want the job, let the employer know that you are willing to go the extra mile. If you fail a test and really want the job, you might consider discussing splitting or paying for the cost of a second test.

Discussing Pregnancy Issues

Critical Thinking

If you are pregnant, what do you need to consider before talking with an employer about it?

When do you tell a new employer that you are pregnant? Even if your job is protected by the Pregnancy Discrimination Act and the Family and Medical Leave Act (FMLA applies if there are 50 or more employees with the company), when do you discuss the pregnancy so that it doesn't interfere with career advancement? Kleiman (1995) reported that waiting a couple of months is okay. She indicated that the "real issues are your comfort level and professionalism."

When you are ready to talk about your pregnancy, be prepared to discuss (1) how long you plan to work, (2) how long you intend to be gone, and possibly (3) how your work will be covered while you are away. Then talk with your coworkers about the pregnancy and enlist their moral support. Expectant mothers may have both good and bad days during the pregnancy; friends can be a great help.

Resignation with Style

Critical Thinking Exercise

Is there a difference between "burning bridges" and "untying the connection"? What is the value of recapping your accomplishments with a resignation letter?

According to Clark (1999), there are times when it pays to quit. In today's job market, employers continue to try to hold down their costs by limiting annual raises to 4% or less. However, in their desperation to staff positions, they will offer job hoppers 10% to 20% over their current salaries. Clark (1999) estimated that approximately 17 million workers quit to take other jobs within that year.

If you are contemplating a change, it is recommended that you look at how long you have been with the employer. If you have worked less than 3 months, you can hop right away, remembering not to list the employer on your résumé. In the event that you have worked longer than three months with the employer, it is recommended that you work a minimum of one year to obtain experience and to demonstrate stability.

If you have made the decision to leave your employer, it is important to leave the job with class. Perhaps the best expression I have heard is "Untie, don't sever, the connection." You never know who may call your former employer as a part of their follow up. You may wish to return to their employ again in the future.

It is strongly recommended that you have a posi-

tion secured prior to leaving. Some employers will let you go the day they are informed even though personnel policy requires a two-week notice (Sixel, 1995). Either way, it is recommended that the employer be given written notice of your intention to leave, allowing adequate time to hire a replacement. It is **resignation courtesy** to give two weeks' notice even if no policy is in place. (It is expensive

---

Box 20–14. Sample Resignation Letter

*September 11, 200_*

Ms. Sivia Hinkkanen, Director of Nursing
Brown County Hospital
1515 Placebo Lane
Minneapolis, Minnesota 55401

Dear Ms. Hinkkanen:

Please accept my resignation as Charge Nurse on Unit 3 to be effective on September 30, 200_. My association with the Brown County Hospital has been rewarding professionally and personally. It is satisfying to have been able to contribute to the positive reputation of client care.

I am especially pleased to have been a member of the Quality Assurance committee, which furthered my professional growth. In addition, I remain appreciative of having been honored as "Employee of the Month."

Please accept my thanks for the support you have provided me during the past one and a half years of employment. I wish the members of this hospital the very best.

Cordially,

Katelyn Bieser, LPN, Alzheimer Unit

for an employer to hire and orient a new person and for the new person to become a productive team member.)

Use a business format and plain paper, and type the letter. Even if you are leaving because of unhappy circumstances on the job, do not vent these feelings in the letter. As mentioned before, you may need this employer as a work reference in the future. Additionally, your current supervisor may also leave in the future, and all that there is to remind the employer about you is your personnel file.

Because resignation is part of your permanent record, it provides you with an opportunity to recap your accomplishments or special recognition. The employer may refer to the letter when he or she is contacted by employers with whom you are seeking employment. See the sample resignation letter in Box 20–14.

Summary

- ☐ To be successful in your job search, it is important to begin it with the first day of classes and not stop from that day on. Opportunities present themselves to those who are willing to put forth a little effort and realize that the world does not owe them a living.
- ☐ The methods presented in this chapter have proved to be successful for graduates, people wishing to make career changes, or those wanting to institute a change in their work. Remember to treat the job search like a job.
- ☐ Make your contacts by telephone or computer, by forwarding résumés or cover letters, or by physically going to the employer to apply and schedule an interview. Explore the **hidden job market** via networking, the Internet, or using the telephone book and then calling employers whether an ad has been placed or not.
- ☐ Actively follow up on all interviews! Let the employer know that you are interested. Remember, the more often the employer hears your name, the better your chances will be. If you are hired, send thank you notes to those who helped you. You may need them again. Remember, you are responsible for making your own luck.

Review Questions

1. What interpersonal style is representative of "talking quickly and finishing other's sentences"?
   A. Friendly-focused
   B. Results-focused
   C. Detailed-focused
   D. Party-focused
2. What method is not typically used to get a job?
   A. Assistance from family and friends
   B. School placement offices
   C. Direct application to an employer
   D. Personal newspaper ad for a position
3. Résumés should include
   A. An objective statement
   B. Salary requirements
   C. Short bulleted sentences
   D. Personal data
4. What is the percentage of prospective job candidates who interview and never follow up with the interviewer?
   A. 90%
   B. 75%
   C. 60%
   D. 50%

5. If participating in a drug screening, you should
   A. Abstain from eating foods with chemical additives.
   B. Do the screening in the early morning hours.
   C. Recall that tests have a 5% to 25% error rate.
   D. Not take your prescription the day before.

References

Anderson M. *Employment Process in Nursing Leadership; Management and Professional Practice for the LPN/LVN.* Philadelphia, F.A. Davis, 1997, p.64.

Clark K. Why it pays to quit. U.S. News & World Report 127(17):74, 1999.

Dahlstrom & Company. *The Job Hunting Handbook: Job Outlook to 2005.* Holliston, MA: Dahlstrom & Company, 1995.

Dixon P. *Choosing Your Electronic Résumé; Job Searching Online for Dummies.* New York: IDG Books Worldwide, 1998.

Ethridge M. Keep ahead of the curve when seeking jobs; Rules for the hunt are evolving. St. Paul Pioneer Press, May 28, 1K, 1995.

Farr J. *America's Top Medical and Human Services Jobs.* Indianapolis: JIST Works, Inc., 1994.

Franklin D. What your voice says about you. Health Magazine 19(2):38, 41, 1995.

Holtorf K. Beware: Drug-test false positives. Bottom Line Personal Publications 21(5):15, 2000.

Kleiman C. Planning leaves for pregnancies eases interim for moms, employers. St. Paul Pioneer Press, June 4, K1, 1995.

Kuntz S. Critical career questions. Twin Cities Employment Weekly 2 (44): 2, 1995.

Meissner J. How to work a room. Twin Cities Employment Weekly 3 (7):2, 8, 1995.

Mercer M. How to make a great impression on anyone. Bottom Line Personal 15(21):1314, 1994.

Messmer M. *Career Search Sites: Job Hunting for Dummies,* 2nd ed. New York: IDG Books Worldwide, 1999.

Sakson S. Positive drug tests post decline. St. Paul Pioneer Press, June 30, B3, 1995.

Seitzer D. Salary negotiations. Twin City Employment Weekly 2(43):23, 1995.

Sixel L. When to tell boss you're planning to quit. St. Paul Pioneer Press, January 22, K1, 1995.

Wischnitzer S, Wischnitzer E. *Health-Care Careers for the 21st Century.* Indianapolis: JIST Works, 2000.

Yeager N, Hough L. *Power Interviews: Job-Winning Tactics from Fortune 500 Recruiters.* New York: John Wiley & Sons, 1990.

State Boards of Nursing

(NOTE: These addresses and websites were current as of July, 2000.)

Alabama

Alabama Board of Nursing
RSA Plaza, Suite 250
770 Washington Avenue
P.O. Box 303900
Montgomery, Alabama 36130-3900
Phone: (334) 242-4060
Fax: (334) 242-4360

http://www.abn.state.al.us/

Alaska

Alaska Board of Nursing
Department of Community and Economic
    Development
Division of Occupational Licensing
3601 C Street, Suite 722
Anchorage, Alaska 99503
Phone: (907) 269-8161
Fax: (907) 269-8196

Mailing address:
P.O. Box 110806
Juneau, Alaska 99811-0806

http://www.dced.state.ak.us/occ/pnur.htm

American Samoa

American Samoa Health Services
    Regulatory Board
LBJ Tropical Medical Center
Pago Pago, American Samoa 96799
Phone: 011-(684) 633-1222
Fax: 011-(684) 633-1869

Arizona

Arizona State Board of Nursing
1651 E. Morten Avenue, Suite 150
Phoenix, Arizona 85020
Phone: (602) 331-8111
Fax: (602) 906-9365

http://azboardofnursing.org/

Arkansas

Arkansas State Board of Nursing
University Tower Building, Suite 800
1123 South University
Little Rock, Arkansas 72204
Phone: (501) 686-2700
Fax: (501) 686-2714

http://www.state.ar.us/nurse

California—RN

California Board of Registered Nursing
400 R Street, Suite 4030
P.O. Box 944210
Sacramento, California 94244-2100
Phone: (916) 322-3350
Fax: (916) 327-4402
NCNET: C.Puri 132:NCZ030

http://www.rn.ca.gov/

California—VN

California Board of Vocational Nurse and Psychiatric
    Technician Examiners
2535 Capitol Oaks Drive, Suite 205
Sacramento, California 95833
Phone: (916) 263-7800
Fax: (916) 263-7859

http://www.bvnpt.ca.gov/

Colorado

Colorado Board of Nursing
1560 Broadway, Suite 880
Denver, Colorado 80202
Phone: (303) 894-2430
Fax: (303) 894-2821

http://www.dora.state.co.us/nursing/

Connecticut

Connecticut Board of Examiners for Nursing
Division of Health Systems Regulation
410 Capital Avenue, MS # 12HSR

P.O. Box 340308
Hartford, Connecticut 06134-0328
Phone: (860) 509-7624
Fax: (860) 509-7553

http://www.state.ct.us/dph/

Delaware

Delaware Board of Nursing
861 Silver Lake Boulevard
Cannon Building, Suite 203
Dover, Delaware 19904
Phone: (302) 739-4522
Fax: (302) 739-2711

District of Columbia

District of Columbia Board of Nursing
Department of Health
825 N. Capitol Street, N.E., 2nd floor
Room 2224
Washington, District of Columbia 20002
Phone: (202) 442-4778
Fax: (202) 442-9431

Florida

Florida Board of Nursing
4080 Woodcock Drive, Suite 202
Jacksonville, Florida 32207
Phone: (904) 858-6940
Fax: (904) 858-6964

http://www.doh.state.fl.us/mqa/nursing/rnhome.htm

Georgia—PN

Georgia State Board of Licensed Practical Nurses
237 Coliseum Drive
Macon, Georgia 31217-3858
Phone: (912) 207-1300
Fax: (912) 207-1633

http://www.sos.state.ga.us/ebd-lpn/

Georgia—RN

Georgia Board of Nursing
237 Coliseum Drive
Macon, Georgia 31217-3858
Phone: (912) 207-1640
Fax: (912) 207-1660

http://www.sos.state.ga.us/ebd-rn/

Guam

Guam Board of Nurse Examiners
P.O. Box 2816
1304 East Sunset Boulevard
Barrgada, Guam 96913
Phone: 011-(671) 475-0251
Fax: 011-(671) 477-4733

Hawaii

Hawaii Board of Nursing
Professional and Vocational Licensing Division
P.O. Box 3469
Honolulu, Hawaii 96801
Phone: (808) 586-3000
Fax: (808) 586-2689

Idaho

Idaho Board of Nursing
280 N. 8th Street, Suite 210
P.O. Box 83720
Boise, Idaho 83720
Phone: (208) 334-3110
Fax: (208) 334-3262

http://www.state.id.us/ibn/ibnhome.htm

Illinois

Illinois Department of Professional Regulation
James R. Thompson Center
100 West Randolph, Suite 9-300
Chicago, Illinois 60601
Phone: (312) 814-2715
Fax: (312) 814-3145

http://www.dpr.state.il.us/

Indiana

Indiana State Board of Nursing
Health Professions Bureau
402 West Washington Street
Room W041
Indianapolis, Indiana 46204
Phone: (317) 232-2960
Fax: (317) 233-4236

http://www.ai.org/hpb

Iowa

Iowa Board of Nursing
RiverPoint Business Park
400 SW 8th Street, Suite B

Des Moines, Iowa 50309-4685
Phone: (515) 281-3255
Fax: (515) 281-4825

http://www.state.ia.us/government/nursing/

Kansas

Kansas State Board of Nursing
Landon State Office Building
900 S.W. Jackson, Suite 551-S
Topeka, Kansas 66612-1230
Phone: (785) 296-4929
Fax: (785) 296-3929

http://www.ksbn.org/

Kentucky

Kentucky Board of Nursing
312 Whittington Parkway, Suite 300
Louisville, Kentucky 40222
Phone: (502) 329-7000
Fax: (502) 329-7011

http://www.kbn.state.ky.us/

Louisiana—PN

Louisiana State Board of Practical Nurse
    Examiners
3421 N. Causeway Boulevard, Suite 203
Metairie, Louisiana 70002
Phone: (504) 838-5791
Fax: (504) 838-5279

Louisiana—RN

Louisiana State Board of Nursing
3510 N. Causeway Boulevard, Suite 501
Metairie, Louisiana 70003
Phone: (504) 838-5332
Fax: (504) 838-5349

http://www/lsbn.state.la.us/

Maine

Maine State Board of Nursing
158 State House Station
Augusta, Maine 04333
Phone: (207) 287-1133
Fax: (207) 287-1149

http://www.state.me.us/nursingbd/

Maryland

Maryland Board of Nursing
4140 Patterson Avenue
Baltimore, Maryland 21215
Phone: (410) 585-1900
Fax: (410) 358-3530

http://dhmh1d.dhmh.state.md.us/mbn/

Massachusetts

Massachusetts Board of Registration in Nursing
Commonwealth of Massachusetts
239 Causeway Street
Boston, MA 02114
Phone: (617) 727-9961
Fax: (617) 727-1630

http://www.state.ma.us/reg/boards/rn/

Michigan

Michigan CIS/Office of Health Services
Ottawa Towers North
611 West Ottawa, 4th floor
Lansing, Michigan 48933
Phone: (517) 373-9102
Fax: (517) 373-2179

http://www.cis.state.mi.us/bhser/genover.htm

Minnesota

Minnesota Board of Nursing
2829 University Avenue SE, Suite 500
Minneapolis, Minnesota 55414
Phone: (612) 617-2270
Fax: (612) 617-2190

http://www.nursingboard.state.mn.us/

Mississippi

Mississippi Board of Nursing
1935 Lakeland Drive, Suite B
Jackson, Mississippi 39216
Phone: (601) 987-4188
Fax: (601) 364-2352

Missouri

Missouri State Board of Nursing
3605 Missouri Boulevard
P.O. Box 656

Jefferson City, Missouri 65102-0656
Phone: (573) 751-0681
Fax: (573) 751-0075

http://www.ecodev.state.mo.us/pr/nursing/

Montana

Montana State Board of Nursing
Arcade Building, Suite 4C
111 North Jackson
P.O. Box 200513
Helena, Montana 59620-0513
Phone: (406) 444-2071
Fax: (406) 444-7759

*http://www.com.state.mt.us/license/pol/pol
    boards/nur board/board page.htm*

Nebraska

Nebraska Health and Human Services System
Department of Regulation and Licensure,
    Nursing Section
301 Centennial Mall South
P.O. Box 94986
Lincoln, Nebraska 68509-4986
Phone: (402) 471-4376
Fax: (402) 471-3577

http://www.hhs.state.ne.us/crl/nns.htm

Nevada

Nevada State Board of Nursing (Las Vegas area)
4330 S. Valley View, Suite 106
Las Vegas, Nevada 89103
Phone: (702) 486-5800
Fax: (702) 486-5803

Nevada State Board of Nursing (Reno/Carson City area)
1755 East Plumb Lane, Suite 260
Reno, Nevada 89502
Phone: (775) 688-2620
Fax: (775) 688-2628

http://www.nursingboard.state.nv.us/

New Hampshire

New Hampshire Board of Nursing
78 Regional Drive, Bldg B
P.O. Box 3898
Concord, New Hampshire 03302
Phone: (603) 271-2323
Fax: (603) 271-6605

http://www.state.nh.us/nursing/

New Jersey

New Jersey Board of Nursing
124 Halsey Street, 6th floor
P.O. Box 45010
Newark, New Jersey 07101
Phone: (973) 504-6586
Fax: (973) 648-3481

http://www.state.nj.us/lps/ca/medical.htm

New Mexico

New Mexico Board of Nursing
4206 Louisiana Boulevard, NE, Suite A
Albuquerque, New Mexico 87109
Phone: (505) 841-8340
Fax: (505) 841-8347

http://www.state.nm.us/clients/nursing

New York

New York State Board of Nursing
State Education Department
Cultural Education Center, Room 3023
Albany, New York 12230
Phone: (518) 474-3845
Fax: (518) 474-3706

http://www.nysed.gov/prof/nurse.htm

North Carolina

North Carolina Board of Nursing
3724 National Drive
P.O. Box 2129
Raleigh, North Carolina 27602
Phone: (919) 782-3211
Fax: (919) 781-9461

http://www.ncbon.com/

North Dakota

North Dakota Board of Nursing
919 South 7th Street, Suite 504
Bismarck, North Dakota 58504
Phone: (701) 328-9777
Fax: (701) 328-9785

http://www.ndbon.org/

Northern Mariana Islands

Commonwealth Board of Nurse Examiners
Public Health Center
P.O. Box 1458

Saipan, MP 96950
Phone: 011-(670) 234-8950
Fax: 011-(670) 234-8930

Ohio

Ohio Board of Nursing
17 South High Street, Suite 400
Columbus, Ohio 43215-3413
Phone: (614) 466-3947
Fax: (614) 466-0388

http://www.state.oh.us/nur/

Oklahoma

Oklahoma Board of Nursing
2915 North Classen Boulevard, Suite 524
Oklahoma City, Oklahoma 73106
Phone: (405) 962-1800
Fax: (405) 962-1821

Oregon

Oregon State Board of Nursing
800 NE Oregon Street, Box 25, Suite 465
Portland, Oregon 97232
Phone: (503) 731-4745
Fax: (503) 731-4755

http://www.osbn.state.or.us/

Pennsylvania

Pennsylvania State Board of Nursing
124 Pine Street
P.O. Box 2649
Harrisburg, Pennsylvania 17101
Phone: (717) 783-7142
Fax: (717) 783-0822

http://www.dos.state.pa.us/bpoa/nurbd/mainpage.htm

Puerto Rico

Commonwealth of Puerto Rico Board of Nurse
  Examiners
800 Roberto H. Todd Avenue
Room 202, Stop 18
Santurce, Puerto Rico 00908
Phone: (787) 725-8161
Fax: (787) 725-7903

Rhode Island

Rhode Island Board of Nurse Registration & Nursing
  Education

105 Cannon Building
Three Capitol Hill
Providence, Rhode Island 02908
Phone: (401) 222-5700
Fax: (401) 222-3352

South Carolina

South Carolina State Board of Nursing
110 Centerview Drive, Suite 202
Columbia, South Carolina 29210
Phone: (803) 896-4550
Fax: (803) 896-4525

Mailing address:
P.O. Box 12367
Columbia, SC 29211

http://www.llr.state.sc.us/bon.htm

South Dakota

South Dakota Board of Nursing
4300 South Louise Avenue, Suite C-1
Sioux Falls, South Dakota 57106-3124
Phone: (605) 362-2760
Fax: (605) 362-2768

http://www.state.sd.us/dcr/nursing/

Tennessee

Tennessee State Board of Nursing
426 Fifth Avenue North
1st floor—Cordell Hull Building
Nashville, Tennessee 37247
Phone: (615) 532-5166
Fax: (615) 741-7899

http://170.142.76.180/bmf-bin/BMFproflist.pl

Texas—RN

Texas Board of Nurse Examiners
William P. Hobby Building, Tower 3
333 Guadalupe, Suite 3-460
Austin, Texas 78701
Phone: (512) 305-7400
Fax: (512) 305-7401

Mailing Address:
P.O. Box 430
Austin, Texas 78716-0430

http://www.bne.state.tx.us/

Texas—VN

Texas Board of Vocational Nurse Examiners
William P. Hobby Building, Tower 3
333 Guadalupe Street, 3-400
Austin, Texas 78701
Phone: (512) 305-8100
Fax: (512) 305-8101

http://link.tsl.state.tx.us/tx/bvne/

Utah

Utah State Board of Nursing
Heber M. Wells Building, 4th floor
160 East 300 South
Salt Lake City, Utah 84111
Phone: (801) 530-6628
Fax: (801) 530-6511

http://www.commerce.state.ut.us/

Vermont

Vermont State Board of Nursing
109 State Street
Montpelier, Vermont 05609-1106
Phone: (802) 828-2396
Fax: (802) 828-2484

Mailing Address:
26 Terrace Street, Drawer 9
Montpelier, Vermont 05609-1101

http://vtprofessionals.org/nurses/

Virginia

Virginia Board of Nursing
6606 West Broad Street, 4th floor
Richmond, Virginia 23230
Phone: (804) 662-9909
Fax: (804) 662-9512

http://www.dhp.state.va.us/

Virgin Islands

Virgin Islands Board of Nurse Licensure
Veterans Drive Station
St. Thomas, U.S. Virgin Islands 00803
Phone: (340) 776-7397
Fax: (340) 777-4003

Washington

Washington State Nursing Care Quality Assurance
Commission
Department of Health
1300 Quince Street SE
Olympia, Washington 98504-7864
Phone: (360) 236-4740
Fax: (360) 236-4738

http://www.doh.wa.gov/nursing/

West Virginia—PN

West Virginia State Board of Examiners for Licensed
Practical Nurses
101 Dee Drive
Charleston, West Virginia 25311
Phone: (304) 558-3572
Fax: (304) 558-4367
(Please indicate for PN Bd)

http://www.lpnboard.state.wv.us/

West Virginia—RN

West Virginia Board of Examiners for Registered
Professional Nurses
101 Dee Drive
Charleston, West Virginia 25311
Phone: (304) 558-3596
Fax: (304) 558-3666

http://www.state.wv.us/nurses/rn/

Wisconsin

Wisconsin Department of Regulation & Licensing
1400 East Washington Avenue
P.O. Box 8935
Madison, Wisconsin 53708
Phone: (608) 266-0145
Fax: (608) 267-0644

http://www.state.wi.us/agencies/drl/

Wyoming

Wyoming State Board of Nursing
2020 Carey Avenue, Suite 110
Cheyenne, Wyoming 82002
Phone: (307) 777-7601
Fax: (307) 777-3519

http://nursing.state.wy.us/

NAPNES Standards of Practice for Licensed Practical/Vocational Nurses

The LP/VN provides individual and family-centered nursing care by:

A. Utilizing appropriate knowledge, skills, and abilities.
B. Utilizing principles of the nursing process in meeting specific patient needs in diversified health care settings.
C. Maintaining appropriate written documentation and utilizing effective communication skills with patients, family, significant others, and members of the health team.
D. Executing principles of crisis intervention to maintain safety.
E. Providing appropriate education to patients, family, and significant others to promote health, facilitate rehabilitation, and maintain wellness.
F. Serving as a patient advocate to protect patient rights.

The LP/VN fulfills the professional responsibilities of the practical/vocational nurse by:

A. Applying the ethical principles underlying the profession.
B. Following legal requirements.
C. Following the policies and procedures of the employing facility.
D. Cooperating and collaborating with all members of the health care team to meet the needs of family-centered nursing care.
E. Assuming accountability for his or her nursing actions.
F. Seeking educational opportunities to improve knowledge and skills.
G. Building skills to assure and increase post-licensure competence.

NAPNES Code of Ethics

The Licensed Practical/Vocational Nurse Shall:

1. Consider as a basic obligation the conservation of life and the prevention of disease.
2. Promote and protect the physical, mental, emotional, and spiritual health of the patient and the family.
3. Fulfill all duties faithfully and efficiently.
4. Function within established legal guidelines.
5. Accept personal responsibility (for his or her acts) and seek to merit the respect and confidence of all members of the health team.
6. Hold in confidence all matters coming to his or her knowledge, in the practice of his or her profession, and in no way and at no time violate this confidence.
7. Give conscientious service and charge just remuneration.
8. Learn and respect the religious and cultural beliefs of his or her patient and of all people.
9. Meet his or her obligation to the patient by keeping abreast of current trends in health care through reading and continuing education.
10. As a citizen of the United States of America, uphold the laws of the land and seek to promote legislation that will meet the health needs of its people.

NFLPN Nursing Practice Standards for the Licensed Practical/Vocational Nurse

Preface

The Standards were developed and adopted by NFLPN to provide a basic model by which the quality of health service and nursing care given by LP/VNs may be measured and evaluated.

These nursing practice standards are applicable in any practice setting. The degree to which individual standards are applied will vary according to the individual needs of the patient, the type of health care agency or services, and the community resources.

The scope of licensed practical nursing has extended into specialized nursing services. Therefore, specialized fields of nursing are included in this document.

The Code for Licensed Practical/Vocational Nurses

The Code, adopted by NFLPN in 1961 and revised in 1979, provides a motivation for establishing, maintaining, and elevating professional standards. Each LP/VN, upon entering the profession, inherits the responsibility to adhere to the standards of ethical practice and conduct as set forth in this Code.

1. Know the scope of maximum utilization of the LP/VN as specified by the nursing practice act and function within this scope.
2. Safeguard the confidential information acquired from any source about the patient.
3. Provide health care to all patients regardless of race, creed, cultural background, disease, or life style.
4. Refuse to give endorsement to the sale and promotion of commercial products or services.
   Uphold the highest standards in personal appearance, language, dress, and demeanor.
   ay informed about issues affecting the practice of
   ing and delivery of health care and, where appro-
   participate in government and policy decisions.
   he responsibility for safe nursing by keeping
   entally and physically fit and educationally
   ractice.

8. Accept responsibility for membership in NFLPN and participate in its efforts to maintain the established standards of nursing practice and employment policies that lead to quality patient care.

Introductory Statement

Definition

Practical/vocational nursing means the performance for compensation of authorized acts of nursing that utilize specialized knowledge and skills and that meet the health needs of people in a variety of settings under the direction of qualified health professionals.

Scope

Practical/vocational nursing comprises the common core of nursing and, therefore, is a valid entry into the nursing profession.

Opportunities exist for practicing in a milieu in which different professions unite their particular skills in a team effort for one common objective—to preserve or improve an individual patient's functioning.

Opportunities also exist for upward mobility within the profession through academic education and for lateral expansion of knowledge and expertise through both academic and continuing education.

Standards

Education

The Licensed Practical/Vocational Nurse:

1. Shall complete a formal education program in practical nursing approved by the appropriate nursing authority in a state.
2. Shall successfully pass the National Council Licensure Examination for Practical Nurses.
3. Shall participate in initial orientation within the employing institution.

Legal/Ethical Status

The Licensed Practical/Vocational Nurse:

1. Shall hold a current license to practice nursing as an LP/VN in accordance with the law of the state wherein employed.
2. Shall know the scope of nursing practice authorized by the Nursing Practice Act in the state wherein employed.
3. Shall have a personal commitment to fulfill the legal responsibilities inherent in good nursing practice.
4. Shall take responsible actions in situations in which there is unprofessional conduct by a peer or other health care provider.
5. Shall recognize and have a commitment to meet the ethical and moral obligations of the practice of nursing.
6. Shall not accept or perform professional responsibilities that the individual knows she or he is not competent to perform.

Practice

The Licensed Practical/Vocational Nurse:

1. Shall accept assigned responsibilities as an accountable member of the health care team.
2. Shall function within the limits of educational preparation and experience as related to the assigned duties.
3. Shall function with other members of the health care team in promoting and maintaining health, preventing disease and disability, caring for and rehabilitating individuals who are experiencing an altered health state, and contributing to the ultimate quality of life until death.
4. Shall know and utilize the nursing process in planning, implementing, and evaluating health services and nursing care for the individual patient or group.

   a. Planning: The planning of nursing includes:

   (1) Assessment of health status of the individual patient, the family, and community groups.
   (2) An analysis of the information gained from assessment.
   (3) The identification of health goals.

   b. Implementation: The plan for nursing care is put into practice to achieve the stated goals and includes:

   (1) Observing, recording, and reporting significant changes that require intervention or different goals.

   (2) Applying nursing knowledge and skills to promote and maintain health to prevent disease and disability and to optimize functional capabilities of an individual patient.
   (3) Assisting the patient and family with activities of daily living and encouraging self-care as appropriate.
   (4) Carrying out therapeutic regimens and protocols prescribed by an RN, physician, or other persons authorized by state law.

   c. Evaluations: The plan for nursing care and its implementations are evaluated to measure the progress toward the stated goals and will include appropriate persons and/or groups to determine:

   (1) The relevancy of current goals in relation to the progress of the individual patient.
   (2) The involvement of the recipients of care in the evaluation process.
   (3) The quality of the nursing action in the implementation of the plan.
   (4) A re-ordering of priorities or new goal setting in the care plan.

5. Shall participate in peer review and other evaluation processes.
6. Shall participate in the development of policies concerning the health and nursing needs of society and in the roles and functions of the LP/VN.

Continuing Education

The Licensed Practical/Vocational Nurse:

1. Shall be responsible for maintaining the highest possible level of professional competence at all times.
2. Shall periodically reassess career goals and select continuing education activities that will help achieve these goals.
3. Shall take advantage of continuing education opportunities that will lead to personal growth and professional development.
4. Shall seek and participate in continuing education activities that are approved for credit by appropriate organizations, such as the NFLPN.

Specialized Nursing Practice

The Licensed Practical/Vocational Nurse:

1. Shall have had at least one year's experience in n ing at the staff level.

2. Shall present personal qualifications that are indicative of potential abilities for practice in the chosen specialized nursing area.
3. Shall present evidence of completion of a program or course that is approved by an appropriate agency to provide the knowledge and skills necessary for effective nursing services in the specialized field.
4. Shall meet all the standards of practice as set forth in this document.

Glossary

authorized (acts of nursing)   Those nursing activities made legal through state nurse practice acts or other laws.

lateral expansion of knowledge   An extension of the basic core of information learned in the school of practical nursing.

LP/VN   A combined abbreviation for licensed practical nurse and licensed vocational nurse. The LVN is the title used in California and Texas for the nurses who are called LPNs in other states.

milieu   One's environment and surroundings.

peer review   A formal evaluation of performance on the job by other LP/VNs.

protocols   Courses of treatment that include specific steps to be performed in a stated order.

specialized nursing practice   A restricted field of nursing in which a person is particularly skilled and has specific knowledge.

therapeutic regimens   Regulated plans designed to bring about effective treatment of disease.

upward mobility   A change of career goal, e.g., licensed practical/vocational nurse to registered nurse.

NLN Entry-Level Competencies of Graduates of Educational Programs in Practical Nursing

Introduction

Licensed practical nurses (LPNs), in some areas called licensed vocational nurses (LVNs), are prepared to function under the definition and framework of the role specified by the nurse practice acts of the states where they are employed. LP/VNs are concerned with basic therapeutic, rehabilitative, and preventive care for people of all ages and diverse cultures in various stages of dependency.

This document was written to describe the entry-level performance expectations of graduates of practical nursing programs. The purpose is to assist the recipients of nursing care, prospective students, employers, and other interested persons in developing an understanding of the importance of the licensed practical nurse as a member of the health care team. Practical/vocational nursing educators can utilize these competencies to formulate program outcomes. The competencies are stated in broad terms rather than specifics, because nurse practice acts differ from state to state.

Role

The graduate of practical/vocational nursing programs is eligible to apply for licensure. Licensed practical/vocational nurses practice under the guidance of a registered nurse or licensed physician/dentist. The primary role of the licensed practical/vocational nurse is to provide nursing care for clients experiencing common, well-defined health problems in structured health care settings. In their roles as members of the discipline of nursing, practical/vocational nurses actively participate in and subscribe to the legal and ethical tenets of the discipline.

Competencies

The graduate practical/vocational nurse demonstrates the following entry-level competencies:

From National League for Nursing, Council of Practical Nursing Programs.

Assessment

- Assesses basic physical, emotional, spiritual, and sociocultural needs of the health care client.
- Collects data within established protocols and guidelines from various sources:
  a. client interviews;
  b. observations/measurements;
  c. health care team members, family, and significant others;
  d. health records.
- Utilizes knowledge of normal values to identify deviations in health status.
- Documents data collection.
- Communicates findings to appropriate health care personnel.

Planning

- Contributes to the development of nursing care plans utilizing **established** nursing diagnoses for clients with common, well-defined health problems.
- Prioritizes nursing care needs of clients.
- Assists in the review and revision of nursing care plans to meet the changing needs of clients.

Implementation

- Provides nursing care according to:
  a. accepted standards of practice;
  b. priority of client needs;
  c. individual and family rights to dignity and privacy.
- Utilizes effective communication in:
  a. recording and reporting;
  b. establishing and maintaining therapeutic relationships with clients, families, and significant others.
- Collaborates with health care team members to coordinate the delivery of nursing care.
- Instructs clients regarding health maintenance based client needs and nurse's knowledge level.

Evaluation

- Seeks guidance as needed in evaluating nursing care.
- Modifies nursing approaches based on evaluation of nursing care.
- Collaborates with other health team members in the revision of nursing care plans.

Member of the Discipline

- Complies with the scope of practice as outlined in the nurse practice act of the state in which licensed.
- Describes the role of the licensed practical/vocational nurse in the health care delivery system.
- Utilizes educational opportunities for continued personal and professional growth.
- Identifies personal potential and considers career mobility options.
- Identifies personal strengths and weaknesses for the purpose of improving performance.
- Adheres to a nursing code of ethics.
- Functions as an advocate for the health care consumer.

Managing/Supervision

- Assumes responsibility for managing his/her own actions when providing nursing care for individuals and groups of clients.
- Is accountable for nursing care delegated to unlicensed health care providers.

Political Activism

- Is aware that the practical nurse, through political, economic, and societal activities, can affect nursing and health.

Definitions

Basic: A word synonymous with fundamental, initial, elementary, essential, and necessary.

Client: A person who is a recipient of nursing care.

Competency: Cognitive, affective, and/or psychomotor capability demonstrated in various roles in the practice setting.

Nursing Care Plan: Written plan incorporating data obtained from utilization of the nursing process.

Nursing Diagnosis: A statement that describes an existing or potential health problem that nurses can treat separately from physician orders.

Nursing Process: The nursing process is the core of the practice of nursing. The four phases of the nursing process—assessment, planning, implementation, and evaluation—are the framework around which competencies have been developed.

Practical Nursing Program: An educational program under the control of a hospital, vocational-technical institute, community college, or in some instances independently incorporated that awards a certificate or diploma in practical nursing and prepares the graduate to be eligible for licensure as a practical/vocational nurse.

Structured Care Setting: An environment in which the policies, procedures, and protocols for provision of health care are established. The amount of structure may vary among individual agencies, such as hospitals, nursing homes, and home health settings.

Learning Exercises for Chapter 4

Time Management: Sample Personal Roles and Activities

Below is an example of one person's listing of personal roles and activities. Using the blank page provided on the next page, list your personal roles and activities for each category. (Explanations for notations appear below.*)

School

A   Be at school 40 hours per week.
A   Be prepared to teach three courses each week (total of 25 hours in class and clinical).

Community

Ⓐ Lector at church.
Ⓑ Member of library board.
Ⓑ Member of homemaker's group.

Recreation

A   Write a book.
A   Attend symphony five times per year.
A   Attend Civic Music five times per year.
B   Periodically attend movies and watch television.
B   Night out with husband.
A   "Special" activities with son.
Ⓑ Selected activities that come up in community during year.

Job

A   School is my job.

Family

A   Principal organizer for family of three.
Ⓐ Spend time with son.
Ⓐ Prepare dinner seven evenings per week.
Ⓑ Prepare one special breakfast on weekend.
Ⓐ Do one load of laundry per day.
Ⓐ Do several loads of laundry on weekend.
Ⓐ Food shop several times a week.
 B   Major housecleaning one time per year.
Ⓐ Daily straightening up of house.
Ⓐ Perform errands as necessary.
Ⓑ Attend PTA.
Ⓑ Attend Boy Scout activities.

---

*A = priority items (These items *have* to be done.);
  B = nonpriority items (These items *do not have* to be done.);
Circled items = delegated items.

My Personal Roles and Activities

School	Job	Family	Community	Recreation

Use of Personal Time

In order to record personal time most accurately, be sure to pick a school day that includes usual activities. A blank page has been provided on page 376 so you can record your activities in chronologic order. When you total up the minutes spent in each activity, they should total 1440, the number found in each 24-hour day. A sample day's activity log has been provided below. This example does not reflect how you actually spend your time. It merely reflects one person's use of time in a 24-hour period. You will see as many different one-day logs as there are students in your personal issues class.

Sample Personal Time and Activity Log for Monday

Time Span	Activity	Total Time
5:45–6:00 AM	Shampoo and blow-dry hair	15 minutes
6:00–6:30 AM	Breakfast and make "to do" list	30 minutes
6:30–6:45 AM	Dress	15 minutes
6:45–7:05 AM	Drive to school	20 minutes
7:05–7:30 AM	Prepare for first class	25 minutes
7:30–9:00 AM	Class	90 minutes
9:00–9:20 AM	Break	20 minutes
9:20–10:20 AM	Class	60 minutes
10:20–10:30 AM	Break	10 minutes
10:30–11:20 AM	Class	50 minutes
11:20–12:30 PM	Lunch	70 minutes
12:30–1:20 PM	Class	50 minutes
1:20–1:30 PM	Break	10 minutes
1:30–2:20 PM	Class	50 minutes
2:20–2:30 PM	Break	10 minutes
2:30–3:30 PM	Study	60 minutes
3:30–3:50 PM	Drive home	20 minutes
3:50–4:30 PM	Start laundry, dinner, "pick up" house	40 minutes
4:30–5:45 PM	Talk to son, study	75 minutes
5:45–6:15 PM	Dinner	30 minutes
6:15–8:00 PM	Study	105 minutes
8:00–8:30 PM	Bathe, set out clothes for tomorrow	30 minutes
8:30–9:45 PM	Watch TV/study	75 minutes
9:45–5:45 AM	Sleep	480 minutes
		1440 minutes

Personal Time and Activity Log for _____

(Day/Date)

Time Span	Activity	Total Time

Setting Personal Priorities

Review all the activities you have listed on page 374 of Appendix E under the five categories of roles you play in everyday life, and rank them according to the following directions:

1. Place an "A" beside the activities you have to do without question. Remember, "A" activities are those you HAVE to do, not necessarily WANT to do. These are your priority activities. For example, you might not want to get up on rainy mornings and go to school, but you have to if you want to graduate.
2. Place a "B" beside those activities that DO NOT have to be done. These are nonpriority items as far as your long-term goal and your well-being are concerned. You might want to do these activities, but you don't have to do them.

Many of you came to the practical/vocational nursing program while filling a variety of roles in your family and community. As much as you hate the idea, you will not be able to do everything you did before starting school. Are all the "A" activities really "A" activities? Can some of them be moved to the "B" category while you are in school? This is like moving them to the back burner for now. Take a few minutes and review the "A" and "B" status of the roles you have listed. The sample roles and activity list on page 373 has examples of setting priorities with activities.

Delegating Activities

Review your list of personal activities on page 374 of Appendix E with the goal of determining whether the activity can be delegated to someone else while you are a student, and make the following notations:

1. Read over all your "A" activities (your "have-to" activities).
2. Circle the activities that can realistically be delegated while you go to school.

Are the "B" activities still on your mind? Can any of these be delegated while you go to school? If so, circle them also. The "Sample Personal Roles and Activities" on page 373 also has examples of activities that were chosen to be delegated. The only thing left to do is to contact the appropriate person to ask about delegating or assigning an activity.

Time Management: Weekly Schedule

Time	Sun	Mon	Tue	Wed	Thur	Fri	Sat
6–7:00 AM							
7–8:00 AM							
8–9:00 AM							
9–10:00 AM							
10–11:00 AM							
11–12:00 noon							
12:00 noon–1:00 PM							
1–2:00 PM							
2–3:00 PM							
3–4:00 PM							
4–5:00 PM							
5–6:00 PM							
6–7:00 PM							
7–8:00 PM							
8–9:00 PM							
9–10:00 PM							
10–11:00 PM							

Internet Resources
(active as of July 2000)

Search Tools

www.altavista.com—search in 25 languages.

www.infoseek.com—search the web.

www.lycos.com—search the web.

www.webcrawler.com—search the web and write a resume, medical information.

www.yahoo.com—search the web. Free e-mail.

www.google.com—search plain and simple.

www.hotbot.com—search the web.

www.dogpile.com—search the web and select a metasearch tool. Investigate healthcare jobs.

Metasearch Tools (Combine the Searching of Several Databases)

www.metacrawler.com—considered by some to be the fastest and most useful tool on the web.

www.stpt.com—Starting point.

Nursing Sites

www.nflpn.org—National Federation of Licensed Practical Nurses.

www.nursingworld.org—The American Nurses' Association.

www.nursingnet.org—Nursing students' webboard and help for nursing students.

www.ncsbn.org—National Council of State Boards of Nursing, Inc. Information about NCLEX-PN, delegation.

www.nln.org—The National League for Nursing, including The Council of Practical Nursing Programs.

Locating Specific Information for SP/VNs

www.usp.org—U.S. Pharmacopoeia establishes standards to ensure quality of medicines for human and veterinary use.

www.factsontap.org—Facts on Tap: Alcohol and Your College Experience.

www.yoursurgery.com—Provides a description of common operations, anatomy of operative area, pathology, diagnostic methods, and postop care.

www.who.org—World Health Organization.

www.mayohealth.org—Drug reference page gives pronunciation of generic drug name.

www.LifeScan.com—LifeScan blood glucose monitoring systems and diabetes information.

www.efa.org—Epilepsy Foundation of America.

www.medscape.com—Provides a link to Medline, where you can search for nursing articles and read abstracts of selected articles. Provides link for drug information.

Personal Health

www.learningmeditation.com—Learn how to relax. Click the text that interests you.

www.wellnessjunction.com—Health information and wellness.

www.CBS.HealthWatch.com—Personal health management.

www.womenshealth.com—Women's Health America.

www.womens-health.com—Interactive site for women's health.

www.wwwomen.com—Search directory for women.

Resources for Clients

www.alz.org—Alzheimer's Association.

www.arthritis.org—Arthritis Foundation.

www.cancer.org—American Cancer Society.

www.choices.org—Choice in Dying/End of Life Decisions.

www.americanheart.org—American Heart Association. Free heart-to-heart e-card.

www.women.americanheart.org—Facts on women's heart disease and stroke.

www.lungusa.org—American Lung Association.

www.ncadd.org—National Council on Alcoholism and Drug Dependence.

www.ama-assn.org/migraine—Journal of the American Medical Association/Migraine Information.

www.acor.org—Association of cancer online resources.

Government Information

www.ahcpr.gov—Agency for Health Care Policy and Research.

www.cdc.gov—Centers for Disease Control and Prevention.

www.fda.gov—U.S. Food and Drug Administration.

http://thomas.loc.gov—Source for legislative information for the U.S. House and Senate.

www.medicare.gov—The official U.S. government site for Medicare information.

www.nih.gov—National Institutes of Health.

Just for Fun

www.epicurious.com—For people who eat. Williams-Sonoma products. Recipes.

www.bluemountain.com—Send a free electronic card to a friend. No strings attached.

www.peapod.com—Thousands of items (food and other items) that can be shipped to your door and eliminate the need to go food shopping. We can dream, can't we?

The Howlett Style of Nursing Leadership

The idea for this management style was found in the *One Minute Manager* and *Putting the One Minute Manager to Work* and was originally written as *The Howlett Theory of Management for Nursing Instructors.*

1. Never assume employees know what is expected of them. Employees are informed of what is expected of them in their job descriptions. They are held accountable for these expectations. Expected performance needs to be stated objectively. This will make employees aware of the appropriate behavior to reach the institution's goals.

2. Reward employees for their "good" behavior (doing what is expected or going beyond the call of duty). This will encourage them to repeat good behavior. But do not ignore bad performance; to do so will have a negative effect. Most employees know what it is like to be caught doing something "bad." Surprise the heck out of them and catch them doing something good. Let them know how you feel about the "good" behavior. Praise them in some way (name on bulletin board, note indicating you caught them doing something "good," and list the behavior).

3. Employees, being human beings, will sometimes make mistakes; for example, they may not follow rules/policies, etc. When these situations arise, determine whether it involves something the employee *cannot* or something he or she *will not* do. If the employee *cannot* do something, it is a training problem. Skill development is the suggested way of handling the situation. If the employee *will not* do something, it is an attitude problem. A reprimand may be in order, according to the policies of your institution. See No. 6.

4. Employees who feel good about themselves produce good results. Let your employees know they are the best group in the world to work with because . . . (identify reason). Wear an apron that says you work with the best staff in the world.

5. Written and oral feedback about behavior and its consequences, whether positive or negative, needs to be objective. Unemotionally, indicate what they did. Relate feedback as closely as possible to the event. Do not save feedback until clinical performance evaluation time. Point out the consequences of positive and negative behavior. For positive behavior, give praise in measurable terms so the behavior can be repeated. Blanchard and Johnson suggest reprimanding negative behavior in such a way that the person will think about the *reprimand* after the episode and *not* the manner in which it was delivered. Offer praise at the end of a reprimand so that the reprimand is heard more clearly and does not ruin the impact of the praising. Focus reprimands on behaviors, not on the individual.

6. Sometimes employees do not respond to support or assistance and need to be disciplined or terminated. Refer to the policies of your institution.

Delegation: Concepts and Decision-Making Process (NCSBN)

Introduction

To meet the public's increasing need for accessible, affordable, quality health care, providers of health care must maximize the utilization of every health care worker and ensure appropriate delegation of responsibilities and tasks. Nurses, who are uniquely qualified for promoting the health of the whole person by virtue of their education and experience, must be actively involved in making health care policies and decisions; they must coordinate and supervise the delivery of nursing care, including the delegation of nursing tasks to others.

Issues related to delegation have become more complex in today's evolving health care environment, creating a need for practical guidelines to direct the process for making delegatory decisions. Accordingly, this paper expands and builds upon the national Council's 1987 and 1990 conceptual and historical papers on delegation by presenting a dynamic decision-making process and practical guidelines for delegation (Hanstem and Washburn, 1992).

Purpose

The purpose of this paper is to provide a resource for Boards of Nursing, health policy makers, and health care providers on delegation and the roles of licensed and unlicensed health care workers. The paper emphasizes and clarifies the responsibility of Boards of Nursing for the regulation of nursing, including nursing tasks performed by unlicensed health care workers, and the responsibility of licensed nurses to delegate nursing tasks in accord with their legal scopes of practice. It provides a decision-making tool that can be used in clinical and administrative settings to guide the process of delegation. This paper also describes the accountability of each person involved in the delegation process and potential liability if competent, safe care is not provided.

National Council Position Paper, 1995

Premises

The following premises constitute the basis for the delegation decision-making process.

1. All decisions related to delegation of nursing tasks must be based on the fundamental principle of protection of the health, safety, and welfare of the public.
2. Boards of Nursing are responsible for the regulation of nursing. Provision of any care that constitutes nursing or any activity represented as nursing is a regulatory responsibility of Boards of Nursing.
3. Boards of Nursing should articulate clear principles for delegation, augmented by clearly defined guidelines for delegation decisions.
4. A licensed nurse must have ultimate responsibility and accountability for the management and provision of nursing care.
5. A licensed nurse must be actively involved in and be accountable for all managerial decisions, policy making, and practices related to the delegation of nursing care.
6. There is a need and a place for competent, appropriately supervised unlicensed assistive personnel in the delivery of affordable quality health care. However, it must be remembered that unlicensed assistive personnel are equipped to assist—not replace—the nurse.
7. Nursing is a knowledge-based process discipline and cannot be reduced solely to a list of tasks. The licensed nurse's specialized education, professional judgment, and discretion are essential for quality nursing care.
8. While nursing tasks may be delegated, the licensed nurse's generalist knowledge of patient care indicates that the practice-pervasive functions of assessment, evaluation, and nursing judgment must not be delegated.
9. A task delegated to an unlicensed assistive person cannot be redelegated by the unlicensed assistive person.
10. Consumers have a right to health care that meets legal standards of care. Thus, when a nursing task is

delegated, the task must be performed in accord with established standards of practice, policies, and procedures.

11. The licensed nurse determines and is accountable for the appropriateness of delegated nursing tasks. Inappropriate delegation by the nurse and/or unauthorized performance of nursing tasks by unlicensed assistive personnel may lead to legal action against the licensed nurse and/or unlicensed assistive personnel.

Definitions

accountability: Being responsible and answerable for actions or inactions of self or others in the context of delegation.

delegation: Transferring to a competent individual the authority to perform a selected nursing task in a selected situation. The nurse retains accountability for the delegation.

delegator: The person making the delegation.

delegatee: The person receiving the delegation. (a.k.a. Delegate)

supervision: The provision of guidance or direction, evaluation, and follow up by the licensed nurse for accomplishment of a nursing task delegated to unlicensed assistive personnel.

unlicensed assistive personnel (UAP): Any unlicensed personnel, regardless of title, to whom nursing tasks are delegated.

Regulatory Perspective: A Framework for Managerial Policies

Boards of Nursing have the legal responsibility to regulate nursing and provide guidance regarding delegation. Registered Nurses (RNs) may delegate certain nursing tasks to Licensed Practical Nurses/Vocational Nurses (LP/VNs) and unlicensed assistive personnel (UAP). In some jurisdictions, LP/VNs may also delegate certain tasks within their scope of practice to unlicensed assistive personnel. The licensed nurse has a responsibility to assure that the delegated task is performed in accord with established standards of practice, policies, and procedures. The nurse who delegates retains accountability for the task delegated.

The regulatory system serves as a framework for managerial policies related to the employment and utilization of licensed nurses and unlicensed assistive personnel. The nurse who assesses the patient's needs and plans nursing care should determine the tasks to be delegated and is

accountable for that delegation. It is inappropriate for employers or others to require nurses to delegate when, in the nurse's professional judgment, delegation is unsafe and not in the patient's best interest. In those instances, the nurse should act as the patient's advocate and take appropriate action to ensure provision of safe nursing care. If the nurse determines that delegation may not appropriately take place, but nevertheless delegates as directed, the nurse may be disciplined by the Board of Nursing.

Acceptable Use of the Authority to Delegate

The delegating nurse is responsible for an individualized assessment of the patient and situational circumstances, and for ascertaining the competence of the delegatee before delegating any task. The practice-pervasive functions of assessment, evaluation, and nursing judgment must not be delegated. Supervision, monitoring, evaluation, and follow up by the nurse are crucial components of delegation. The delegatee is accountable for accepting the delegation and for his/her own actions in carrying out the task.

The decision to delegate should be consistent with the nursing process (appropriate assessment, planning, implementation, and evaluation). This necessarily precludes a list of nursing tasks that can be routinely and uniformly delegated for all patients in all situations. Rather, the nursing process and decision to delegate must be based on careful analysis of the patient's needs and circumstances. Also critical to delegation decisions are the qualifications of the proposed delegatee, the nature of the nurse's delegation authority set forth in the law of the jurisdiction, and the nurse's personal competence in the area of nursing relevant to the task to be delegated.

Delegation Decision-Making Process

In delegating, the nurse must ensure appropriate assessment, planning, implementation, and evaluation. The delegation decision-making process, which is continuous, is described by the following model:

I. Delegation criteria

    A. Nurse Practice Act

        1. Permits delegation

        2. Authorizes task(s) to be delegated or authorizes the nurse to decide delegation

    B. Delegator qualifications

        1. Within scope of authority to delegate

2. Appropriate education, skills, and experience
3. Documented/demonstrated evidence of current competency

C. Delegatee qualifications

1. Appropriate education, training, skills, and experience
2. Documented/demonstrated evidence of current competency

Provided that this foundation is in place, the licensed nurse may enter the continuous process of delegation decision-making.

II. Assess the situation

A. Identify the needs of the patient, consulting the plan of care

B. Consider the circumstances/setting

C. Assure the availability of adequate resources, including supervision

If patient needs, circumstances, and available resources (including supervisor and delegatee) indicate patient safety will be maintained with delegated care, proceed to III.

III. Plan for specific task(s) to be delegated

A. Specify the nature of each task and the knowledge and skills required to perform it

B. Require documentation or demonstration of current competence by the delegatee for each task

C. Determine the implications for the patient, other patients, and significant others

If the nature of the task, competence of the delegatee, and patient implications indicate patient safety will be maintained with delegated care, proceed to IV.

IV. Assure appropriate accountability

A. As delegator, accept accountability for performance of the task(s)

B. Verify that delegatee accepts the delegation and the accountability for carrying out the task correctly

If delegator and delegatee accept the accountability for their respective roles in the delegated patient care, proceed to V.

V. Supervise performance of the task

A. Provide directions and clear expectations of how the task(s) is to be performed

B. Monitor performance of the task(s) to assure compliance to established standards of practice, policies, and procedures

C. Intervene if necessary

D. Ensure appropriate documentation of the task(s)

VI. Evaluate the entire delegation process

A. Evaluate the patient

B. Evaluate the performance of the task(s)

C. Obtain and provide feedback

The Five Rights of Delegation provide an additional resource to facilitate decisions about delegation.

The Five Rights of Delegation

- **Right Task**
One that is delegable for a specific patient.
- **Right Circumstances**
Appropriate patient setting, available resources, and other relevant factors considered.
- **Right Person**
Right person is delegating the right task to the right person to be performed on the right person.
- **Right Direction/Communication**
Clear, concise description of the task, including its objective, limits and expectations.
- **Right Supervision**
Appropriate monitoring, evaluation, intervention, as needed, and feedback.

Conclusion

The guidelines presented in this paper provide a decision-making process that facilitates the provision of quality care by appropriate persons in all health care settings. The National Council of State Boards of Nursing believes that this paper will assist all health care providers and health care facilities in discharging their shared responsibility to provide optimum health care that protects the public's health, safety, and welfare.

Reference

Hansten R, Washburn M. Delegation: How to deliver care through others. American Journal of Nursing 92(8):87, 88, 90, 1992.

accountability. Obligation to answer for your actions.

acculturate. To adopt the culture of a different group.

active learner. Takes charge of his or her own education.

active listener. A person who hears sounds and searches for information relevant to those sounds so that the sounds may be understood.

ADPIE. The five steps in the nursing process as revised in 1977: Assessment (data collection), Diagnosis, Planning, Intervention, and Evaluation. RNs are responsible for all five steps; Diagnosis is not an LP/VN responsibility.

adult ADD. Adult form of attention deficit disorder (ADD).

advanced practice. Post-registered nurse (RN) degree or special education resulting in an expanded role (e.g., clinical nurse specialist, nurse practitioner, certified nurse midwife, nurse anesthetist).

affective communication. Sending or receiving information through feeling tone.

aggressiveness. An attacking type of behavior that occurs in response to frustration and hostile feelings.

alliances. New partnerships among hospitals, clinics, laboratories, health care systems, and physicians. They coordinate the delivery of care, contain costs, and attempt to provide a seamless system.

ALPNA. American Licensed Practical Nurses Association.

APIE. The four steps in the nursing process as originally designed in the 1950s: Assessment (data collection), Planning, Intervention, and Evaluation. LP/VNs are responsible for these four steps.

assault. An unjustified attempt or threat to touch someone.

assertiveness. A way of accepting responsibility for oneself by expressing thoughts and feelings directly and honestly without blaming oneself or others.

assessment. Step 1 of the nursing process, which involves gathering as much significant information about a client as is possible. See Data Collection.

assigning. Allotting tasks that are in the job description of workers. Assigned tasks are those that these workers are hired and paid to perform.

associate degree nurse. An RN who has received his or her education in a two-year community college or technical school program.

auditory learner. Talks to himself or herself or hears sounds when he or she thinks. Learns best by hearing.

automatic responses. Both passive and aggressive responses result from being caught by an emotional hook, and these responses are not based on choice.

autonomy. Control over personal decisions.

baccalaureate nurse. An RN who has received his or her education in a four-year college or university program.

battery. Acute physical harm to someone.

beneficence. Doing good.

biomedicine (Western medicine). Belief that abnormalities in structure and function of body organs are caused by pathogens, biochemical alterations, and/or environmental factors.

bodily/kinesthetic learner. Learns best by touching, moving, and processing knowledge through bodily sensations.

body language. Nonverbal communication of one's thoughts and feelings.

bucket theory. Suggests that merely by lecturing, the teacher can transfer knowledge from the teacher's mind to the student's mind.

CAI. Computer aided instruction.

CALPN. Certification in Addiction for LP/VNs; post-licensure education.

capitation. Set fee for health care, paid annually regardless of the number of health services provided.

career ladder. Nursing program planned to avoid duplication of content. The student may progress from a position as a nursing assistant to a practical/vocational nurse to an associate degree nurse to a baccalaureate nurse in about four years.

case management method. A method of client care that uses care pathways or critical paths with an interdisciplinary staff, with a focus on quality, service, and cost.

case method. A method of client care in which one nurse is assigned to give total care to one patient.

certification. Certificate awarded to an RN or LP/VN after passing a comprehensive examination in a select area of practice.

Certification in Pharmacology. A continuing education course offered by NAPNES.

charting by exception (CBE). Normal events charted by placing a check mark on a flowsheet. Abnormal events or changes are charted in narrative form.

civil action related to individual rights. Involves the relationships between individuals and the violation of those rights.

closed-ended. A question that requires a specific answer from a client.

CLTC. Certification in Long-Term Care.

CMCN. Certification in Managed Care.

codependency. Situation in which a person allows another person's behavior to affect him or her and is obsessed with controlling that person's behavior.

common law. Judge-made law, which has its origins in the courts.

communication. Conveying a thought or idea from a sender to a receiver or from one person to another.

compensation. A coping/mental mechanism in which the individual covers for a real or imagined inadequacy by developing or exaggerating what some consider to be a desirable trait.

computer simulation. Learning activities on a computer that make use of an imaginary client situation. The student uses the nursing process as he or she would in an actual clinical situation.

confidentiality. A client's right to privacy.

constructive evaluation. Critique directed toward performance and behavior; has no bearing on one's value as a person.

continuous quality improvement (CQI). Searches for new ways to improve client care, prevent errors, and identify and fix problems.

cooperative learning. Emphasis on individual accountability for learning a specific academic task while working in small groups.

co-payment. Percentage of the bill that is paid by a subscriber who is enrolled in a health insurance plan.

copyright laws. These laws permit a single copy of an article for personal use. Instructors may not make copies of articles, chapters, or books for distribution to each student.

cost containment. Holding costs within fixed limits.

criminal action. Involves persons and society as a whole; for example, murder.

critical pathways. Also called care maps and care guides. They show a sequence of care to be delivered within a definite time frame, include potential problems and expected outcomes. They help the client to be discharged from the hospital in the fastest time possible.

critical thinking. Used to resolve problems and find ways to make improvements even when no problem exists.

cross-training. Health care workers trained to provide specific skills outside their area of education when needed by clients in an attempt to use workers more efficiently and reduce costs.

cultural bias. Prejudice.

cultural sensitivity. Learning about other cultures and being respectful of their customs, rites, and beliefs.

culture. The total of all the ideas, beliefs, values, attitudes, and objects that a group of persons possesses. Culture includes ways of doing things.

custom. Ways of doing things that are common to a group of people of the same culture.

data collection. Step 1 of the nursing process for practical/vocational nurses, which involves gathering significant information about the client to assist the RN in the assessment process.

decentralized. The idea to locate centralized service departments, such as the x-ray department and the laboratory, on client units. Health care workers are cross-trained to provide a variety of services for the client. The goal is client-focused care.

deductible. Amount the subscriber must pay before health insurance begins to cover costs.

delegating. Generally, tasks and duties within your job description that can be given to another worker to perform. Duties that are part of your *legal* scope of practice cannot be delegated. Check your nurse practice act to confirm authority to delegate in your state.

diagnosis. Step 2 in the nursing process. RN determines the client's response to the medical diagnosis.

diagnostic-related groups (DRGs). Prospective payment system. Specifies number of days for which Medicare will pay.

diploma nurse. RN who has received his or her education in a three-year hospital-based program.

distance learning. A course in which the teacher and student are separated by physical distance, utilizing such tools as two-way television, videotapes, audiotapes, and the World-Wide Web.

durable power of attorney (DPOA). In this case, durable medical power of attorney. Written while the person is mentally competent. Identifies who will make decisions regarding future care, extent of treatment, and kinds of treatment if the person is unable to make his or her own decisions.

effectiveness. Choosing the most important thing to do and doing it as soon as possible.

efficiency. Getting tasks done in the shortest time possible.

empathy. Respectful, detached concern.

ethics. Rules or principles that govern correct conduct.

ethnic group. Special type of cultural group composed of people who are members of the same race, religion, or nation or who speak the same language.

ethnocentrism. The belief that one's own culture is best; the belief that one's way of doing things is best.

evaluation. Step 5 of the nursing process; involves taking a critical look at the effectiveness of a nursing action.

external distractions. Interruptions in concentration from outside oneself, such as background sounds, lighting, peers, and so forth.

facilitator. Teacher who creates a learning environment by arranging for a variety of activities and experiences. The student is expected to participate actively in his or her own learning.

fee-for-service. Client pays a fee to the physician for each service provided.

fidelity. In nursing, to be faithful to the charge of acting in the client's best interest when the capacity to make free choice is no longer available.

focused. A question that requires definitive, precise information from a client.

functional method. A method of client care that is task-oriented and involves dividing the tasks to be done among staff members according to their abilities.

generalizations. Broad, sweeping statements made about a group.

goals. Realistic, measurable, time-limited statements of resolution of a problem or need.

harassment. Any unwanted, deliberate, or repeated unsolicited comments, gestures, graphic materials, physical contacts, or solicitation of favors that affects the person's work or work environment.

Health Care Financing Administration (HCFA). A federal agency that administers Medicare, Medicaid, and state children's health insurance programs.

health care team. The various individuals who provide the services needed for the comprehensive care of clients.

health maintenance organization. A comprehensive care system of medical services based on a set, prepaid fee.

idea sketch. Representing a verbal concept with a picture.

impaired nurse. One who is addicted to alcohol or other drugs.

implementation. Step 3 of the nursing process, which uses the client care plan as a guideline for daily care and carrying out planned activities.

incremental changes. Changes that occur here and there without affecting the system as a whole.

informational interview. By appointment, meet with an administrator to learn about a facility. This is not a job interview, although it is treated with the same courtesy.

intentional tort. Intent to do a wrongful act.

internal distractions. Interruptions in concentration from inside oneself, such as daydreaming and boredom.

Internet. Physical infrastructure that allows the electronic circulation of vast amounts of information to computer users. This information is unregulated and cannot always be taken at face value.

interpersonal learner. Learns best by sharing, comparing, cooperating, and interviewing.

interpersonal style. Four major styles: (1) results-focused, (2) detail-focused, (3) friendly-focused, and (4) party-focused.

intervention. Step 4 of the nursing process: actions, activity, treatment for the client.

intrapersonal learner. Learns best by working alone, self-paced instruction, and having own space.

Joint Commission of Accreditation of Health Care Organizations (JCAHCO). Sets the standards of care for hospitals and long-term care agencies. Agencies receive accreditation if they elect to be reviewed and meet standards.

justice. Giving clients their due and treating them fairly.

leadership. Manner in which the leader gets along with coworkers, with the goal of producing workplace changes to meet the goals of the employing agency.

learning resource center. The library.

left brain dominant. A person who is more orderly; logical; reads and writes well; and excels at analytical thinking.

liability. Legal responsibility of a person to account for wrongful acts by making financial restitution.

libel. Damage to someone's reputation through written communication or pictures.

linguistic learner. Learns best by reducing the number of words included in class notes.

living will. Written directive stating personal wishes regarding future health care. Not recognized as a legal document everywhere.

logical learner. Learns best by using an organized method of study.

long-term goal. A general realistic statement of what one hopes to attain ultimately.

long-term memory. A function of the brain that allows one to store information over time; for example, knowledge of what one wore on one's first date (synonym: permanent memory).

malpractice. A part of negligence that relates to lack of skill or misconduct by professional persons.

managed care. A system of controlling cost of health care by arranging health care at predetermined rates. An HMO is an example of managed care.

management. Organization of all care required for clients in a health care setting for a specific period of time.

mandatory licensure. Protects the nursing role.

manipulation. An indirect way of dealing with issues that may be positive or negative. Negative (maladaptive) manipulation occurs if the feelings of others are disregarded or other people are treated as objects.

mapping. A form of note making in which information and its relationships are put in a visual pattern.

Medicaid. Financial assistance provided by the federal government for states and counties to pay for medical services for eligible poor.

Medicare. Federally sponsored and supervised health insurance plan for persons 65 years of age and older and persons under 65 years who are totally and permanently disabled.

message. Idea being conveyed or the question being asked.

minitask. Simple to do and takes no more than five minutes of time. An unpleasant, difficult, time-consuming task can be divided into a series of minitasks.

mission statement. A statement that defines the purpose and goals of a health care organization.

mnemonic device. Memory aid such as rhymes or acronyms.

morals. Ethical habits of a person.

multistate licensure. Legislation in some states that renders a nursing license obtained in that state valid for practice in other states with multistate legislation.

Each state's individual regulations must still be followed.

musical learner. Learns best by humming, singing, or playing an instrument.

NANDA. North American Nursing Diagnosis Association.

NAPNES. National Association for Practical Nurse Education and Service.

naturalistic system. Beliefs developed from the traditional medical practices of the ancient civilizations of China, India, and Greece.

NCLEX-PN. National Council Licensing Examination—Practical Nursing.

negligence. Conduct that falls below the standard of care established by law for the protection of others.

networking. Building relationships with instructors, employers, and peers, for the purposes of finding new jobs, better pay, faster promotions, and greater job satisfaction.

NFLPN. National Federation of Licensed Practical Nurses.

NIC. Nursing Interventions Classification.

Nightingale, Florence. Founder of modern nursing, who is often known as "The Lady with the Lamp" because of her after-hours rounds with her lamp during the Crimean War.

NLN. National League for Nursing.

NOC. Nursing Outcomes Classification.

nonmaleficence. First, do no harm.

nonverbal communication. Sending or receiving information by facial expressions or body language.

nurse practice act. Governs the practice of nursing. Developed by each state and provincial board of nursing.

nursing. The diagnosis and treatment of human responses to actual or potential health problems (ANA definition). Assisting sick or well individuals in performing activities that contribute to health or its recovery (Henderson's definition).

nursing process. An orderly way of developing a plan of care for the individual client. Usually broken down into five steps: assessment, nursing diagnosis, planning, implementation, and evaluation. The LP/VN assists the RN in four steps of the nursing process: gathering data (assessment), planning, implementation, and evaluation.

nursing team. The individuals who carry out the client's plan of care 24 hours a day, seven days a week. This team includes registered and practical/vocational nurses, nursing assistants, ward clerks, unit managers, and unlicensed persons.

objective. Data that can be observed and verified. Data

obtained by seeing, hearing, touching, smelling, tasting, measuring, counting, etc. Does not include subjective judgment.

Omnibus Budget Reconciliation Act of 1987 (OBRA). Federal law that regulates how nursing homes provide for residents' quality of life, health, and safety.

one-way communication. When the sender controls a situation and offers no opportunity for feedback from the receiver; used to give a command.

on-line catalog. Computerized card catalog in the library.

open-ended. A question that permits the client to respond in a way most meaningful to him or her. This type of question often begins with what, where, when.

outcome. Identifies the degree of progress or not, made by the client toward reaching a goal.

passive listener. A person who receives sounds with little recognition or personal involvement.

passive (nonassertive) behavior. Dishonest, self-defeating behavior that is an attempt to avoid conflict by not dealing with issues.

pastoral care team. Members of the health team who assist nurses in meeting the spiritual needs of the clients.

patient-focused care. Attempt to improve the quality of care by using hospital resources more efficiently to meet the client's needs (e.g., decentralizing services).

performance evaluation. Evaluation of clinical performance that involves both the teacher and the student.

permissive licensure. May practice nursing without a license, but cannot use the title of LPN or LVN.

personalistic system. Belief that the sick person is being punished by a deity, ghost, god, evil spirit, witch, or angry ancestor.

planning. Step 3 of the nursing process, which involves setting priorities, establishing goals, determining approaches to achieve the goals, and documentation of a plan of care. A blueprint for action.

PQRST. A method of reading to increase understanding by developing comprehension. (Preview, Question, Read, State, Test.)

practical/vocational nurse. A person who performs for compensation any simple acts in the care of convalescent, subacutely or chronically ill, injured, or infirm persons, or any act or procedure in the care of the acutely ill, injured, or infirm under the specific direction of a registered nurse, physician, podiatrist, or dentist.

preferred provider organization (PPO). Similar to HMOs, except that physicians maintain their own practice and continue to be part of their own physician group. Part of the day is spent treating clients enrolled in a PPO.

prejudice. The opinion that a person has about something, even though facts dispute the opinion.

primary care. The point at which a person enters the health care system.

primary method. A method of client care in which one nurse is responsible and accountable for care given to clients on all shifts from admission to discharge.

private health care agencies. Agencies that are generally proprietary (for profit) and that charge a fee for service. The primary focus is curing illness.

private pay. The client pays out of pocket for services received.

procrastination. Putting off tasks that must be done.

progression program. A nursing program for LP/VNs who wish to become an associate degree nurse.

projection. A coping or mental mechanism in which an individual attributes his or her own weaknesses to others.

rapport. A harmonious relationship.

rationalization. A coping or mental mechanism in which the individual offers a logical but untrue reason as an excuse for his/her behavior.

receiver. Person receiving the message, idea, or question.

recycled adult learner. Starting a new career by enrolling in practical/vocational nursing.

reference hierarchy. Potential employers rate references this way, from best to least: (1) current and former supervisors from work and volunteer experiences, unit managers, and teachers; (2) workers who have seen your work; and (3) personal references or friends.

registered nurses. A member of the nursing team who has gone to nursing school for two, three, or four years and has passed an examination to be registered. The person on the nursing team who functions independently in decision making regarding the nursing care of clients.

religious denomination. An organized group of persons with a philosophy that supports their particular concept of God.

résumé. Summary of what you have accomplished—work, skills, education, experience, and sometimes personal achievements. Used to persuade an employer that you are the right person for the job. Limited to one or two pages.

returning adult learner. A learner in the age bracket of the mid-20s or older who has entered an educational program and has not experienced formal education for a period of time.

right brain dominant. The person shows more advanced spatial relationships, recognizes negative emotions more quickly, is less verbal, adds tone and inflection to voice, sees total picture.

self-directed learner. Takes responsibility for own learning and performance.

sender. Person conveying an idea or asking a question.

short-term goal. A smaller, more reasonable, and manageable unit of a long-term goal; that is, the small step toward attaining a long-term goal.

short-term memory. A function of the brain that allows one to store information for a short time; for example, a telephone number (synonym: temporary memory).

slander. Damage to someone's reputation by verbalizing untrue or confidential information.

spatial learner. Learns best by studying diagrams, boxes, and special lists.

spirituality. Pertaining to the soul, one's life force.

spiritual needs. Requirements that arise out of the desire of human beings to find meaning in life, suffering, and death.

standards of care. Nursing standard of care is based on what an ordinary prudent nurse with similar education and experience would do or not do in similar circumstances (an important legal implication).

statutory law. Law developed by the legislative branch of state and federal governments.

stereotyping. The fixed notion that all individuals in a cultural group are the same.

stress management. Maintenance of stress at a moderate level. The reaction to both high and low levels of stress may be overwhelming.

subjective. Information based on a client's opinion.

syllabus. Up-to-date course document distributed at the beginning of a course. This document usually includes a course description, course objectives, course require-

ments, required text, grading scale, and instructor information.

tactual learner. Learns best by doing.

team method. A method of client care in which small teams of nursing personnel are assigned to give total care to groups of patients.

therapeutic. Having healing properties, results of treatment.

therapeutic communication. Between the client and the nurse. The focus is on the client.

time management. The effective use of time to meet goals.

total quality management (TQM). A method by which continuous quality improvement (CQI) is carried out.

traditional adult learner. A learner who comes to an educational program directly from high school or from another program of study, usually in the late teens or early 20s.

two-way communication. When there is feedback or discussion between the sender and receiver; the usual form of conversation.

universal coverage. Health insurance coverage for all persons; usually paid through taxes.

unlicensed assistive personnel. Trained by health care organizations to function in an assistive role to RNs and LP/VNs. Also known as patient care technicians, patient care associates, nurse extenders, multiskilled workers, and so on.

verbal communication. Sending or receiving communication through the spoken or written word.

visual learner. Generates visual images; that is, thinks primarily in pictures. Learns best by watching a demonstration first.

voluntary health care agencies. Not-for-profit nonofficial health care agencies that complement official health agencies and meet the needs of persons with a specific disease.

Index

Note: Page numbers in *italics* refer to Figures. Page numbers followed by the letter t refer to tables.